Critical Sources
Gynecology

This innovative text analyses 45 Scientific Impact Papers produced by the Royal College of Obstetricians and Gynaecologists and tests readers on their knowledge in detail of the contents via single best answers. Any candidate for professional examination or certification/recertification will want to use this resource as a way to revise and strengthen their knowledge.

Volumes in *Critical Sources in Gynecology*

Critical Sources in Gynecology

Volume 2

RCOG Scientific Impact Papers

Rhythm Bhalla

MBBS, MD OBGYN, FMAS(ICOG), DNB, MRCOG
Consultant Obstetrician and Gynecologist
CloudNine Hospital Panchkula
Haryana, India

CRC Press
Taylor & Francis Group
Boca Raton London New York

CRC Press is an imprint of the
Taylor & Francis Group, an **informa** business

Designed cover image: Shutterstock

First edition published 2026

by CRC Press
2385 NW Executive Center Drive, Suite 320, Boca Raton FL 33431

and by CRC Press
4 Park Square, Milton Park, Abingdon, Oxon, OX14 4RN

CRC Press is an imprint of Taylor & Francis Group, LLC

© 2026 Rhythm Bhalla

ISBN: 9781041094845 (hbk)
ISBN: 9781041094821 (pbk)
ISBN: 9781003650355 (ebk)

DOI: 10.1201/9781003650355

Typeset in Palatino
by Deanta Global Publishing Services, Chennai, India

Contents

1 SIP – Acupuncture and Chinese Herbal Medication for Chronic Pelvic Pain (CPP)

Source: Acupuncture and Chinese Herbal Medicine for Women with Chronic Pelvic Pain Scientific Impact Paper No. 30 February 2012. www.rcog.org.uk/guidance/browse-all-guidance/scientific-impact -papers/acupuncture-and-chinese-herbal-medicine-for-women-with-chronic-pelvic-pain-scientific -impact-paper-no-30/

IMPORTANT POINTS FROM THE GUIDELINE (SIP)

- Chronic pelvic pain (CPP) is characterized by intermittent or persistent discomfort in the lower abdomen or pelvis lasting a minimum of 6 months, not solely linked to menstruation or sexual activity, and not related to pregnancy.

- Approximately one in six adult females may experience CPP, which can be indicative of various conditions presenting with pelvic symptoms, including gynecological issues such as endometriosis, urinary tract disorders such as interstitial cystitis, digestive conditions such as irritable bowel syndrome (IBS), and musculoskeletal disorders.

- Psychological aspects significantly contribute to CPP, with numerous women disclosing experiences of physical, mental, and sexual abuse.

- The standard treatment for CPP may be ineffectual, prompting women with CPP to pursue other methods for symptom management.

- While traditional medicine seeks to evaluate new treatments via controlled clinical trials, some complementary and alternative medicine methods, such as acupuncture and herbal therapy, have been practiced extensively for centuries.

- China has conducted approximately 20,000 randomized controlled trials examining Chinese herbal medicine (CHM).

- Nevertheless, a significant percentage of this research has been compromised by inadequate techniques, resulting in most of the findings remaining inconclusive.

- Alongside clinical trials, there is an expanding corpus of research investigating biologically plausible mechanisms that may alleviate CPP by anti-inflammatory and other actions.

- Acupuncture is a medical system that originated in China about 2000 years ago.

- It entails the insertion of slender needles into precise, designated spots over the body's surface.

- Stimulation of these sites is believed to elicit both local and systemic healing responses.

- The frequency of treatment ranges from acute problems necessitating two to three sessions per week to more stable chronic disorders that may require acupuncture only once a month.

- Treatment is often administered weekly.

- The length of treatment is variable.

- In many cases, two to three sessions may be adequate; nevertheless, for more intricate and resistant problems, treatment may necessitate several months.

- Generally, significant favorable effects should be seen after three to four sessions.

- Patients contemplating acupuncture treatment should verify that their practitioner is registered with a prominent acupuncture association, such as the British Acupuncture Council, the Association of Traditional Chinese Medicine, or the British Medical Acupuncture Society.

- The literature review did not identify any trials of acupuncture explicitly pertaining to CPP.

- It did, however, identify studies on acupuncture for dysmenorrhea, pelvic inflammatory disease (PID), and IBS, all of which are recognized contributors to CPP.

- Two minor trials featured in this Cochrane review demonstrated that acupuncture treatment markedly alleviated menstruation symptoms in comparison to typical nonsteroidal anti-inflammatory drugs (NSAIDs).

DOI: 10.1201/9781003650355-1

- NSAIDs are fundamental in the management of dysmenorrhea and other pelvic inflammatory disorders, including endometriosis.

- The application of acupuncture as a potentially efficacious and safe method for pain management, devoid of the harmful gastrointestinal effects associated with NSAIDs, necessitates additional examination.

- A Cochrane analysis of acupuncture for IBS indicated minimal distinction between authentic and sham acupuncture treatments, but both demonstrated clinically significant enhancements.

- A Cochrane analysis of acupuncture for IBS revealed minimal distinction between genuine and sham acupuncture treatments, but both demonstrated clinically significant benefits.

- Chinese research has examined the efficacy of acupuncture in treating chronic PID relative to CHM and antibiotic therapy.

- These were unblinded trials that exhibited insufficient methodological rigor and presented a significant risk of bias.

- During a consultation with a CHM practitioner, a comprehensive case history is obtained, the tongue is examined, and the pulse is palpated.

- The data from this technique is utilized to delineate a conventional pattern or syndrome of illness.

- A herbal formulation is subsequently produced to target this pattern and to alleviate both the symptoms and the root cause of the ailment.

- In the UK, exclusively plant-based products are utilized, and a CHM practitioner normally selects between 8 to 15 herbs from a repertoire of over 400 widely employed plants.

- Treatment may be delivered through several methods, including cooked decoctions, herbal soups, concentrated powders, herbal pills, or alcoholic tinctures.

- It is advised that individuals exclusively seek treatment from members of the Register of Chinese Herbal Medicine or the Association of Traditional Chinese Medicine.

- A Cochrane review of CHM for endometriosis indicated that CHM administered post-surgery exhibited benefits comparable to the anti-progestin gestrinone, and a significantly greater efficacy in alleviating dysmenorrhea and reducing pelvic lesions compared to danazol, while also presenting fewer adverse reactions than conventional treatments.

- There is a distinct necessity for more stringent trials to evaluate the possible advantages of CHM in the management of endometriosis, as a factor in CPP treatment.

- A Cochrane review of complementary and alternative medicine for dysmenorrhea encompassed 39 randomized controlled trials and indicated favorable outcomes for complementary and alternative medicine relative to pharmacological interventions such as NSAIDs and oral contraceptives.

- This review demonstrated that CHM was linked to substantial enhancements in pain alleviation and a decrease in the consumption of supplementary analgesics.

- Nonetheless, the study is constrained by the incorporation of trials with poor methodological rigor and restricted sample numbers, necessitating cautious interpretation of these results.

- A Cochrane review of herbal remedies for the management of IBS encompassed 75 randomized controlled studies assessing the efficacy of herbal medications compared to placebo controls and other conventional treatments. Nevertheless, the methodological rigor of these experiments was inadequate.

- A meticulously executed and well-powered trial identified a considerable disparity between CHM and placebo.

- In this experiment, 76% of participants receiving standard CHM intervention reported improvements during therapy, in contrast to only 33% of the placebo group.

- Chinese reports also exist on the effects of CHM on PID when delivered orally or by an herbal enema.

- Numerous investigations juxtapose various CHM regimes and indicate significant pain and symptom alleviation, despite the substandard quality of these trials.

- Current research delineates the biologically plausible immunological and anti-inflammatory effects of CHM, including the suppression of cytokines (TNF-α, IL-6, IL-8), inhibition of COX-2, antioxidant activity, and analgesia through opioid, dopaminergic, and GABAergic pathways, which align with potential clinical advantages in pelvic inflammation.

- Acupuncture performed with disposable needles by a qualified, certified, and trained practitioner is regarded as a highly safe practice.

- Recent years have raised concerns over the safety of CHM, mainly due to adulteration with prescription medications or contamination with hazardous plant species.

- Although major adverse outcomes from CHM seem few, further rigorous investigation is necessary.

- The new EU rule for over-the-counter (OTC) herbal goods will mandate adherence to good manufacturing practice (GMP) standards to safeguard against adulteration or unintentional contamination.

- Acupuncture and CHM may contribute to the management of CPP related to dysmenorrhea, endometriosis, IBS, and PID, either as a supplementary or alternative approach to conventional therapies.

- Regrettably, the existing data is deficient in rigor, and the available studies are often limited in size, poorly structured, and improperly documented.

- Consequently, this area necessitates more careful examination.

- Women seeking acupuncture or CHM should be apprised of the highly tentative nature of the research underpinning these modalities.

QUESTIONS

1. Acupuncture is a traditional Chinese technique to treat various conditions depending on the flow of which of the following through the body?

    A. Energy called 'yao'

    B. Energy called 'shenti'

    C. Energy called 'qi'

    D. Energy called 'bing'

2. A 36-year-old patient who has a known case of CPP presents to you in the outpatient department (OPD) in extreme distress. She has tried multiple therapies, but all have failed. She has read about the role of acupuncture in chronic pain conditions and wants to go ahead with this treatment. Regarding acupuncture, which of the following statements is incorrect?

    A. It entails the insertion of slender needles into designated points on the body (termed acupoints) and operates on the principle of energy flow, or 'qi,' throughout the body.

    B. It has demonstrated substantial evidence in alleviating chronic pain conditions, such as CPP, and is endorsed by numerous guidelines.

    C. It is regarded as a secure technique with little hazards when conducted by a licensed and trained practitioner.

    D. It can induce the production of endogenous analgesics such as endorphins and opioids to diminish the sense of pain.

3. In general, regarding the frequency of sessions of acupuncture in different painful conditions, all of the following statements are true, except?

   A. Acute conditions may need sessions two to three times per week.

   B. Stable chronic conditions need sessions once every 10 days.

   C. A typical session is mostly offered once a week.

   D. Beneficial effect is generally noticed in about three to four sessions.

4. According to available evidence, which of the following is not a potential benefit of acupuncture in patients with CPP?

   A. Causes pain relief even if used as a monotherapy

   B. Improves quality of life in patients with CPP

   C. Produces long-lasting pain relief not requiring additional therapy for >3–6 months

   D. Reduces need for pain relief medications

5. What is regarded as a mechanism of action in patients receiving acupuncture for pain alleviation?

   A. Acupuncture activates endogenous analgesics such as endorphins and opioids.

   B. It is recognized for its ability to diminish inflammation and enhance blood circulation to the affected region.

   C. It regulates the operation of the neuro-endocrine system and adheres to the gate control theory for analgesia.

   D. All of the above.

   E. A and B.

6. All of the following are examples of specific Chinese herbal medications for CPP relief, except?

   A. Guizhi Fuling Wan

   B. Qian-Yu decoction

   C. Herbal retine enemas

   D. Burdock fruit/Shi Zhen tea

7. Regarding the role of moxibustion in patients with CPP, which of the following statements is not true?

   A. It is a thermal therapy that entails the combustion of Chinese herbs at designated acupoints on the patient's dermis.

   B. The heat expands blood vessels and enhances blood circulation to the affected region.

   C. It elevates the release of inflammatory cytokines in the affected region.

   D. The evidence supporting the efficacy of moxibustion in individuals with CPP still remains limited.

8. According to the comprehensive research by Chinese journals, what percentage of drug-induced hepatotoxic events are caused by herbal-based supplements?

   A. <1%

   B. 5%

   C. 10%

   D. 20%

9. Which of the following drugs used as an herb in CHM is a cause of direct liver injury?

   A. Anthraquinones

   B. *Aristolochia contorta* Bunge

   C. *Aristolochia manshuriensis* Kom

   D. *Dioscorea bulbifera* L.

10. For clinical diagnosis of drug-induced liver injury (DILI), which of the following symptoms is most commonly seen in affected patients?

   A. Fatigue and jaundice

   B. Fever

   C. Clay-colored stools

   D. Rash and pruritis

ANSWERS

1. C	5. D	9. D
2. B	6. D	10. A
3. B	7. C	
4. C	8. D	

2 SIP – Adhesion Prevention Agents

Source: The Use of Adhesion Prevention Agents in Obstetrics and Gynaecology Scientific Impact Paper No. 39 May 2013. https://www.rcog.org.uk/guidance/browse-all-guidance/scientific-impact-papers/the-use-of-adhesion-prevention-agents-in-obstetrics-and-gynaecology-scientific-impact-paper-no-39/

IMPORTANT POINTS FROM THE GUIDELINE (SIP)

- Adhesions are fibrous bands that form between and within organs due to abnormal healing, typically occurring post-surgery and/or infection as a result of inflammation.

- Any abdominal surgery may result in the formation of adhesions and possible complications.

- Evidence supports the utilization of hyaluronic acid derivatives, PEG (polyethylene glycol)-based derivatives, and solid barrier agents from oxidized regenerated cellulose, specifically Interceed, in laparoscopy or laparotomy for benign gynecological surgery to diminish the incidence, severity, and extent of adhesion formation.

- Evidence exists to endorse the application of hyaluronic acid derivatives in hysteroscopic surgery to diminish the occurrence of intrauterine adhesion development.

- Nonetheless, there is scant data to substantiate the utilization of pharmacological and hydro-flotation medicines, including Icodextrin, in gynecological surgery.

- In the United Kingdom, the incidence of cesarean sections has risen markedly.

- Any technique that diminishes the occurrence of lower segment cesarean sections (LSCS) or inhibits adhesion formation during LSCS might mitigate the maternal morbidity linked to subsequent LSCS.

- The use of adhesion prevention medicines during cesarean section shows no discernible advantage.

- Additional proof is necessary prior to endorsing anti-adhesion agents in contemporary gynecological practice.

- Post open gynecological surgery, 4.5% of patients are hospitalized due to adhesion-related complications.

- Surgical methods such as laparoscopic surgery and microsurgery diminish the likelihood of adhesion formation, although do not completely eradicate it.

- Following surgical excision, adhesions frequently reoccur.

- A variety of agents exist to mitigate the repercussions of surgery.

- Various pharmacological medications have been proposed to facilitate complete healing and prevent adhesion development.

- The application of steroids, historically prevalent in fertility-preserving pelvic surgery, lacks support from published studies.

- The administration of steroids may hinder the healing process and inhibit the hypothalamic–pituitary axis.

- Antihistamines, heparin, and nonsteroidal anti-inflammatory drugs (NSAIDs) have been ineffective in preventing adhesions.

- Barrier agents function by separating opposing wounded peritoneal surfaces throughout the healing period to minimize adhesion formation.

- The investigation encompassed various liquid agents, including crystalloids, icodextrin (ADEPT®, Baxter Healthcare), and hyperosmotic solutions.

- A meta-analysis of 350 trials did not demonstrate a decrease in postoperative adhesion development with the administration of crystalloids.

DOI: 10.1201/9781003650355-2

- It is unsurprising that 1000 mL of crystalloid is entirely absorbed from the peritoneal cavity after 24 hours.

- Dextran is a polysaccharide (Hyskon Pharmacia, Sweden) that promotes the transudation of fluids into the peritoneal cavity. The meta-analysis indicated no significant difference in the average adhesion score or pregnancy rate associated with the administration of dextran during second-look laparotomy (SLL). The substantial transudate is expected to be entirely absorbed before the completion of full healing, which is not unexpected. Documented adverse effects encompass allergy, pleural effusion, and peritonitis.

- Icodextrin, exemplified by ADEPT®, is a high-molecular-weight iso-osmolar alpha-1,4-glucose polymer that is gradually absorbed from the peritoneal cavity. Research has demonstrated incongruent findings.

- Hyaluronic acid is a linear polysaccharide consisting of disaccharide units formed from sodium D-glucuronate and N-acetyl-D-glucosamine. It is absorbed from the peritoneal cavity within 7 days. Multiple compounds of hyaluronic acid are or have been commercially accessible. They manufacture a gel-based barrier.

- A meta-analysis of four randomized controlled trials revealed a significant decrease in the incidence of adhesions with the application of hyaluronic acid derivatives (Intergel: 0.5% ferric hyaluronate gel; Hyalobarrier Gel: auto crosslinked hyaluronic acid gel; and Sepracoat: dilute hyaluronic acid solution) in comparison to placebo or no intervention.

- A recent meta-analysis of five randomized controlled trials revealed a substantial decrease in intrauterine adhesions following hysteroscopic surgery and intraperitoneal adhesions after laparoscopic surgery.

- Seprafilm® (Genzyme Corporation, Cambridge, MA) consists of chemically synthesized sodium hyaluronate and carboxymethylcellulose. It is absorbed from the peritoneal cavity within 7 days.

- A meta-analysis of six randomized controlled trials shown a significant decrease in the incidence, extent, and severity of peritoneal adhesions in non-gynecological abdominal surgery with the use of hyaluronic acid and carboxymethyl membrane.

- Nonetheless, a similar decrease in the occurrence of intestinal obstruction requiring surgical intervention was not observed.

- PEG-based liquid precursors (SprayGel™, Confluent Surgical, Waltham, MA) produce a gel barrier within seconds upon application to target tissue. It is absorbed from the peritoneal cavity within 30 days. A meta-analysis of three randomized controlled trials indicates a decrease in the occurrence of adhesion development with the application of PEG in fertility-preserving gynecological surgery.

- Gynecare Interceed® (Ethicon Inc, Somerville, NJ), an oxidized regenerated cellulose, serves as a synthetic barrier that creates a gelatinous protective layer over exposed areas. Careful hemostasis and the application of this membrane are crucial, as layering or contact with neighboring organs and blood may enhance adhesion formation.

- A meta-analysis of 12 randomized controlled trials at SLL indicated that the application of Interceed correlated with a reduced occurrence of adhesions compared to no therapy, for both de novo adhesions and the reformation of adhesions in the laparoscopy cohort. The laparotomy subgroup showed a decrease in the occurrence of adhesion reformation after adhesiolysis and ovarian surgery.

- The Gore-Tex® surgical inert membrane (W. L. Gore & Associates, AZ) is a non-absorbable adhesion prevention product that necessitates suturing and a subsequent surgical procedure for extraction. It exerts little influence on coagulation. Evidence of its efficacy as an anti-adhesive agent is minimal. Moreover, the requirement for suturing and subsequent removal renders Gore-Tex an improbable option.

- A general result indicates that cost-effectiveness can be attained if agents are utilized at the minimal expense of approximately £110 each application, contingent upon a 25% reduction in adhesions.

QUESTIONS

1. What percentage of patients after open gynecological surgery are readmitted with adhesion-related concerns in the UK?

    A. 1 in 1000

    B. 1%

    C. 4.5%

    D. 10%

2. Which of the following is considered the gold standard method to prevent post-surgery adhesion formation?

    A. Use of minimally invasive surgical techniques

    B. Using meticulous surgical techniques with minimal tissue handling and ensuring optimal hemostasis

    C. Use of physical barriers between peritoneal surfaces

    D. Use of anti-inflammatory agents such as steroids post-surgery

3. Which of the following are direct clinical consequences of adhesion formation after any surgery?

    A. Subfertility and pain

    B. Intestinal obstruction

    C. Difficulty in future surgical procedures

    D. A and C

    E. All of the above

4. Regarding icodextrin as an agent for post-surgery adhesion prevention, which of the following statements is incorrect?

    A. It is a polymer of alpha-1,4-glucose.

    B. It is rapidly absorbed from the peritoneal cavity.

    C. It is a high-molecular-weight and iso-osmolar solution.

    D. Research has yielded inconsistent findings concerning its efficacy in diminishing de novo adhesion development post-surgery.

5. All of the following are examples of hydroflotation agents for the prevention of post-surgery adhesion formation except?

    A. Crystalloids

    B. Icodextrin

    C. Dextran

    D. Hyaluronic acid

6. Among gels including hyaluronic acid derivatives used for prevention of post-surgery adhesion formation, which of the following is most slowly absorbed from the peritoneal cavity?

    A. Seprafilm

    B. Hyaluronic acid

    C. PEG

    D. Sepracoat

7. Which of the following post-surgery anti-adhesive agents is most quickly absorbed from the peritoneal cavity?

   A. Seprafilm

   B. Hyaluronic acid

   C. PEG

   D. Crystalloids

8. Which of the following statements regarding Seprafilm as a post-surgery adhesion prevention agent is incorrect?

   A. It is composed of sodium hyaluronate and carboxymethylcellulose.

   B. It is absorbed from the peritoneal cavity within 7 days.

   C. It significantly reduces the incidence and extent of peritoneal adhesions post-surgery.

   D. It is a solid barrier anti-adhesive agent.

9. All of the following post-surgery anti-adhesive agents are absorbable agents except?

   A. Seprafilm

   B. Interceed

   C. Gore-Tex

   D. PEG

10. Regarding the use of Gynecare Interceed as an anti-adhesive agent post-surgery, which of the following statements is NOT true?

   A. It is an oxidized regenerated cellulose.

   B. It is a synthetic barrier that creates a gelatinous protective layer over the raw areas.

   C. Meticulous hemostasis and the application of this membrane are crucial, as layering or contact with neighboring organs and blood may exacerbate adhesion formation.

   D. It is a gel-based anti-adhesive barrier.

11. Which of the following anti-adhesive agents has shown evidence to reduce the incidence of intra-uterine adhesions after operative hysteroscopic procedures?

   A. Seprafilm

   B. Hyaluronic acid

   C. Interceed

   D. Dextran

12. Which of the following statements is not correct regarding the use of Gore-Tex as a post-surgery anti-adhesive agent?

   A. It is a surgically inert membrane.

   B. It is a delayed absorbable anti-adhesive drug that is absorbed from the peritoneal cavity within 30 days.

   C. It requires suturing and a subsequent surgical procedure for its removal.

   D. It is regarded as an unlikely agent of choice for use as an anti-adhesive agent.

13. Which of the following is the only adhesion prevention agent approved by the FDA in the United States for prevention of adhesions during gynecological laparoscopic surgery?

   A. Hyaluronic acid gel

   B. Seprafilm

   C. 4% Icodextrin (ADEPT)

   D. Coseal/SprayGel

14. Which of the following adhesion agents are approved by the FDA in the United States for prevention of adhesions for open surgeries?

    A. Interceed

    B. Hyaluronic acid sheets

    C. Hyaluronic acid gel

    D. All of the above

    E. A and B

15. All of the following are examples of solid physical barrier anti-adhesion agents used in laparoscopic surgery except?

    A. Gore-Tex

    B. Interceed

    C. Seprafilm

    D. Hyalobarrier

16. Which of the following anti-adhesion agents is not correctly matched with their mechanism of action in the prevention of adhesions?

    A. Icodextrin solution – a solution retained in the peritoneal cavity to separate peritoneal surfaces

    B. Coseal – it is applied to the peritoneum to create a gel barrier

    C. Oxidized regenerated cellulose – it is a non-absorbable solid membrane sutured to the peritoneum

    D. Hyalobarrier — it is a highly viscous gel that coats the peritoneum

17. Based on recent studies, which of the following medications lack current evidence for preventing postoperative adhesion formation?

    A. Use of corticosteroids

    B. Low-molecular-weight heparin

    C. Unfractionated heparin

    D. All of the above

    E. B and C

ANSWERS

1. C	7. D	13. C
2. B	8. D	14. E
3. E	9. C	15. D
4. B	10. D	16. C
5. D	11. B	17. D
6. C	12. B	

3 SIP – Air Travel in Pregnancy

Source: Air Travel and Pregnancy Scientific Impact Paper No. 1 May 2013. https://www.rcog.org.uk/guidance/browse-all-guidance/scientific-impact-papers/air-travel-and-pregnancy-scientific-impact-paper-no-1/

IMPORTANT POINTS FROM THE GUIDELINE (SIP)

- The primary alteration in the environment linked to commercial air travel is the cabin altitude.

- Despite the pressurization of cabins, the cabin altitude will correspond to an elevation of between 4000 and 8000 feet during cruising altitude.

- Consequently, the barometric pressure is markedly lower than at sea level, leading to a corresponding decrease in the partial pressure of oxygen, which subsequently results in a fall of blood oxygen saturation by around 10%.

- This reduction does not present an issue for healthy persons, and this holds true during pregnancy.

- Due to the elevated levels of red blood cells in fetal circulation and the advantageous characteristics of fetal hemoglobin, it is believed that there is minimal, if any, alteration in fetal oxygen pressures.

- The humidity in aircraft cabins is approximately 15%, indicative of the reduced ambient humidity at high altitudes.

- This results in an elevation of insensible fluid loss, which is inadequate to induce dehydration, although mucous membrane desiccation occurs.

- Concerning the potential negative effects of air travel on pregnancy, there is insufficient data to indicate that commercial airline travel correlates with an elevated risk of unfavorable pregnancy outcomes, such as preterm labor, preterm rupture of membranes, or placental abruption.

- While there is no evident direct danger of pregnancy issues for passengers, alterations in cabin conditions may correlate with heightened discomfort and medical complications for the mother.

- As altitude increases and barometric pressure decreases, gases undergo expansion. This often results in ear issues, especially when accompanied by nasal congestion, which is more prevalent due to pregnancy-induced vasodilation.

- For certain women, motion sickness may exacerbate morning sickness.

- The flight's duration will result in considerable immobility and heightened risk of leg edema and deep vein thrombosis (DVT).

- Moreover, when combined with the physiological alterations in the coagulation system during pregnancy, this may exacerbate the risk of thrombosis, especially in the presence of additional risk factors, such as a history of DVT or obesity.

- The heightened exposure to cosmic radiation from flying is deemed negligible regarding risk to the mother or fetus during infrequent flights.

- Aircrew face limitations on radiation exposure, and numerous airlines prohibit pregnant aircrew from flying to minimize radiation exposure to the lowest practically achievable amount due to its cumulative effects.

- Women are increasingly inquiring about the utilization of body scanners, including backscatter devices and millimeter wave units, which employ ionizing radiation for security screenings before air travel.

- The cumulative radiation exposure from an examination with body scanners, which may consist of two or three scans, is inferior than that experienced during 2 minutes of flight at cruising altitude or 1 hour at ground level.

DOI: 10.1201/9781003650355-3

- It is indicated that little radiation doses are absorbed by the body during pregnancy, resulting in a significantly lower fetal dose compared to that received by the pregnant woman.

- This aligns with information from US authorities, which contextualize radiation exposure by indicating that backscatter machines emit radiation equivalent to 2 minutes of air travel, whereas millimeter wave units, which generate three-dimensional images, have emission levels 10,000 times lower than those of a mobile phone.

- This exposure level is deemed to pose no major risk; hence, there is no evidence indicating that a pregnant woman should refrain from such security scans.

- The primary issue preventing airlines from permitting pregnant women as passengers pertains to the potential onset of labor, which could interrupt or necessitate the diversion of the trip, coupled with the absence of suitable medical personnel and facilities to address labor or any obstetric complications during the flight.

- Due to the fact that most pregnancies reach a minimum of 37 weeks of gestational age, several airlines prohibit women from flying beyond 36 completed weeks of gestation due to this danger.

- Women with strong risk factors for preterm labor, such as those with multiple pregnancies, should refrain from flying after 32 completed weeks of gestation.

- This aligns with International Air Transport Association (IATA) recommendations; nevertheless, variations across airlines exist, and the woman should verify with the specific carrier prior to flying.

- The woman should be instructed to secure the seat belt snugly beneath her abdomen and across the upper portion of her thighs.

- Numerous airlines will mandate a letter from a midwife or physician affirming the absence of predicted problems during flights occurring after the 28th week of gestation, along with verification of the planned delivery date.

- While commercial air travel does not pose specific risks to pregnancy, it is crucial for the obstetrician to be cognizant of conditions that may complicate the pregnancy and potentially elevate the chance of complications.

- Examples of pertinent medical issues that may arise during pregnancy and contraindicate commercial flight travel include:
  - Severe anemia with hemoglobin below 7.5 g/dL
  - Recent hemorrhage
  - Otitis media and sinusitis
  - Severe cardiac or respiratory conditions
  - Recent sickle cell crisis
  - Recent gastrointestinal surgery, including laparoscopic procedures, where intestinal suture lines may be compromised due to pressure reduction and gas expansion
  - A fracture, which may lead to considerable limb swelling during flight, poses a particular risk in the initial days following the application of a cast

- Pregnancy poses a considerable risk of venous thrombosis.

- Despite the minimal absolute risk, this risk is likely exacerbated by air travel due to immobility and occasionally confined settings for taller women.

- The actual incidence of DVT during long-haul flights in pregnancy remains uncertain and challenging to ascertain, especially since the illness may be asymptomatic.

- Prolonged air travel is acknowledged to elevate the absolute incidence of venous thromboembolism (VTE) by almost 3-fold, with an 18% increased risk of VTE for every additional 2 hours of flight duration.

- Flights over 4 hours in duration are linked to a slight elevation in the relative risk of VTE; nevertheless, the total absolute risk remains minimal.

- The absolute incidence of symptomatic VTE is minimal, occurring at a rate of 1 in 4600 flights within the month following a flight lasting 4 hours.

- The risk will undoubtedly fluctuate based on the individual's thrombosis risk factors.

- For instance, there is a heightened prevalence among individuals with thrombophilia and users of combination oral contraceptives.

- In non-pregnant populations, it is predicted that approximately 4–5% of those at high risk will exhibit signs of DVT related to travel.

- Evidence suggests that wearing graduated elastic compression stockings during a flight mitigates the risk of asymptomatic DVT, with a relative risk of 0.10.

- This corresponds to an absolute risk reduction of 4.5 fewer symptomatic DVT cases per 10,000 individuals in a low-risk population, and 16.2 fewer symptomatic DVT cases per 10,000 individuals in a high-risk population.

- For women experiencing an uncomplicated pregnancy without medical or obstetric risk factors that would contraindicate air travel, there is no basis for advising against commercial air travel.

- In cases where a woman is at risk of miscarriage or ectopic pregnancy, particularly if she has a history of recurrent miscarriage or a previous ectopic pregnancy, it is advisable to verify the location and/or viability of the pregnancy through ultrasound before traveling.

- It is essential to secure suitable travel insurance that encompasses pregnancy-related coverage, including repatriation expenses in the event of a significant issue.

- Administering inactivated viral vaccinations, bacterial vaccines, or toxoids to pregnant women is deemed safe.

- Live vaccines, including yellow fever, should be avoided.

- To mitigate the risk of DVT, the following general recommendations are advised:

  - Opt for an aisle seat to enhance mobility

  - Engage in regular ambulation within the cabin

  - Perform in-seat exercises approximately every 30 minutes during medium-to-long-haul flights

  - Ensure adequate hydration while limiting caffeine and alcohol consumption to prevent dehydration

  - Conduct a tailored risk assessment for thrombosis in pregnant women traveling by air

- No specific actions are anticipated for short-haul journeys.

- For medium- to long-haul flights over 4 hours, it is recommended that all pregnant women wear appropriately fitted graded elastic compression stockings. This aligns with recent global directives.

- Women may possess supplementary risk factors for thrombosis, including a history of DVT, symptomatic thrombophilia (such as antiphospholipid syndrome or hereditary thrombophilia), morbid obesity, or medical conditions including nephrotic syndrome.

- For these women, targeted pharmacological prophylaxis using low-molecular-weight heparin (LMWH) at the standard prenatal prophylactic doses should be contemplated on the day of travel and for several subsequent days, provided she is not already receiving LMWH.

- The optimal length of thromboprophylaxis remains undefined and is up to professional judgment, contingent upon the assessed level and duration of risk for each individual woman.

- Consultation with an expert is advisable regarding the necessity of thromboprophylaxis.

- Low-dose aspirin is contraindicated during pregnancy for thromboprophylaxis related to air travel.

QUESTIONS

1. What is the cruising altitude at which most commercial flights fly?

    A. 2000 to 4000 feet

    B. 4000 to 8000 feet

    C. 8000 to 10,000 feet

    D. 10,000 to 12,000 feet

2. To what extent does blood oxygen saturation fall during commercial air travel at 4000 to 8000 feet cruising altitude?

    A. By 5%

    B. By 10%

    C. By 15%

    D. By 20%

3. All of the following changes occur in commercial flight cabins during air travel, except?

    A. Barometric pressure diminishes with rising altitude

    B. The gases in the cabin undergo expansion

    C. Humidity declines to around 15%

    D. Fetal oxygen levels drastically fall

4. Which of the following medical concerns can occur in pregnant patients during routine commercial air travel?

    A. Increase in motion sickness

    B. Increased nasal congestion

    C. Increased risk of DVT in long flights

    D. All of the above

    E. A and C

5. A 30-year-old primigravida patient presents to your outpatient department (OPD) for her routine check-up. Her pregnancy has been uncomplicated so far. All her blood tests and scans are normal. She is currently 16 weeks into her pregnancy and wants to discuss if she can fly to Scotland for a baby-moon holiday with her husband. She is very concerned about the exposure to body scanners at the airports. What is your recommendation regarding exposure to body scanners for pregnant women?

    A. Body scanners at airports ought to be entirely avoided.

    B. There is no evidence indicating that a pregnant woman should refrain from undergoing such security screenings.

    C. Exposure to two to three body scans must be strictly prohibited.

    D. Fetal exposure significantly exceeds mother exposure.

6. Up to what gestation do airlines allow most uncomplicated pregnant women carrying singleton pregnancies to travel?

    A. 28 completed weeks of pregnancy

    B. 32 completed weeks of pregnancy

    C. 34 completed weeks of pregnancy

    D. 36 completed weeks of pregnancy

7. Up to what gestation do airlines allow pregnant women carrying uncomplicated multiple pregnancies (twins) to travel?

  A. 28 completed weeks of pregnancy

  B. 32 completed weeks of pregnancy

  C. 34 completed weeks of pregnancy

  D. 36 completed weeks of pregnancy

8. After what gestation do some airlines require a medical certificate from the concerned midwife or physician stating that the pregnancy is uncomplicated, and the patient is 'fit to travel'?

  A. After 20th week of pregnancy

  B. After 24th week of pregnancy

  C. After 28th week of pregnancy

  D. After 32nd week of pregnancy

9. What is the overall absolute incidence of symptomatic VTE in pregnant women during the month after traveling on a 4-hour duration flight?

  A. 1 in 1000 flights   C. 1 in 3400 flights

  B. 1 in 2500 flights   D. 1 in 4600 flights

10. To what extent does prolonged air travel increase the absolute incidence of VTE?

  A. 2-fold   C. 5-fold

  B. 3-fold   D. 10-fold

11. For each 2-hour increase in flight duration, by what percentage does the absolute incidence of VTE increase?

  A. 5%   C. 18%

  B. 10%   D. 25%

12. An uncomplicated primigravida patient at 18 weeks of gestation presents to your OPD for a routine check-up before her upcoming holiday. She is traveling with her husband from London to Paris for a 2-week trip. What is your recommendation regarding her DVT prophylaxis?

  A. No specific measures are required other than routine measures

  B. Recommended to wear graduated compression stockings in addition to routine prophylactic measures

  C. Recommended to take low-molecular-weight heparin

  D. Recommended to take low-dose aspirin

13. An uncomplicated primigravida patient at 14 weeks of gestation presents to your OPD for a routine check-up before her upcoming holiday. She is traveling with her husband from the UK to Thailand for a 2-week trip. What is your recommendation regarding her DVT prophylaxis?

  A. No specific measures required

  B. Recommended to wear graduated compression stockings in addition to routine prophylactic measures

  C. Recommended to take low-molecular-weight heparin

  D. Recommended to take low-dose aspirin

14. An uncomplicated primigravida patient at 22 weeks of gestation presents to your OPD for a routine check-up before her upcoming holiday. She is traveling with her husband from London to Bali for a 2-week trip. Her body mass index (BMI) is >40 kg/m². What is your recommendation regarding her DVT prophylaxis?

    A. No specific measures required

    B. Recommended to wear graduated compression stockings in addition to routine prophylactic measures

    C. Recommended to take low-molecular-weight heparin after expert advice

    D. Recommended to take low-dose aspirin

15. All of the following are medical complications that contraindicate commercial air travel, except?

    A. Anemia with hemoglobin less than 9.5 g/dL

    B. Serious cardiac or respiratory disease

    C. Recent sickling crisis

    D. Recent gastrointestinal surgery, including laparoscopic surgery

ANSWERS

1. B	6. D	11. C
2. B	7. B	12. A
3. D	8. C	13. B
4. D	9. D	14. C
5. B	10. B	15. A

4 SIP – Alternative Therapies for Hormone Replacement Therapy (HRT)

Source: Alternatives to HRT for the Management of Symptoms of the Menopause Scientific Impact Paper No. 6 September 2010. https://www.rcog.org.uk/guidance/browse-all-guidance/scientific-impact -papers/alternatives-to-hrt-for-the-management-of-symptoms-of-the-menopause-scientific-impact -paper-no-6/

IMPORTANT POINTS FROM THE GUIDELINE (SIP)

- Evidence indicates that aerobic exercise can enhance psychological well-being and quality of life in women with vasomotor symptoms.

- Moreover, numerous randomized controlled trials have demonstrated that aerobic exercise can lead to substantial enhancements in various prevalent menopause-related symptoms (e.g. mood, health-related quality of life, and insomnia) compared to non-exercise control groups.

- Low-intensity exercise, such as yoga, may alleviate vasomotor symptoms and enhance psychological well-being in menopausal women.

- Not all forms of activity result in symptom enhancement.

- Infrequent high-intensity exercise may exacerbate symptoms.

- Regular prolonged aerobic exercise, such as swimming or jogging, seems to be the most beneficial activity.

- The minimization or elimination of alcohol and caffeine use may alleviate the intensity and occurrence of vasomotor symptoms.

- Lubricants typically comprise a mixture of protectants and thickening agents inside a water-soluble matrix. They are typically employed to alleviate vaginal dryness during coitus. Consequently, they do not offer a sustainable solution.

- Moisturizers may incorporate a bio-adhesive polymer based on polycarbophil that adheres to mucin and epithelial cells on the vaginal wall, thereby retaining moisture. Moisturizers are advertised as offering prolonged alleviation of vaginal dryness and require less frequent application.

- Progestogens have become a prevalent alternative to combined hormone replacement therapy (HRT) in women experiencing severe vasomotor symptoms and possessing contraindications to estrogen, such as breast and uterine malignancy or venous thromboembolism.

- Nevertheless, certain studies, including the Women's Health Initiative, have raised concerns over the safety of progestogens, as the elevated risk of breast cancer associated with HRT is attributed to the combination of estrogen and progestogen, rather than estrogen in isolation.

- Consequently, it is likely unsuitable to administer progestogens to women at heightened risk of breast cancer, especially those with progesterone-receptor-positive tumors.

- Clonidine, a centrally acting alpha-2 agonist, has emerged as a prominent alternative treatment for vasomotor symptoms. Regrettably, it is among the medications for which the least evidence of efficacy is available.

- A systematic review and meta-analysis demonstrated a slightly significant advantage of clonidine compared to placebo; nonetheless, the efficacy of clonidine was inferior to that of estrogen, and unpleasant effects may limit its applicability for numerous women.

- A substantial body of evidence supports the effectiveness of selective serotonin reuptake inhibitors (SSRIs) and selective noradrenaline reuptake inhibitors (SNRIs) in alleviating vasomotor symptoms.

- While there exists some evidence for SSRIs such as fluoxetine and paroxetine, the most compelling results pertain to the SNRI venlafaxine administered at a dosage of 37.5 mg twice daily.

- The primary disadvantage of these preparations, particularly the SNRIs, is the elevated occurrence of nausea, frequently resulting in premature discontinuation of therapy before optimal symptom alleviation is attained.

DOI: 10.1201/9781003650355-4

- Recent research on an analog of venlafaxine, desvenlafaxine succinate, has demonstrated that symptom alleviation can be sustained while minimizing unwanted effects.

- The antiepileptic medication gabapentin has demonstrated effectiveness in reducing hot flushes compared to a placebo.

- A study utilizing gabapentin at a dosage of 900 mg/day revealed a 45% decrease in hot flush frequency and a 54% reduction in symptom severity. The adverse impact profile, including drowsiness, dizziness, and fatigue, may limit its usage.

- Assertions have been made that steroids (diosgenin) in yams (*Dioscorea villosa*) can be metabolized in the human body into progesterone; however, this is biochemically unfeasible in humans.

- Consequently, it is unsurprising that brief application of topical wild yam extract seems to exert minimal influence on menopausal symptoms.

- To mitigate the detrimental consequences of progestogens, certain ladies undergoing systemic estrogen therapy utilize transdermal progesterone cream for endometrial safeguarding.

- Nonetheless, the evidence regarding the efficacy of transdermal progesterone creams in inhibiting mitotic activity or inducing secretory changes in an estrogen-primed endometrium is inconsistent.

- Consequently, the use of natural progesterone cream as progestogenic opposition is not advised.

- Current evidence suggests that women should be informed about the potential increase in their risk of endometrial cancer associated with such combinations.

- Women regard complementary therapies as safer and more natural alternatives to conventional hormone therapies.

- Nevertheless, the effectiveness and safety of several of these formulations have not been adequately assessed.

- Women utilize a range of botanicals.

- The information from clinical trials regarding the efficacy on menopausal symptoms is scarce and contradictory.

- A significant problem is that herbal medicines include pharmacological properties, which may lead to adverse effects and potentially hazardous interactions with other medications, both herbal and conventional.

- Furthermore, as most herbal medicinal goods are unlicensed, they are exempt from adhering to quality and good manufacturing practice laws.

- Phytoestrogens are botanical compounds that exhibit actions analogous to those of estrogens. The primary groups are referred to as isoflavones and lignans.

- Isoflavones are present in soybeans, chickpeas, and red clover, as well as likely in other legumes such as beans and peas.

- Oilseeds such as flaxseed are abundant in lignans, which are also present in cereal bran, whole grains, vegetables, legumes, and fruits.

- The significance of phytoestrogens has garnered much attention, as populations with a diet rich in isoflavones, such as the Japanese population, seem to exhibit reduced incidences of menopausal vasomotor symptoms, cardiovascular disease, osteoporosis, and malignancies of the breast, colon, endometrium, and ovaries.

- A review determined that isoflavone supplementation may yield a mild to moderate decrease in the frequency of daily flushes in menopausal women, with more pronounced benefits shown in those having a high incidence of flushes daily.

- Due to the estrogenic properties of phytoestrogens, there are apprehensions over their safety in hormone-sensitive tissues, including the breast and uterus, as well as their interactions with selective estrogen receptor modulators such as tamoxifen and aromatase inhibitors such as letrozole.

- Black cohosh (*Actaea racemosa*, previously *Cimicifuga racemosa*) is a herbaceous perennial plant indigenous to North America, extensively utilized to mitigate menopausal symptoms. No unanimity exists about the method by which it alleviates hot flushes.

- Findings from placebo-controlled trials or comparisons with alternative medicines, such as tibolone or estrogen, provide mixed results about the efficacy of black cohosh, whether utilized independently or in conjunction with other botanicals.

- The long-term safety of black cohosh remains mostly unknown.

- Liver toxicity has been documented, prompting certain regulatory bodies, notably those in the UK, to advise cautionary labels.

- Evening primrose oil is abundant in gamma-linolenic acid and linoleic acid.

- Despite its widespread use, there is little data supporting its efficacy in menopause. It has been demonstrated to be ineffective in treating hot flushes.

- Dong quai (*Angelica sinensis*) is a perennial herb indigenous to southwest China, frequently utilized in traditional Chinese medicine. Interactions with warfarin have been documented, elevating the risk of hemorrhage and photosensitivity.

- Ginseng is a perennial herb indigenous to Korea and China, widely utilized throughout East Asia.

- Case studies have linked ginseng to postmenopausal hemorrhage and mastalgia; interactions with warfarin (resulting in a diminished international normalized ratio), phenelzine, and alcohol have been noted.

- St John's wort (*Hypericum perforatum*) has demonstrated efficacy in mild to moderate depression in both peri- and premenopausal women due to its SSRI-like effect; however, its effectiveness for vasomotor symptoms has yet to be established. t interacts with numerous other pharmaceuticals.

- For instance, it reduces the plasma levels of cyclosporin, midazolam, tacrolimus, amitriptyline, digoxin, indinavir, warfarin, phenprocoumon, and theophylline.

- Concurrent usage with oral contraceptives may result in breakthrough bleeding and contraceptive failure.

- There is a paucity of data about the impact of Agnus Castus (*Vitex agnus-castus*) on menopausal symptoms.

- Ginkgo biloba, hops, sage leaf, liquorice, and valerian root are widely recognized; nevertheless, substantial evidence supporting their efficacy in alleviating menopausal symptoms is lacking.

- Kava kava (*Piper methysticum*), formerly utilized extensively for anxiety, particularly related to menopause, has been prohibited in the UK due to allegations of hepatic damage associated with the herb.

- Additional complementary therapies encompass acupressure, acupuncture, the Alexander technique, ayurveda, osteopathy, hypnosis, reflexology, magnetism, and reiki. Additional investigation is required to comprehend their potential impacts.

- Vitamins, including E and C, and minerals, such as selenium, are found in several supplements. The research supporting their benefits for postmenopausal women is exceedingly sparse.

- The stellate ganglion blockade, entailing the injection of a local anesthetic into the stellate ganglion, has lately surfaced as a novel approach for managing hot flushes and sweating that are resistant to alternative therapies or in cases where HRT is contraindicated, such as in women with breast cancer. Initial trials indicate promising effectiveness with negligible problems.

- Notwithstanding additional investigations into alternate formulations, their effectiveness remains inferior to that of conventional HRT (maximally 50–60% symptom alleviation compared to 80–90% with traditional HRT).

- Alternatives possess inherent harmful effects and hazards, prompting regulatory organizations to issue warnings for certain items.

- Legislation has been proposed that will require herbal preparations to be registered (but not licensed) with the Medicines and Healthcare products Regulatory Authority in the UK.

- This will facilitate regulation of over-the-counter sales. This directive is presently applicable solely in EU countries.

- Significant uncertainty and discord exist in the literature concerning the efficacy and safety of soy, red clover, and black cohosh; further trials are necessary.

QUESTIONS

1. To what extent does traditional HRT reduce menopausal symptoms?

   A. By 30–40%

   B. By 40–50%

   C. By 50–60%

   D. By 80–90%

2. To what extent do alternative therapies (other than traditional HRT) help to reduce menopausal symptoms?

   A. By 30–40%

   B. By 40–50%

   C. By 50–60%

   D. By 80–90%

3. Which of the following menopause-related symptoms can be improved by aerobic exercise?

   A. Vasomotor symptoms

   B. Psychological health problems

   C. Sleep-related issues such as insomnia

   D. All of the above

   E. A and B

4. Low-intensity exercise such as yoga can improve which of the following menopause-related symptoms?

   A. Vasomotor symptoms

   B. Psychological health problems

   C. Bleeding irregularities

   D. All of the above

   E. A and B

5. Which of the following can make menopausal-related symptoms worse?

   A. Aerobic exercise

   B. Low-intensity exercise such as yoga

   C. Occasional high-impact exercises

   D. Regular exercise such as swimming

6. Regarding vaginal lubricants, which of the following statements is false?

   A. Lubricants typically comprise a combination of protectants and thickening agents.

   B. They predominantly have a water-soluble base.

   C. They are used to alleviate vaginal dryness during intercourse.

   D. They offer a long-term sustainable solution and need to be applied less frequently.

7. Regarding vaginal moisturizers, all of the following statements are true, except?

   A. Moisturizers may contain a bioadhesive polymer derived from polycarbophil.

   B. These polymers adhere to mucin and epithelial cells on the vaginal wall.

   C. They possess the capacity to retain water.

   D. They do not offer sustained alleviation of vaginal dryness and require more frequent use.

8. What is the mechanism of action of clonidine?

   A. Beta-1 agonist

   B. Beta-2 agonist

   C. Alpha-1 agonist

   D. Alpha-2 agonist

9. Which of the following have convincing evidence as an alternative to HRT for treatment of menopausal symptoms?

   A. Fluoxetine   C. Paroxetine

   B. Citalopram   D. Venlafaxine

10. What is the mechanism of action of Venlafaxine?

    A. SSRIs

    B. SNRIs

    C. Selective progesterone receptor modulator (SPRM)

    D. Selective estrogen receptor modulator (SERM)

11. What is the most significant side effect of SNRIs which leads to withdrawal of therapy?

    A. Dry mouth   C. Nausea

    B. Constipation   D. Reduced libido

12. All of the following food groups are rich sources of isoflavones, except?

    A. Soybeans   C. Red clover

    B. Chickpeas   D. Flaxseeds

13. Which of the following is an important safety concern regarding the use of black cohosh for menopausal symptoms?

    A. Renal toxicity

    B. Hepatotoxicity

    C. Brain fogging

    D. Gastrointestinal cancer

14. Regarding stellate ganglion blockade, which of the following statements is false?

    A. It entails the administration of a local anesthetic into the stellate ganglion.

    B. It is applicable for people experiencing refractory vasomotor symptoms.

    C. It is applicable for women with breast cancer in whom HRT is contraindicated.

    D. It has demonstrated minimal efficacy and several complications, raising doubts about its therapeutic application.

15. Which of the following correctly explains the drug interactions of St John's Wort?

    A. Augments the efficacy of alprazolam.

    B. Reduces the efficacy of oral contraceptive pills, hence elevating the risk of contraceptive failure.

    C. Enhances the efficacy of warfarin, hence elevating the risk of hemorrhage.

    D. May reduce the risk of seizures due to its interaction with phenytoin and phenobarbital.

16. Regarding the role of black cohosh in menopausal women, which of the following statements is incorrect?

    A. It is a natural supplement occasionally employed to mitigate menopausal symptoms, including hot flashes and night sweats.

    B. The mechanism is described as an interaction with the body's opioid receptors, so potentially relieving pain and affecting mood.

    C. The FDA has now formally cleared it for routine use in menopausal women.

    D. It is not intended for prolonged use, and experts recommend employing it for a period of less than 6 consecutive months.

17. Which of the following does not correctly explain the beneficial effects of Korean red ginseng as an alternative therapy in menopausal women?

    A. It is known to reduce symptoms of fatigue

    B. It does not have any beneficial effect on female sexual function

    C. It enhances antioxidant activity

    D. It enhances overall quality of life in menopausal women

18. Which of the following chemicals is the active component of red clover that is potentially beneficial in menopausal women?

    A. Saponins

    B. Isoflavones

    C. Malonyl-ginsenoside

    D. Nucleic acids and amino acids

19. Regarding the role of evening primrose oil (EPO) in menopausal women, all of the following statements are true, except?

    A. It is often employed as a natural remedy for menopausal symptoms, particularly hot flashes, and may also mitigate other symptoms such as night sweats and vaginal dryness.

    B. EPO contains eicosapentaenoic acid (EPA), an omega-3 fatty acid that promotes the production of prostaglandins, hormone-like substances that aid in the regulation of physiological functions, including hormonal balance.

    C. EPO may assist in alleviating supplementary menopausal symptoms, including arthralgia and insomnia.

    D. The recommended dosage for menopausal women typically varies from 500 mg to 1000 mg daily, frequently administered in capsule form.

20. Which of the following Chinese herbal medicines has a phytoestrogen-like chemical named *Angelica sinensis*, which is potentially useful in menopausal women?

    A. Shugan Yidan fang

    B. Huangbai

    C. Dong quai

    D. Zhimu

ANSWERS

1. D	8. D	15. B
2. C	9. D	16. C
3. D	10. B	17. B
4. E	11. C	18. B
5. C	12. D	19. B
6. D	13. B	20. C
7. D	14. D	

5 SIP – Analgesia

Source: Antenatal and Postnatal Analgesia Scientific Impact Paper No. 59 December 2018. https://www
.rcog.org.uk/guidance/browse-all-guidance/scientific-impact-papers/antenatal-and-postnatal-analge-
sia-scientific-impact-paper-no-59/

IMPORTANT POINTS FROM THE GUIDELINE (SIP)

■ Insufficient pain management may result in the onset of anxiety and sadness, adversely affecting a woman's physical and psychological health, as well as her capacity to care for her infant.

ANTENATAL ANALGESIA

■ Acetaminophen:

- The precise mechanism of action of paracetamol remains incompletely elucidated.

- It is typically regarded as a poor inhibitor of prostaglandin synthesis, while a report indicates that it functions as a selective cyclooxygenase (COX)-2 inhibitor.

- Paracetamol is commonly employed as a primary analgesic in pregnant and lactating
women, owing to its superior safety profile and minimal medication interactions.

- Administered orally, it can elicit an analgesic response within 40 minutes; however, bioavailability may vary.

- When administered intravenously, the discrepancies in bioavailability are mitigated, resulting in an analgesic effect onset of merely 5 minutes.

- It is accessible as an over-the-counter medicine and is deemed safe during pregnancy.

- Reported adverse effects include a heightened prevalence of childhood asthma and behavioral issues, as well as delays in gross motor and communicative development in children
with prolonged prenatal exposure to paracetamol.

- Current guidance indicates that paracetamol is deemed safe for use during pregnancy and
lactation, and its administration in any trimester does not seem to elevate the risk of significant congenital anomalies.

■ Nonsteroidal anti-inflammatory agents (NSAIDs):

- Arachidonic acid is metabolized by the isoenzymes COX-1 and COX-2 into prostaglandins,
which serve as mediators of pain and inflammation.

- NSAIDs alleviate pain by peripheral inhibition of COX enzymes, thereby obstructing prostaglandin synthetase, with their therapeutic efficacy contingent upon their selectivity for
these enzymes.

- Conflicting information exists concerning the relationship between NSAID usage and the
heightened risk of first-trimester miscarriage.

- The FDA advises that, when feasible, the use of NSAIDs should be circumvented during
pregnancy.

- Nevertheless, when clinically warranted (as in cases when other analgesics may be ineffective, such as severe migraine and ankylosing spondylitis), it is recommended to administer
the lowest effective dose for the minimal duration necessary.

- The FDA advises against the use of NSAIDs after 30 weeks of gestation due to the risk of
newborn pulmonary hypertension and premature closure of the ductus arteriosus.

- NSAIDs diminish fetal renal blood flow, thereby decreasing urine production and resulting
in a reduced volume of amniotic fluid.

- Consequently, the administration of NSAIDs should be prohibited beyond 30 weeks of
gestation.

DOI: 10.1201/9781003650355-5

- Codeine:
  - Codeine is a natural opioid with a modest affinity for opioid receptors, resulting in little analgesic efficacy in its unaltered state.
  - It depends on its transformation into active metabolites, namely morphine.
  - Numerous genetic variables affect the conversion of codeine to morphine. Polymorphisms exist in the cytochrome P450 isoenzyme CYP2D6, a primary route for the conversion of codeine to morphine.
  - The pharmacokinetics of codeine in a person are variable due to genetic diversity in this route.
  - Individuals may be categorized as poor, intermediate, extensive, or ultrarapid metabolizers.
  - Approximately 7–10% of Caucasians are categorized as poor metabolizers, characterized by their minimal conversion of codeine into morphine, resulting in negligible pain alleviation.
  - The ultrarapid metabolizer phenotype results from duplications of the CYP2D6 gene, with prevalence differing by ethnic background.
  - Ultrarapid metabolizers of codeine may have plasma concentrations of its active metabolite morphine that are up to 50% more than those of extensive metabolizers, resulting in a heightened risk of severe toxicity even at therapeutic doses of codeine in these persons.
- Dihydrocodeine (DHC):
  - DHC exhibits comparable analgesic efficacy to codeine.
  - In contrast to codeine, which is a pro-drug exhibiting minimal analgesic characteristics on its own, the analgesic effect of DHC seems to mostly stem from the parent molecule.
  - It is predominantly uninfluenced by an individual's metabolic capacity.
  - DHC is converted to dihydromorphine (DHM) by CYP2D6, although only a minor fraction of DHC is transformed into DHM.
- Tramadol:
  - Tramadol is efficacious for mild to moderate pain relief.
  - It operates via both opioid and monoaminergic pathways.
  - It is additionally metabolized by CYP2D6 to yield an active O-desmethyl metabolite.
  - Tramadol exhibits less conventional opioid side effects, such as respiratory depression and constipation, although it can induce psychological problems, potentially linked to elevated plasma concentrations of the metabolite O-desmethyltramadol.
  - It is noteworthy that over 10% of the general population cannot tolerate tramadol due to the unpleasant effects encountered.
- Morphine:
  - Morphine is utilized for the management of moderate to severe pain.
  - It is an agonist of opioid receptors and functions in its parent form.
  - Its primary impact is the binding to and activation of opioid receptors in the central nervous system.
  - Its principal therapeutic effects are analgesia and sedation.
  - Peak plasma concentrations are attained about 15–20 minutes following parenteral dosing and within 30–90 minutes after oral administration.
  - It undergoes first-pass metabolism via the cytochrome P450 pathway, rendering an oral dose approximately half as effective as an intramuscular dose.
  - Morphine has been widely utilized during pregnancy and the postoperative period and is approved for use.

- It is easily absorbed via all methods of administration.
- Opioid analgesics may be utilized during pregnancy and lactation for the short-term management of moderate to severe pain when paracetamol proves ineffective.
- They should be administered solely upon evaluation and subsequently prescribed by a licensed medical professional or midwife.
- The use of opioids was associated with a minor increase in neural tube abnormalities; however, the data is inadequate, necessitating further investigation.
- The indiscriminate administration of opioids during pregnancy should be prohibited.
- The use of opioids, particularly during delivery, might result in neonatal respiratory depression; thus, the neonatology team must be notified if a woman in labor has been on long-term opioid therapy.
- Prolonged administration of opioid analgesics may result in neonatal withdrawal symptoms and maternal dependence; hence, the minimal therapeutic dosage should be utilized for the briefest duration feasible.
- Opioids might intensify constipation, nausea, and vomiting, which may already provide challenges for pregnant women.

- Gabapentin:
  - Gabapentin is employed in the management of chronic pain syndromes, particularly neuropathic pain.
  - The mechanism of action is not well comprehended.
  - Evidence concerning the use of gabapentin during pregnancy is scarce, and no association has been established between gabapentin and specific congenital anomalies.
  - The current advice is for women on gabapentin to additionally consume substantial doses of folic acid preconceptually and during the first trimester.
  - Gabapentin is not linked to a heightened risk of miscarriage.
  - Evidence concerning gabapentin use at 30 weeks of gestation or beyond is exceedingly scarce.
  - If gabapentin is administered near the time of delivery, more monitoring may be necessary during the neonatal period because of the potential risk of neonatal withdrawal.
  - Consequently, the neonatology team must be notified if an intrapartum woman has been administered gabapentin.
- Numerous women endure discomfort during pregnancy, encompassing headaches, lower back pain, and pelvic pain.
- Nonpharmacological therapies should be prioritized, including sufficient rest, hot and cold compresses, massage, acupuncture, physiotherapy, relaxation techniques, and exercise.
- Certain women consider aromatherapy to be calming and beneficial for relaxation; thus, it may be recommended to assist with pain relief following evaluation and consultation with a healthcare expert.
- Before administering medications to pregnant women, it is essential to evaluate the risk–benefit ratio and to use them judiciously to minimize detrimental effects on the growing fetus.
- All teratogenic medications should be avoided throughout the first trimester, as the embryo is particularly susceptible to teratogenic effects during organogenesis (4–10 weeks of gestation).

POSTPARTUM ANALGESIA

- Insufficiently managed pain can result in decreased mobility in women, so elevating their risk of venous thromboembolism and increasing susceptibility to shallow breathing, which heightens the likelihood of pneumonia development.

- It may adversely affect the woman's capacity to breastfeed or care for her newborn and may contribute to sadness or mental fatigue.

- Postnatal analgesia should not be contingent upon a woman's nursing status.

- Units must implement a standardized policy consistent with Medicines and Healthcare products Regulatory Agency (MHRA) advice.

- A unified approach for nursing and non-breastfeeding women is preferable to prevent confusion among professionals.

- Paracetamol, supplemented with NSAIDs (barring contraindications), should serve as the primary analgesic for all women.

- Alongside analgesic medications, women should receive guidance on nonpharmacological pain reduction techniques, such as the application of heat and cold compresses, as well as recommendations for suitable sitting and resting positions.

- Nonsteroidal anti-inflammatory drugs (NSAID)s:

  - Information about the use of NSAIDs while breastfeeding is exceedingly scarce.

  - Nonetheless, ibuprofen and diclofenac remain the favored options.

  - Ibuprofen is the preferred NSAID because of concerns with the long-term use of diclofenac and its association with elevated cardiovascular risk.

  - Ibuprofen is deemed safe for breastfed infants, as relatively minimal amounts are excreted into breast milk following maternal use.

  - A single administration of rectal diclofenac may be provided to women post-delivery.

  - NSAIDs may negatively impact renal function, platelet activity, and can aggravate asthma in around 10% of asthmatic patients.

  - Furthermore, they may induce stomach inflammation or ulcers.

  - Diclofenac and ibuprofen are contraindicated for individuals with a known hypersensitivity and should be avoided in the following conditions:

    - If there has been substantial hemorrhage, the woman is hypovolemic, and/or there exists a risk of further hemorrhage.

    - In females with compromised renal function or pre-eclampsia.

    - In females with severe asthma.

    - In women with asthma worsened by NSAIDs, especially aspirin.

    - In females with a history of stomach ulcers.

- Opioids:

  - If women endure more intense pain and require supplementary analgesia, opioid analgesics should be used.

- Codeine:

  - Until recently, codeine was regarded as the recommended painkiller for breastfeeding women.

  - A lethal instance of morphine intoxication in a breastfed newborn due to maternal codeine use prompted the MHRA and European Medicines Agency (EMA) to contraindicate its use in nursing women.

  - The woman in the newborn fatality case report was an ultrarapid metabolizer, resulting in the accelerated synthesis of morphine.

  - This is an exceedingly uncommon complication of codeine usage, and genetic testing to assess an individual's reaction to gene variations is presently unfeasible, as there is little information to determine if it would facilitate optimal codeine administration.

- Even at prescribed dosage regimens, ultrarapid metabolizers may encounter life-threatening or fatal respiratory depression or exhibit signs of overdose.

- Numerous reports indicate harmful consequences in breastfed infants subsequent to maternal administration of codeine.

- These encompass bradycardia, respiratory depression, lethargy, somnolence, inadequate feeding, cyanosis, and neonatal mortality.

- Research indicates that it is not solely the maternal CYP2D6 metabolizer status, but rather the interplay of mother genotype, neonatal clearance ability, and the administration of codeine for over 4 days that results in the accumulation of potentially dangerous morphine levels in breastfed neonates.

- Given the impracticality of genotyping all breastfeeding moms and newborns, mild opioids, particularly dihydrocodeine (DHC) or tramadol, may be recommended for breastfeeding mothers in lieu of codeine.

- The minimal effective dosage must be given for the briefest period, and continuous use of any opioid beyond 3 days should occur under stringent medical oversight.

- In instances where enhanced analgesia is necessary, DHC should be favored over codeine due to toxicity concerns.

- All breastfed newborns must be observed for opioid side effects, irrespective of the maternal dosage.

- Current guidance indicates that tramadol may be utilized (with caution) when nursing.

- The majority of women necessitating analgesia upon discharge should be administered paracetamol and ibuprofen, barring any contraindications to NSAIDs.

- Should supplementary analgesia be necessary, for instance, if a woman is discharged 1–2 days following a lower segment cesarean section as part of an enhanced recovery protocol and continues to require oral morphine solution in the hospital or is unable to take NSAIDs, she should be discharged with a restricted supply of DHC to be taken as needed (maximum of four doses per day).

- Tramadol may be deemed appropriate if a woman is intolerant to DHC.

- Given that tramadol is categorized as a Schedule 3 Controlled Substance, its supplementary stipulations must be verified during the prescribing process.

QUESTIONS

1. Which of the following analgesic agents is contraindicated in breastfeeding mothers due to increased risk to the infant?

    A. Paracetamol

    B. Ibuprofen

    C. Naproxen

    D. Codeine

2. Which of the following statements regarding paracetamol as an analgesic is NOT true?

    A. It is a selective COX-2 inhibitor.

    B. The analgesic effect manifests within 40 minutes when administered orally.

    C. When administered intravenously, the analgesic effect manifests within 20 minutes.

    D. It is regarded as a first-line analgesic owing to its superior safety profile and minimal medication interactions.

3. What is the mechanism of action of NSAIDs?

   A. Inhibits COX enzymes

   B. Inhibits prostaglandin synthetase

   C. Certain drugs disrupt cell adhesion and signaling pathways

   D. All of the above

   E. A and B

4. Regarding the analgesic action of codeine, which of the following statements is false?

   A. It is a naturally occurring opioid.

   B. It exhibits a high affinity for opioid receptors and possesses potent analgesic effects.

   C. Genetic variation exists in the cytochrome P450 isoenzyme CYP2D6, which metabolizes codeine into morphine.

   D. Individuals are categorized as poor, intermediate, extensive, or ultrarapid metabolizers of codeine.

5. Regarding the analgesic action of DHC, which of the following statements is true?

   A. It is a more potent analgesic than codeine.

   B. It is metabolized by cytochrome P450 CYP2E1 from DHC to DHM.

   C. Its analgesic effect is independent of the individual's metabolic capacity.

   D. DHC is entirely converted to DHM during metabolism.

6. Discussing tramadol as an analgesic agent, which of the following statements is false?

   A. It is efficacious in alleviating severe pain.

   B. It operates via both opioid and monoaminergic pathways.

   C. It is also metabolized by CYP2D6 to yield an active O-desmethyl metabolite.

   D. It may induce psychiatric problems, potentially linked to elevated plasma concentrations of the metabolite O-desmethyltramadol.

7. All of the following statements regarding morphine and its mechanism of action are true, except?

   A. It is utilized for the management of moderate-to-severe pain.

   B. It is an agonist of opioid receptors, primarily stimulating receptors in the central nervous system.

   C. It does not experience first-pass metabolism via the cytochrome P450 pathway.

   D. Peak plasma concentrations are attained about 15–20 minutes following parenteral dosing and within 30–90 minutes after oral administration.

8. Which of the following phases of pregnancy is the fetus most vulnerable to the teratogenic effects of medications?

   A. First 4 weeks

   B. 4–10 weeks

   C. 10–14 weeks

   D. 20–28 weeks

9. Which of the following drugs is the first-choice analgesic for mild-to-moderate pain in pregnant and breastfeeding women?

    A. Ibuprofen

    B. Paracetamol

    C. Codeine

    D. Tramadol

10. All of the following are reported to have adverse effects in children with long-term antenatal exposure to paracetamol, except?

    A. Childhood asthma

    B. Behavioral problems

    C. Major congenital birth defects

    D. Delay in gross motor and communication development

11. First-trimester use of opioids during pregnancy has been linked to which of the following birth defects?

    A. Heart defects

    B. Cleft lip and palate

    C. Clubfoot

    D. Neural tube defects

12. Which of the following are absolute contraindications for diclofenac and ibuprofen?

    A. Severe asthma

    B. Pre-eclampsia

    C. Gastrointestinal ulcers

    D. All of the above

13. All of the following are proven risks of using nonsteroidal anti-inflammatory drugs after 30 weeks of pregnancy, except?

    A. Pulmonary hypertension in newborn

    B. Premature closure of patent ductus arteriosus

    C. Decreased renal blood flow causing oligohydramnios

    D. Neonatal bradycardia and cyanosis

ANSWERS

1. D	6. A	11. D
2. C	7. C	12. D
3. D	8. B	13. D
4. B	9. B	
5. C	10. C	

6 SIP – Bariatric Surgery

Source: The Role of Bariatric Surgery in Improving Reproductive Health Scientific Impact Paper No. 17 October 2015. https://www.rcog.org.uk/guidance/browse-all-guidance/scientific-impact-papers/bariatric-surgery-in-the-management-of-female-fertility-the-role-of-scientific-impact-paper-no-17/

IMPORTANT POINTS FROM THE GUIDELINE (SIP)

- Obesity is a prevalent issue among women of childbearing age.

- In the UK, 26% of women possess a body mass index (BMI) exceeding 30 kg/m^2.

- Women are 3-fold more likely than males to be hospitalized with a main diagnosis of obesity.

- Female patients desiring bariatric surgery exceed male patients by a ratio of around 3:1, with around 70% of these women being of reproductive age.

- In a study, 25% of women seeking bariatric surgery experienced infertility.

- Obesity adversely affects natural conception, pregnancy, and the long-term health of both mother and child, resulting in a heightened incidence of congenital anomalies, pregnancy complications, and potential metabolic diseases in later life; additionally, the risk of miscarriage is elevated in obese women who conceive.

- Obese women exhibit a diminished response to pharmacological agents employed for ovarian stimulation in the management of anovulation and assisted reproductive techniques.

- Obesity may directly impact the technical feasibility of clinical operations, such as ovarian visualization by ultrasound or oocyte retrieval.

- Obesity impacts oocyte and embryo viability and may also influence endometrial receptivity.

- Obesity mostly impacts the quality of the oocyte rather than the reproductive environment.

- Obesity in pregnant women can trigger metabolic disorders and is linked to obstetric complications.

- A maternal BMI exceeding 30 kg/m^2 was linked to a heightened risk of gestational diabetes, gestational hypertension, pre-eclampsia, and fetal macrosomia in comparison to those with a BMI below 30 kg/m^2.

- Obese women exhibit a higher prevalence of induced labor, cesarean birth, anesthetic problems, perioperative morbidity, and extended hospital stays.

- The National Institute for Health and Care Excellence (NICE) guidelines advise considering bariatric surgery for those with a BMI of 40 kg/m^2 or more, or for those with a BMI between 35 and 40 kg/m^2 who have additional comorbidities and have not succeeded with conventional nonsurgical interventions.

- Bariatric surgery can be either restrictive, designed to diminish caloric intake by decreasing stomach capacity, or malabsorptive.

- Restrictive techniques encompass laparoscopic adjustable gastric banding (LAGB), silastic ring gastroplasty (SRG), vertical banded gastroplasty (VBG), and sleeve gastrectomy (SG).

- An example of a malabsorptive bariatric intervention is biliopancreatic diversion (BPD).

- The Roux-en-Y gastric bypass (RYGB) is a technique that is both restrictive and malabsorptive.

- Bariatric surgery leads to a sustained loss of 15–25% of body weight over the long term, along with considerable reductions in healthcare expenses and comorbidities linked to obesity, including diabetes, hypertension, and specific malignancies.

- The rates of serious complications linked to laparoscopic bariatric surgery are equivalent to those of standard elective operations, such as laparoscopic cholecystectomy, when conducted in big centers.

DOI: 10.1201/9781003650355-6

- In LAGB, an adjustable silicone band is positioned around the upper portion of the stomach to form a tiny upper stomach pouch, which restricts hunger and food consumption while facilitating an early sensation of satiety post-meals. The complication rate is approximately 13%, whereas the reoperation rate is 12%. The most common complication of LAGB are proximal gastric pouch expansion (10%) and port site infection (2.6%).

- In RYGB, a diminutive stomach pouch is segregated from the remainder of the stomach and discharges directly into the distal jejunum, thereby postponing the amalgamation of food with bile and pancreatic secretions. The outcome is an initial feeling of fullness that diminishes the inclination to continue eating. Complications encompass hemorrhage, anastomotic leakage accompanied by peritonitis, deep vein thrombosis, and internal hernias.

- In SG, a partial gastrectomy is conducted to diminish stomach capacity while preserving the normal anatomy of the remaining gastrointestinal tract. The metabolic effects and weight loss initially resemble those of RYGB surgery, although RYGB demonstrates superiority after 3 years.

- Calorie malabsorption does not seem to be a symptom of LAGB, SG, and RYGB; however, BPD and BPD with duodenal switch (DS) are malabsorptive procedures that diminish nutrient absorption by circumventing a significant portion of the small intestine, potentially resulting in deficiencies of iron, calcium, folate, thiamine, B12, and fat-soluble vitamins.

- Additional consequences of BPD and DS encompass steatorrhea, protein deficiency, anastomotic leakage, deep vein thrombosis, and internal hernia.

- Numerous prospective and randomized controlled studies have demonstrated that short-term remission of diabetes can be attained in 40% of patients following bariatric surgery.

- Numerous patients may experience relapse over the long term yet maintain much improved long-term glycemic control.

- Bariatric surgery improves the indicators of polycystic ovarian syndrome (PCOS) that affect fertility, such as anovulation, hirsutism, hormonal fluctuations, insulin resistance, sexual activity, and libido.

- There is a scarcity of research about miscarriage rates subsequent to bariatric surgery.

- Bariatric surgery is expected to decrease the risk of miscarriage.

- Concerning assisted conception, it was reported that 80% of IVF treatments after bariatric surgery resulted in live newborns; nevertheless, there is a potential heightened risk of ovarian hyperstimulation syndrome, which may cause ascites and considerable morbidity.

- Moreover, skin laxity combined with reduced adipose tissue may restrict the bioavailability of subcutaneously administered gonadotrophin hormones necessary for treatment.

- Numerous studies have shown enhanced maternal and fetal outcomes in women who have undergone bariatric surgery compared to untreated obese mothers.

- SG has demonstrated a reduction in anemia and a decrease in vitamin and mineral deficiencies during pregnancy compared to RYGB and BPD.

- Although RYGB does not cause malabsorption of macronutrients, the maintenance of sufficient nutrition during pregnancy may be affected by decreased absorption of fat-soluble vitamins.

- All patients are recommended to continue lifetime vitamin supplementation after bariatric surgery.

- Current guidelines advocating for the postponement of conception for 12–18 months post-surgery are founded on theoretical risks rather than empirical facts.

- It necessitates a more individualized strategy, considering maternal age and weighing the theoretical nutritional risks against the potential detriment to older women who have undergone bariatric surgery in delaying conception, which may further jeopardize their likelihood of conceiving a healthy kid.

- Expert opinion advises that postoperative bariatric patients should be regarded as a specialized obstetric population with distinct requirements.

- Intensive dietary support should be provided, ideally by dietitians experienced in addressing the nutritional issues following bariatric surgery, with careful monitoring for deficits and supplementation administered as necessary.

- All patients, irrespective of the type of operation, should have monitoring of ferritin, vitamins A, D, B1, B12, K1, and folate.

- Furthermore, weight must be meticulously managed, and weight gain should adhere to standard recommendations based on the BMI at conception.

- Continuous observation and systematic evaluation of fetal growth and development during pregnancy must be conducted, alongside surveillance for gestational diabetes.

- The deflation of the gastric band results in the concerning outcomes of weight regain, increased risk of gestational diabetes, and return of diabetes.

- Moreover, delayed stomach emptying may hinder the assessment of glucose tolerance testing, and the diagnosis of gestational diabetes is likely more accurately conducted using a diurnal blood glucose profile rather than through formal glucose tolerance testing.

- Surgical difficulties in pregnant individuals may be overlooked and misidentified as medical issues of pregnancy.

- The potential causes of stomach pain during pregnancy in women who have undergone bariatric surgery may include, band slippage or erosion, bowel herniation, or intussusception.

- The degree to which various surgical procedures differ in effectiveness and unfavorable impacts on pregnancy, as well as the long-term risk of obesity and cardiometabolic diseases in children, requires additional research, considering their distinct modes of action.

- The long-term effects on the progeny of women who have bariatric surgery should be investigated.

- A personalized strategy for selecting bariatric surgery and timing subsequent pregnancies should be adopted in the management of fertility and female reproduction.

QUESTIONS

1. What percentage of patients opting for bariatric surgery are suffering from infertility?
   A. 10%
   B. 25%
   C. 40%
   D. 50%

2. How does obesity affect fertility in women?
   A. Affects oocyte quality and embryo health
   B. Affects endometrial receptivity
   C. Obese women respond poorly to medications given for ovarian stimulation
   D. All of the above
   E. A and C

3. All of the following are restrictive bariatric procedures except?
   A. LAGB
   B. VBG
   C. SG
   D. BPD

4. Which of the following bariatric procedures is both restrictive and malabsorptive?

    A. LAGB

    B. RYGB

    C. VBG

    D. BPD

5. What is the reported weight loss that occurs with bariatric procedures that is sustained in the long term?

    A. 5–10% of body weight

    B. 15–25% of body weight

    C. 30–40% of body weight

    D. >50% of body weight

6. Which of the following is the most common complication of LAGB?

    A. Proximal gastric pouch enlargement

    B. Port site becoming infected

    C. Perforation

    D. Bleeding

7. Calorie and nutrient malabsorption are reported to be maximum with which of the following bariatric procedures?

    A. LAGB

    B. RYGB

    C. SG

    D. BPD

8. What percentage of patients achieve short-term remission of diabetes mellitus after bariatric surgery?

    A. 10%

    B. 20%

    C. 40%

    D. 60%

9. According to the guidelines, what is the minimum timeframe after which women who have undergone bariatric surgery should start planning pregnancy?

    A. 3 months after surgery

    B. 6 months after surgery

    C. 12–18 months after surgery

    D. 24 months after surgery

10. Which of the following tests is the best way to diagnose gestational diabetes in women who have undergone bariatric surgery?

    A. Fasting blood glucose and HbA1c levels

    B. Diurnal blood glucose profile

    C. Glucose tolerance test with 75 gm glucose

    D. 2-hour oral glucose challenge test (OGCT)

11. All patients who have undergone bariatric surgery must undergo monitoring of all of the following nutrients during pregnancy, except?

   A. Vitamins A, D, K1

   B. Vitamins B1, B12, and folate

   C. Serum ferritin

   D. Serum calcium

12. All of the following are reported complications of the RYGB procedure, except?

   A. Risk of hemorrhage and internal hernias

   B. Anastomotic leakage accompanied by peritonitis

   C. Deep vein thrombosis

   D. Proximal gastric pouch enlargement

13. All of the following factors are increased by vertical SG (bariatric surgery), except?

   A. GLP-1

   B. Ghrelin

   C. Peptide YY (PYY)

   D. Fibroblast growth factor 19 (FGF19)

14. Which of the following correctly describes the mechanism of action by which bariatric surgery induces weight loss?

   A. Increases bile acid release and hence enhances fatty acid oxidation

   B. Improves satiety

   C. Suppresses appetite by increasing GLP-1 and Peptide YY

   D. All of the above

   E. B and C

15. Which of the characteristic effects of bariatric surgery is the most important factor that improves clinical outcomes for patients with PCOS?

   A. Decreases fasting blood glucose and HbA1c levels

   B. Decreases systolic and diastolic blood pressure

   C. Decreases visceral adipose tissue and hence reduces androgenic fat distribution

   D. Decreases low-density lipoprotein levels

16. Which of the following is considered to have a protective role in folliculogenesis in patients with PCOS?

   A. Ghrelin

   B. PYY

   C. FGF19

   D. Adiponectin

17. Which of following mechanisms correctly explains the positive effect of bariatric surgery on menstrual function in patients with PCOS?

   A. Increases levels of sex hormone-binding globulin (SHBG)

   B. Reduces total testosterone levels

   C. Reversal of hyperandrogenism

   D. All of the above

18. What is the clinically significant conclusion of the multicenter, randomized control trial 'BAMBINI' that compared bariatric surgery versus medical care in PCOS patients?

    A. Significant improvement in clinical hyperandrogenism in the surgical group

    B. No significant improvement in cardiometabolic risk factors in the surgical group

    C. Significant increase in spontaneous ovulation rates in the surgical group

    D. No significant improvement in biochemical hyperandrogenism in the surgical group

ANSWERS

1. B	7. D	13. B
2. D	8. C	14. D
3. D	9. C	15. C
4. B	10. B	16. D
5. B	11. D	17. D
6. A	12. D	18. C

7 SIP – Biomarkers for Ovarian Cancer

Source: The Use of Biomarkers to Stratify Surgical Care in Women with Ovarian Cancer Scientific Impact Paper No. 69 May 2022. https://www.rcog.org.uk/guidance/browse-all-guidance/scientific -impact-papers/the-use-of-biomarkers-to-stratify-surgical-care-in-women-with-ovarian-cancer-scien-tific-impact-paper-no-69/

IMPORTANT POINTS FROM THE GUIDELINE (SIP)

- The prognosis for advanced-stage epithelial ovarian cancer (EOC) remains unfavorable, with a 5-year overall survival rate of 46.2%, despite advancements in chemotherapy and more aggressive surgical interventions aimed at achieving cancer stem cells.

- Surgery and platinum-based chemotherapy constitute the standard of care in the UK; nonetheless, there is considerable variability in their application.

- Cytoreductive surgery is generally acknowledged to confer a survival advantage among gynecological oncologists; nonetheless, subsequent relapse is prevalent, primarily due to the emergence of chemotherapy resistance, with 80% of women with advanced EOC developing resistance to first-line chemotherapy.

- The presence of residual disease at surgery correlates with a diminished prognosis; thus, biomarkers capable of forecasting surgical outcomes would enhance standards.

- Until recently, all women received platinum and/or taxane-based chemotherapy, with or without the incorporation of newer biological agents.

- This comprehensive regimen of chemotherapy and surgery disregarded tumor biology and was administered quite indiscriminately until the introduction of personalized biological agents.

- Customized therapy, using poly-ADP ribose polymerase inhibitors for women with germline or somatic BRCA1 or BRCA2 mutations (BRCAmut), is fundamentally transforming the landscape of medical treatment for EOC by precisely addressing the tumor's distinct biology.

- Surgery for EOC is conducted either prior to adjuvant chemotherapy (primary debulking surgery [PDS]) or midway through neoadjuvant chemotherapy (delayed debulking surgery [DDS]).

- The histological diagnosis of epithelial ovarian carcinoma is established prior to neoadjuvant treatment, and image-guided sampling of a solid tumor region may be supplemented by cytological sampling of ascitic fluid.

- This preoperative sampling allows for the identification of tissue-specific biomarkers that may affect surgical decision-making.

- Biomarkers indicating which individuals will respond to surgical cytoreduction have demonstrated potential.

- Epigenetic markers have been investigated to demonstrate responses to chemotherapy using MSX1 and to identify which optimally cytoreduced patients exhibit the poorest survival outcomes.

- Computed tomography (CT) imaging biomarkers, along with tumor-derived genetic and regulatory biomarkers, have been demonstrated to predict CSC.

- Phospholipid biomarkers can quickly ascertain tissue histology in both in vivo and ex vivo environments, enabling real-time surgical adjustments based on histological findings.

- The fundamental surgical intervention for epithelial ovarian carcinoma entails total abdominal hysterectomy accompanied by bilateral salpingo-oophorectomy and omentectomy; yet, this may be inadequate in cases with more advanced illness.

- Advanced disease may require a multi-visceral surgical strategy, including lymphadenectomy, splenectomy, bowel resection, diaphragmatic stripping, and hepatic capsule resection.

- Significant complications from extensive surgery were observed in 19% of women; nonetheless, this surgical method is endorsed by the National Institute for Health and Care Excellence

DOI: 10.1201/9781003650355-7

(NICE) under specific criteria, emphasizing that the current evidence about its safety and efficacy for advanced EOC is insufficient.

- The determination of surgical radicality disregards cancer biology; yet, tumor biology may serve as a predictive indicator of surgical success.

- A single DNA methylation biomarker aids in identifying high-risk women who may not get a satisfactory survival benefit from PDS.

- The DNA methylation of a cytosine-guanine pair in the myosin light chain kinase 3 (MYLK3) gene was strongly correlated with survival, even when limited to women who attained CSC.

- This biomarker has not been verified in a prospective clinical trials; however, it may potentially identify women who would benefit most from surgery.

- Serum CA-125 values exceeding 420 U/mL, significant ascites, and hepatic metastases are indicative of inadequate surgical cytoreduction, with an 80% probability if any of these characteristics are present.

- A triad of biomarkers related to gene expression (POSTN, CXCL14, phosphorylated Smad 2/3) has been correlated with the capacity to attain CSC, accurately categorizing 92.8% of cases into high or low risk for suboptimal cytoreduction.

- A systematic review indicated that fluorodeoxyglucose-18 positron emission tomography, CT, and diffusion-weighted magnetic resonance imaging (MRI) exhibited high specificity and moderate sensitivity for predicting CSC; however, there was inadequate evidence to endorse its routine application.

- The Risk of Malignancy Index (RMI) is routinely computed in the UK, derived from the blood CA-125 level, menopausal status, and ultrasound scan score.

- NICE presently advises that all women with an RMI score exceeding 250 should be referred to secondary care for additional evaluation.

- ROCkeTS (Refining Ovarian Cancer Test Accuracy Scores) is a phase III study designed to evaluate diagnostic test accuracy, with the objective of enrolling 2450 patients across 15 sites in the UK.

- ROCkeTS will evaluate and ascertain the precision of many diagnostic techniques within the same cohort, including ultrasonography, HE4 (human epididymis protein 4), ROMA, and RMI.

- Preoperative CT is widely employed to strategize surgical intervention.

- Alongside preoperative radiological diagnosis, numerous novel biomarkers have been documented. Cell-free circulating tumor cells and circulating tumor DNA have demonstrated potential in diagnosis, with DNA methylation patterns in cell-free DNA offering prospects for the early detection of EOC.

- Proton magnetic resonance spectroscopy has been suggested as a non-invasive biomarker for tumor metabolism; nevertheless, it has demonstrated inadequate ability to differentiate EOC from benign lesions.

- The sampling of ascitic fluid and pleural effusions yields a relatively precise diagnosis for adnexal masses.

- These fluids may provide significant biological insights on tumors and assist in preoperative diagnosis.

- Numerous high-throughput methodologies, such as as microarray-based gene expression profiling, next-generation sequencing, and proteomic analyses, are increasingly accessible for investigating the cellular and acellular constituents of ascites.

- New approaches cannot be integrated into everyday practice and will remain merely intriguing research concepts until they demonstrate diagnostic credibility.

- The sole recognized method for intraoperative histological diagnosis is the frozen section technique.

- A meta-analysis of frozen section accuracy indicated a sensitivity range of 65–97% for benign tumors and 71–100% for malignant tumors.

- A Cochrane analysis indicated that borderline ovarian tumors identified after frozen section are misclassified as EOC in 21% of instances.

- The frozen section procedure is time-intensive, expensive, susceptible to misinterpretation, and constrained by the capacity to obtain only a limited number of samples.

- Intraoperative misdiagnosis results in excessively radical surgery for some women or necessitates two surgical procedures if EOC is subsequently detected.

- Abnormal metabolism in malignancy has long been acknowledged as a defining characteristic of cancer, particularly characterized by elevated glycolysis and enhanced cellular lipogenesis.

- The distinct lipid metabolism in normal and malignant tissues is utilized by the surgical intelligent knife (iKnife) and the MasSpec pen.

- The iKnife integrates quick evaporative ionization mass spectrometry with a conventional handheld surgical diathermy instrument and multivariate statistical methodologies.

- This study examines lipid profiles in tissue-derived aerosols during tissue diathermy and provides histological diagnoses to the surgeon in near real-time.

- This method differentiates EOC from normal tissues with remarkable precision (97.4% sensitivity and 100% specificity).

- This approach can identify borderline histology with a sensitivity of 90.5% and specificity of 89.7%, far surpassing intraoperative methods such as frozen section.

- Desorption electrospray ionization mass spectrometry (DESI-MS) integrates mass spectrometry techniques with multivariate statistical approaches to analyze a microdroplet solution applied to a biological surface.

- The DESI-MS approach is non-destructive to tissue and offers remarkable predictions of tumor histology, along with forecasting the aggressiveness of serous EOC.

- These technologies produce diagnostic results rapidly, with the majority of systems capable of delivering a diagnosis in under 2 seconds.

- Intraoperatively, plasma, serum, and ascitic fluid have been evaluated via Raman microspectroscopy.

- This technique quantifies vibrational alterations in biomolecules generated by infrared radiation and has demonstrated potential as an intraoperative instrument for oncological diagnosis, achieving approximately 80% accuracy, sensitivity, and specificity.

- In the interval surgical cytoreduction context, following neoadjuvant chemotherapy, distinguishing live tumor from post-chemotherapy scar tissue might be difficult.

- Tumors exhibit morphological alterations such as fibrosis, calcification, and lymphocytic infiltration.

- The EOC cells have demonstrated the expression of folate receptor α (FRα).

- This tumor feature has facilitated the creation of technology that use FRα as a tumor-specific biomarker, tagging FRα with a bioluminescent dye that is visualized via near-infrared fluorescence.

- This green luminescence can be observed during surgery to assist the surgeon in identifying regions requiring resection.

- Unpublished data suggest that the surgical iKnife may effectively identify viable tumor deposits in neoadjuvant damaged tissue.

- Should these tentative findings be validated, employing the lipidome as an intraoperative tumor biomarker may allow the surgeon to guide surgical dissection.

- Hence, regions of neoadjuvant scar tissue containing live tumor cells may be removed, whereas portions of benign fibrosis can be safely retained.

QUESTIONS

1. What is the overall 5-year survival rate of women with advanced-stage EOC?

   A. 16%

   B. 26%

   C. 46%

   D. 56%

2. What percentage of patients with EOC develop resistance to first-line chemotherapy agents?

   A. 20%

   B. 40%

   C. 60%

   D. 80%

3. Which of the following drug therapies is incorrectly matched with the respective tumors that they treat according to the tumor biology?

   A. Poly-ADP ribose polymerase inhibitors for BRCA mutant tumors

   B. Human epidermal growth factor receptor 2 (HER2) antagonists for HER2-driven tumors

   C. Nipocalimab for BRAF mutant melanoma

   D. DNA methylation of MGMT for glioblastoma

4. A three-biomarker panel of gene expression which has the ability to correctly classify cases into high or low risk for suboptimal cytoreduction, includes all of the following except?

   A. POSTN

   B. CXCL14

   C. Phosphorylated Smad 2/3

   D. HE4

5. In a patient diagnosed with EOC, all of the following features are predictive of suboptimal surgical cytoreduction, except?

   A. Serum CA-125 levels greater than 420 U/mL

   B. Massive ascites

   C. Liver metastases

   D. Bilateral complex ovarian mass

6. RMI score, is calculated as a product of all of the following, except?

   A. IOTA score

   B. CA-125 level

   C. Menopausal status

   D. Ultrasound scan score

7. Which of the following preoperative tests is proposed as a non-invasive biomarker of metabolism in tumors?

   A. DNA methylation

   B. Proton magnetic resonance spectroscopy

   C. RMI

   D. IOTA (International Ovarian Tumor Analysis) rules

8. Regarding the role of frozen section as an intraoperative biomarker to decide the extent of surgery, which of the following statements is NOT true?

   A. It exhibits an accuracy range of 65–97% for benign tumors and 71–100% for malignant tumors.

   B. Borderline ovarian tumors identified after frozen section are misclassified as epithelial ovarian tumors in 21% of instances.

   C. The frozen section procedure is comparatively less time-intensive and cost-effective.

   D. Intraoperative misdiagnosis results in unreasonably radical surgical procedures.

9. What is the mechanism by which iKnife differentiates malignant from non-malignant tissues intraoperatively?

   A. Analyzes lipid patterns in tissue-derived aerosols during tissue diathermy and provides histological diagnoses to the surgeon in near real time

   B. Evaluates glycolysis rates during the operation

   C. Intraoperative analysis of the aberrant metabolism of malignant cells

   D. Evaluates DNA methylation in malignant cells during surgery

10. What is the accuracy (sensitivity/specificity) of iKnife to distinguish between EOC cells and normal tissue?

    A. 60%/75%   C. 90%/90%

    B. 70%/85%   D. 97%/100%

11. What is the accuracy (sensitivity/specificity) of iKnife to determine borderline histology intraoperatively?

    A. 60%/75%   C. 90%/90%

    B. 70%/85%   D. 97%/100%

12. All of the following are true regarding the mechanism of DESI-MS technique to differentiate malignant from non-malignant tissues intraoperatively, except?

    A. It integrates mass spectrometry with multivariate statistical methodologies

    B. It examines a microdroplet solution applied to a biological surface

    C. The reporting time is significantly slower than that of frozen section

    D. It is non-destructive to tissue and offers remarkable predictions of tumor histology

13. What is the mechanism by which Raman microspectroscopy differentiates malignant from non-malignant tissues intraoperatively?

    A. Evaluates glycolysis rates during surgery

    B. Assesses abnormal metabolism of malignant cells during surgery

    C. Examines DNA methylation in malignant cells during surgery

    D. Analyzes vibrational alterations in biomolecules generated by infrared radiation

14. What is the accuracy (sensitivity/specificity) of Raman microspectroscopy to determine an intraoperative oncological diagnosis?

    A. 60%/75%

    B. 70%/85%

    C. 80%/80%

    D. 97%/100%

15. In patients after neoadjuvant chemotherapy, which of the following receptors expressed by EOC cells can intraoperatively differentiate viable malignant cells from post-chemotherapy scarred tissue to guide tumor resection?

   A. FRα

   B. HER2

   C. Estrogen receptors (ER)

   D. G-protein-coupled receptors (GPCRs)

16. The multivariate quantitative assay OVA1 includes all of the following serum proteins as a biomarker for detection of ovarian cancer, except?

   A. CA-125 levels

   B. Transthyretin and transferrin

   C. Apolipoprotein A1 and beta-2-microglobulin

   D. Osteopontin

17. Which of the following serum biomarkers has shown substantial evidence in differentiating benign from malignant ovarian tumors?

   A. Osteopontin

   B. Kallikreins (KLKs)

   C. Human epididymis protein 4 (HE4)

   D. Mesothelin

18. ROMA quantitative assay includes all of the following as biomarkers for detection of ovarian cancer, except?

   A. CA-125 levels

   B. HE4 concentration

   C. Menopausal status

   D. Transthyretin

19. Which of the following statements regarding osteopontin as a biomarker for early diagnosis of ovarian cancer is incorrect?

   A. It is an extracellular glycoprotein.

   B. It is secreted by vascular endothelial cells and osteoblasts.

   C. Can be quantified in urine samples of women with high-grade (advanced) ovarian cancer.

   D. It is not independently associated with unfavorable outcomes in women with ovarian cancer.

20. Regarding the use of KLKs as a potential biomarker for ovarian cancer, which of the following statements is true?

   A. KLKs are a family of 15 serine proteases, encoded by a gene cluster located on chromosome 19q13, that participate in several cellular processes and pathways by influencing proteolytic cascades.

   B. They are expressed in epithelial and endocrine tissues governed by hormones in cancer and are secreted and detected in human bodily fluids.

   C. Certain KLKs are linked to poor prognosis and advanced disease stages (4–7, 10, and 15), in addition to chemoresistance (KLK 4 and 7) to first-line paclitaxel therapy.

   D. The sensitivity of these biomarkers is augmented through their combinations.

   E. All of the above.

ANSWERS

1. C	8. C	15. A
2. D	9. A	16. D
3. C	10. D	17. C
4. D	11. C	18. D
5. D	12. C	19. D
6. A	13. D	20. E
7. B	14. C	

8 SIP – Botulinum Toxin for Overactive Bladder (OAB)

Source: Botulinum Toxin for an Overactive Bladder Scientific Impact Paper No. 42 February 2014. https://www.rcog.org.uk/guidance/browse-all-guidance/scientific-impact-papers/botulinum-toxin-for-an-overactive-bladder-scientific-impact-paper-no-42/

IMPORTANT POINTS FROM THE GUIDELINE (SIP)

- Botulinum toxin type A (BoNT-A) preparations have gained recognition as a therapeutic alternative for detrusor overactivity (DO) and overactive bladder (OAB).

- DO can be neurogenic (NDO), such as following spinal injury or multiple sclerosis, or idiopathic (IDO), with no discernible underlying cause.

- Nonetheless, the function of BoNT-A in therapeutic protocols remains to be definitively determined.

- Typically, individuals with OAB are first managed with conservative strategies, including lifestyle modifications, reduction of caffeine consumption, pelvic floor exercises, and bladder training, prior to the initiation of various anticholinergic pharmacotherapies, such as oxybutynin, tolterodine, solifenacin, or trospium.

- The majority of clinicians will administer two or more oral drugs before progressing to second-line treatments, which presently encompass implantable sacral nerve stimulators or botulinum toxin.

- After a multidisciplinary team evaluation, BoNT-A may be deemed appropriate for women with OAB resulting from documented DO, in cases when conservative therapy, including pharmaceutical interventions, has proven futile.

- Botulinum toxin is delivered using a cystoscope and injected into the detrusor muscle at around 20–30 locations over the bladder dome, typically avoiding the trigone.

- The procedure may be performed under local or general anesthesia using rigid or flexible cystoscopy.

- Flexible cystoscopy with local anesthesia is rapid, straightforward, and entails little hazards.

- BoNT-A inhibits the presynaptic release of acetylcholine, resulting in complete or partial paralysis and attenuation of hyperactive muscular activity.

- Randomized controlled trials have shown substantial effectiveness in alleviating neurogenic DO, decreasing detrusor pressure, enhancing bladder capacity, diminishing incontinence episodes, and improving quality of life in individuals with neurogenic incontinence.

- Nonetheless, these enhancements are typically counterbalanced by a certain degree of compromised bladder evacuation.

- The mechanism of action is more complex than mere paralysis of the detrusor muscle.

- The mechanism of action may not only restore the expression of neuronal sensory receptors to normal levels in bladder biopsies from effectively treated patients but may also involve a complex inhibitory effect on the vesicular release of excitatory neurotransmitters and the axonal expression of additional proteins.

- These are considered significant in mediating the intrinsic or spinal reflexes believed to induce NDO. This indicates the involvement of the sensory afferent pathway.

- An additional impact on efferent (motor) pathways is likely, as impairment or deterioration of bladder emptying commonly occurs in individuals with NDO and, to a lesser degree, in those with IDO.

- Onabotulinumtoxin A (onaBoNT-A) (Botox®, Allergan, Marlow, UK) is now licensed for the treatment of IDO and OAB in the United States and most European nations, including the United Kingdom.

- The alternative preparations have not yet received licensure for NDO.

    DOI: 10.1201/9781003650355-8

- Multiple uncontrolled case studies have documented the effects of BoNT-A in individuals with IDO, and the findings are largely consistent.

- The results of these research generally show significant enhancements in OAB symptoms, including urgency, frequency of urination, incontinence, utilization of continence pads, and disease-specific quality of life metrics.

- OAB is a symptom complex characterized by urgency, frequency, nocturia, with or without incontinence.

- OAB is linked to the urodynamic assessment of DO.

- Currently, most UK doctors do not regularly provide BoNT-A to women lacking a urodynamic diagnosis of DO.

- Parkinson's disease is linked to urine disturbances in up to 30% of patients and has conventionally been managed with anticholinergic medications.

- Nevertheless, the effectiveness of this treatment has been demonstrated to be inadequate.

- Preliminary findings indicate that BoNT-A may be effective in managing bladder symptoms in Parkinson's disease via altering afferent nerve activity.

- BoNT-A injections were shown to enhance the likelihood of sexual intercourse and reduce levator ani EMG hyperactivity in women diagnosed with vaginismus, as well as alleviate symptoms of bladder pain.

- In patients with neurogenic NDO, the dosage of onaBoNT-A prescribed has decreased, as current studies indicate that smaller doses are comparably efficacious.

- Recent data from two trials indicate that a dosage of 100 units for IDO treatment may be as efficacious as 150 or 200 units, while exhibiting a reduced incidence of side effects, including a notably low rate of urine retention.

- An algorithm for determining an initial dose, as well as the timing and criteria for administering a greater dose, is not fully established.

- There is scant evidence comparing various doses of the alternative formulations.

- Various preparations possess units of activity that are not comparable; therefore, caution is necessary to ensure equivalence is attained.

- To our knowledge, there is limited data regarding rimabotulinumtoxin B (rimaBoNT-A) (Myobloc®) and incobotulinum toxin A (incBoNT-A) (Xeomin®).

- The ideal period between injections remains to be determined, and it is presently uncertain whether patients will have lifelong repeat injections or if a subset of patients will attain a cure post-treatment.

- The data suggest that onaBoNT-A may offer substantial alleviation of OAB symptoms and DO, with a median duration of approximately 6 months.

- Patients should be cautioned about potential side effects, including urinary tract infections in around one in six patients and voiding dysfunction (either complete or partial) in up to 10% of women, typically treated with self-catheterization.

QUESTIONS

1. Which of the following parts of the bladder should be spared while injecting botulinum toxin for OAB?

    A. Dome of the bladder

    B. Trigone of the bladder

    C. Body of the bladder

    D. Apex of the bladder

2. Regarding the technique of injecting botulinum toxin for DO, which of the following statements is incorrect?

    A. It is administered through a cystoscope.

    B. It is administered into the detrusor from within.

    C. It is typically injected at 20 to 30 locations within the trigone of the bladder.

    D. Flexible cystoscopy under local anesthesia is efficient, straightforward, and entails little hazards.

3. In NDO, all of the following are significant improvements demonstrated by randomized controlled trials, except?

    A. Increasing detrusor pressure

    B. Increasing bladder capacity

    C. Reducing episodes of incontinence

    D. Improving quality of life of patients

4. Which of the following preparations of botulinum toxin is licensed for treatment of DO (both idiotpathic and neurogenic) and OAB?

    A. Abobotulinumtoxin A (aboBoNT-A)

    B. onaBoNT-A

    C. rimaBoNT-A

    D. incBoNT-A

5. OAB syndrome includes all of the following symptoms, except?

    A. Urgency and frequency of urination

    B. Nocturia, with or without incontinence

    C. Urodynamic observation of DO

    D. Overflow incontinence

6. What percentage of adults diagnosed with Parkinson's disease have urinary disturbance?

    A. 10%

    B. 30%

    C. 50%

    D. 70%

7. What is the incidence of urinary tract infections in patients with DO treated by botulinum toxin injection?

    A. One in two

    B. One in four

    C. One in six

    D. One in ten

8. What is the incidence of voiding dysfunction in patients with DO treated by botulinum toxin injection?

    A. Up to 5%

    B. Up to 10%

    C. Up to 20%

    D. Up to 30%

9. What is the median duration of symptom relief for patients with OAB after treatment with botulinum toxin injection?

    A. 6 weeks

    B. 3 months

    C. 6 months

    D. 12 months

10. What is the preferred dose (in units) of botulinum toxin in treatment of IDO for good symptom relief with minimal adverse effects?

    A. 50 units

    B. 100 units

    C. 150 units

    D. 200 units

ANSWERS

1. B	5. D	9. C
2. C	6. B	10. B
3. A	7. C	
4. B	8. B	

9 SIP – Chemical Exposures in Pregnancy

Source: Chemical Exposures during Pregnancy: Dealing with Potential, But Unproven, Risks to Child Health Scientific Impact Paper No. 37 May 2013. https://www.rcog.org.uk/guidance/browse-all-guidance/scientific-impact-papers/chemical-exposures-during-pregnancy-dealing-with-potential-but-unproven-risks-to-child-health-scientific-impact-paper-no-37/

IMPORTANT POINTS FROM THE GUIDELINE (SIP)

- The notion that maternal exposure to specific chemicals and pharmaceuticals during gestation and lactation may adversely affect the fetus or infant is well-established.

- The detrimental impacts of cigarette smoking and alcohol intake during pregnancy on fetal development and long-term health are extensively documented.

- This has resulted in the issuance of guidelines and recommendations for pregnant women regarding the implications of these lifestyle choices on unborn infants.

- Conversely, there are no official antenatal recommendations or guidelines that advise pregnant or breastfeeding women about the possible risks that certain chemical exposures may cause to their infants.

- Instead, they encounter frequent media reports on 'chemical scares' that are often erroneous or overstated.

- These narratives cause discernible worry for women who are pregnant or lactating.

- The mother is the custodian of her infant's growth and future well-being; any external factors affecting the infant mostly originate from the mother.

- The predisposition to some adult health conditions is increasingly acknowledged to be influenced by the quality of fetal development and the immediate postnatal period.

- Modified susceptibility to adult ailments, including obesity, type II diabetes, and cardiovascular disease, exemplifies the impact of prenatal development on health.

- Proactive measures to provide the infant with an optimal beginning in life, minimizing the likelihood of future ailments, can be implemented through healthy lifestyle modifications and decisions during the planning and duration of pregnancy and breastfeeding.

- Examples include abstaining from smoking and alcohol consumption, as well as maintaining a balanced diet during pregnancy.

- Epidemiological studies have associated exposure to certain chemicals during pregnancy with negative birth outcomes, including pregnancy loss, preterm birth, low birth weight, congenital anomalies, childhood morbidity, obesity, cognitive impairment, compromised immune system development, asthma, early onset of puberty, adult diseases, and mortality (specifically cardiovascular effects and cancer).

- Moreover, exposure to common environmental toxins has been linked to diminished fertility and fecundity in women, as well as impaired testicular development and reproductive function in men.

- Nearly all pregnant women are exposed to specific chemicals present in common items.

- Bisphenol A (BPA) is present in beverages and food containers, while phthalate esters are located in plastics, carpets, textiles, personal care items, and adhesives.

- This complicates the identification of any potential effects of such exposures, as there is no unexposed 'control' group for comparative analysis.

- To minimize exposure to environmental toxins, women must first comprehend when such exposures take place.

- Humans are universally exposed to some environmental chemicals through various channels, some of which are beyond our control.

DOI: 10.1201/9781003650355-9

- Phthalates are utilized in various polymers as well as in numerous everyday household items, including adhesives, flooring materials, and automobiles.

- Additional compounds exist in the air we inhale, including combustion byproducts referred to as polycyclic aromatic hydrocarbons (PAHs).

- While it is challenging to entirely evade these exposures, one can mitigate them by steering clear of direct and secondary cigarette smoke, as well as barbecues and bonfires.

- Food serves as a significant conduit for exposure to environmental toxins, manifesting in various forms.

- Dichlorodiphenyltrichloroethane (DDT) and polychlorinated biphenyls (PCBs) accumulate in adipose tissue, exhibiting lipophilic properties.

- These substances accumulate throughout the food chain and are transmitted along it, notwithstanding their current prohibition.

- Research has linked human fetal exposure to certain substances with negative birth outcomes previously enumerated.

- Fortunately, exposure to these substances is gradually diminishing.

- Nevertheless, supplementary preventative measures can further mitigate this.

- Such chemicals tend to bioaccumulate in oily fish, which are otherwise regarded as 'nutritious.'

- Limiting the ingestion of such fish to once per week is a prudent measure.

- This approach is further motivated by the fact that certain species, including tuna, acquire heavy elements such as mercury and lead.

- Mercury and lead are conclusively associated with issues in fetal and child development.

- Consequently, current UK guidelines recommend that pregnant women diminish or cease their intake of oily fish during pregnancy.

- Consuming an abundance of fruits and vegetables during pregnancy is highly advised, even with the potential presence of pesticide residues.

- Such exposure to pesticides is commonly regarded as a significant health hazard.

- Pesticides are subject to stringent regulations, resulting in limited human exposure through food residues, even in non-organic products.

- The majority of individuals are oblivious to the fact that food may also be tainted by chemicals from the handling equipment utilized in food processing.

- Chemicals may seep into food packaging and containers, such as food and beverage cans.

- Fresh food typically contains fewer non-food chemicals and/or lower concentrations than processed oven-ready or microwave meals.

- This can be exemplified by citing two prevalent chemicals utilized in diverse plastics and other applications, specifically phthalate esters and bisphenol A.

- When participants were transitioned for 3 days from their regular food sources to freshly sourced and unpackaged meals, the concentrations of BPA and a significant phthalate in their urine diminished by 65% and 53%, respectively.

- The exposure of an individual's internal tissues to chemicals is likely influenced by differences in gut microbiota, which are probably contingent upon the individual's diet and health.

- Another significant form of chemical exposure for women is cosmetics and personal care items, particularly those applied to extensive skin areas to enhance absorption, including moisturizers, sunscreens, cosmetics, scents, shower gels, and hairspray.

- The consumption of these items by women has surged significantly in recent decades.

- Current legislation stipulates that manufacturers are not supposed to disclose all potentially dangerous compounds in the ingredients list if they are not classified as active components.

- A product endorsed and evaluated by a prominent environmental health website, designed for infants, children, and adults with sensitive skin, was also analyzed.

- Phthalates were the predominant component identified in the inactive constituents of this product.

- Heightened utilization of infant care items, including lotions, powders, and shampoos, correlates with elevated exposure to phthalates in infants.

- These instances underscore the inadequacies of product labeling and illustrate how women could erroneously conclude that a product is 'safe' for use during pregnancy, despite the omission of certain elements from consideration.

- Compiling a list of such concealed compounds is unfeasible, as they are exclusively known to the manufacturer of the particular product.

- Women are similarly subjected to toxins from a range of household goods.

- This encompasses cleaning solutions, air fresheners, furniture, carpets, and fabrics, as well as DIY agents such as paint and glue.

- Polybrominated diphenyl ethers (PBDEs) are chemicals utilized in household products as flame retardants in furniture, electronics, and automobiles.

- Another category includes perfluorinated compounds (PFCs), utilized in the production of materials that exhibit resistance to stains, oils, and water.

- Certain analgesics, including paracetamol, are advised as safe for use during early pregnancy.

- Recent studies indicate that prolonged paracetamol usage during early pregnancy may elevate the incidence of incomplete testis descent (cryptorchidism) and asthma in kids.

- Numerous pharmaceutical prescriptions and dietary supplements have phthalates in their tablet coatings, categorizing them as inactive substances or excipients.

- Consequently, phthalates are not mandated to be disclosed on product labels.

- Over-the-counter medications serve as a common avenue for inadvertent chemical exposure.

- It is particularly alarming when 'herbal' or alternative 'natural' therapies are advertised as 'safe' for pregnant women.

- Alarmingly, these have not undergone any safety testing for use.

- Consequently, it is crucial for women who are planning to conceive or are pregnant to recognize that 'natural' products do not guarantee safety for usage during pregnancy.

- Vitamin A and retinoids are crucial for human health, although excessive consumption can significantly produce prenatal abnormalities.

- Consequently, it is prudent for pregnant women to limit their intake of liver, as it is a repository for vitamin A.

- The increasing apprehension regarding the impacts of ordinary chemical exposure derives from the potential of many of these chemicals to disrupt one or more hormonal systems in the body, which are crucial for appropriate fetal development.

- Endocrine disruptors, such as BPA plastics, PBDEs, and phthalates, can imitate or obstruct the function of endogenous endocrine hormones, so interfering with normal embryonic development.

- An illustrative example of this is 'anti-androgenic' chemicals, such as certain phthalates, which can disrupt the masculinization of male fetuses, a developmental process dependent on the adequate secretion of androgenic hormones by the fetal testis during early pregnancy.

- Under typical lifestyle and dietary circumstances, the exposure level of most women to certain environmental toxins is likely to present negligible harm to the developing fetus or infant.

- Pregnant women are exposed to numerous substances at low concentrations.

- This exposure may function additively or interactively, suggesting the potential for 'mixed' effects.

- Current evidence renders it impossible to evaluate the risk, if any, associated with such exposures.

- Acquiring more conclusive guidelines is expected to require several years; significant ambiguity persists regarding the dangers associated with chemical exposure.

- The following measures would, nonetheless, mitigate total chemical exposure:

  - Opt for fresh meals instead of processed items wherever feasible.

  - Minimize the consumption of canned and plastic container foods/beverages, including their application for food storage.

  - Reduce the utilization of personal care items such as moisturizers, cosmetics, shower gels, and scents.

  - Reduce the acquisition of newly manufactured household furnishings, textiles, non-stick cookware, and automobiles during pregnancy and nursing.

  - Refrain from utilizing garden, household, or pet pesticides or fungicides, including fly sprays, rose sprays, and flea powders.

  - Eliminate paint vapors.

  - Administer over-the-counter analgesics or pain relievers just as required.

  - Do not presume the safety of products just due to the absence of 'dangerous' substances in their ingredient list or the designation 'natural' (herbal or otherwise).

- While it is improbable that these exposures are genuinely detrimental to most infants, given the prevailing uncertainty on dangers, particularly for 'mixtures,' these measures will mitigate environmental chemical exposures.

QUESTIONS

1. Which of the following chemicals are unavoidable exposures to women on a day-to-day basis as these are present in everyday products?

    A. Bisphenol A

    B. Phthalate esters

    C. PAHs

    D. All of the above

    E. B and C

2. Oily fish can accumulate which of the following heavy metals that are considered to be associated with adverse effects on fetal and childhood development?

    A. Mercury

    B. Lead

    C. Arsenic

    D. All of the above

3. According to recommendations, which of the following fish should be avoided by pregnant and lactating women due to risk of heavy metal accumulation causing adverse fetal outcomes?

    A. Sardines

    B. Salmon

    C. Tuna

    D. Trout

4. According to research, which of the following chemicals in plastics are found to be high in oven-ready/microwave-type meals?

   A. Bisphenol A

   B. Phthalate esters

   C. PAHs

   D. All of the above

   E. A and B

5. According to studies, which of the following lipophilic chemicals accumulate in the adipose tissue and are passed on in the food chain?

   A. Phthalate esters

   B. PAHs

   C. DDT and PCB

   D. All of the above

6. In products such as baby lotions and shampoos, which of the following chemicals is most commonly found and considered to have adverse effects?

   A. Bisphenol A

   B. Phthalate esters

   C. PAHs

   D. DDT

7. Which of the following compounds are found in household products such as materials that are resistant to stains and water, to which pregnant women are exposed daily?

   A. PAHs   C. Bisphenol A

   B. DDT   D. PFCs

8. Which of the following compounds are found in household products such as materials to make flame retardants in furniture, electronics, and cars, to which pregnant women are exposed daily?

   A. PAHs   C. PBDEs

   B. DDT   D. Bisphenol A

9. Which of the following food options should women planning pregnancy avoid due to risk of excessive intake of vitamin A, which is a known cause of fetal malformations?

   A. Salmon

   B. Liver

   C. Chicken

   D. Turkey

10. Of the following chemicals, which one is known to be 'anti-androgenic' and interferes with masculinization of male fetuses?

   A. BPA plastics

   B. PBDEs

   C. Phthalates

   D. Bisphenol A

11. Prenatal exposure of male fetuses to paracetamol can increase the risk of which of the following conditions?

A. Premature closure of ductus arteriosus

B. Fetal anemia

C. Undescended testes (cryptorchidism)

D. Renal impairment and oligohydramnios

12. Which of the following chemical compounds is not an example of an 'endocrine disruptor'?

A. BPA plastics

B. PBDEs

C. Phthalates

D. Essential oils used in aromatherapy/fragrances

13. According to research, organochlorine pesticide exposure in pregnant women has all of the following potential adverse effects on the fetus, except?

A. Alters cognitive and behavioral development

B. Causes endocrine disruption

C. Causes immune suppression

D. Exacerbates asthma

14. What is the half-life of phthalates in the human body?

A. 12–24 hours

B. 48 hours

C. 1 week

D. 1 month

15. Which of the following statements does not correctly describe phthalates?

A. Phthalates are regarded as persistent chemicals within the human body.

B. They possess shorter half-lives of approximately 12–24 hours, so the detected levels indicate recent exposures.

C. Factors such as younger age, increased utilization of cleaning and personal care products, and a high-fat diet correlate with elevated phthalate levels in pregnant women.

D. Early life exposure to phthalates correlates with the onset of allergy disorders, modified neurodevelopment, and endocrine disruption, including reduced anogenital distance in male babies and premature birth.

16. Regarding exposure of pregnant women to phenols, which of the following statements is false?

A. They possess a prolonged half-life in the human body, ranging from 1 to 2 weeks and hence are considered as persistent chemicals.

B. Phenols, such as BPA, triclosan, and parabens, are utilized in various consumer products, including food can linings, plastic bottles, dental sealants, antimicrobials, and preservatives.

C. Early life exposure to BPA is linked to compromised neurodevelopment, endocrine disruption, pediatric asthma, and potentially cardiometabolic diseases.

D. Elevated prenatal BPA levels have been correlated with factors such as younger age, lower socioeconomic status, African American ethnicity, and the increased intake of canned vegetables.

17. All of the following are examples of non-persistent chemicals in the human body, except?

    A. BPA

    B. Phthalates

    C. Triclosan and parabens

    D. Perfluorinated chemicals

18. Exposure to which of the following endocrine-disrupting chemicals during pregnancy is potentially linked to small-for-gestational-age babies?

    A. Dioxins

    B. PFCs

    C. PCBs

    D. All of the above

19. What is the half-life of PBDE flame retardants in an adult human body?

    A. 48 hours

    B. 1 week

    C. 2 weeks

    D. Several months to over a decade

20. Which of the following statements regarding exposure to PCBs is incorrect?

    A. They are extremely persistent, lipophilic compounds that accumulate in humans and the environment.

    B. They possess half-lives of 3–6 months in the human adipose tissue.

    C. Due to the bioaccumulation of PCBs, maternal concentrations correlate with age and year of birth.

    D. Women consuming substantial amounts of fatty fish, particularly northern Norwegian mothers, are significantly exposed.

ANSWERS

1. D	8. C	15. A
2. D	9. B	16. A
3. C	10. C	17. D
4. E	11. C	18. D
5. D	12. D	19. D
6. B	13. D	20. B
7. D	14. A	

10 SIP – Clamping of Umbilical Cord and Placental Transfusion

Source: Clamping of the Umbilical Cord and Placental Transfusion Scientific Impact Paper No. 14 February 2015. https://www.rcog.org.uk/guidance/browse-all-guidance/scientific-impact-papers/clamping-of-the-umbilical-cord-and-placental-transfusion-scientific-impact-paper-no-14/

IMPORTANT POINTS FROM THE GUIDELINE (SIP)

- Postpartum, blood circulation in the umbilical arteries and veins typically persists for many minutes.

- The supplementary blood volume conveyed to the infant during this period is referred to as placental transfusion.

- Immediate clipping of the umbilical cord has conventionally been advised as a component of active treatment during the third stage of labor, with a prophylactic uterotonic agent and controlled cord traction, to mitigate postpartum hemorrhage.

- The administration of a prophylactic uterotonic agent significantly diminishes the chance of substantial hemorrhage.

- The timing of cord clamping does not seem to significantly affect blood loss during birth.

- The term 'immediate cord clamping' refers to the procedure being performed within 30 seconds of the infant's delivery.

- 'Deferred cord clamping' is defined as the practice of postponing the clamping of the umbilical cord for a minimum of 2 minutes following delivery.

- The function of 'immediate' versus 'delayed' cord clamping has not been consistently acknowledged in the active management of the third stage of labor, and the best timing for cord clamping remains ambiguous.

- The International Federation of Gynecology and Obstetrics and the World Health Organization (WHO) have ceased to endorse immediate cord clamping as part of active management.

- The RCOG currently advises that 'The cord should not be clamped sooner than necessary, according to clinical evaluation of the circumstances.'

- The WHO recommends late cord clamping, conducted 1 to 3 minutes post-birth, for all deliveries while simultaneously commencing crucial infant care.

- The National Institute for Health and Care Excellence (NICE) advises that, for healthy mothers with term deliveries, umbilical cord clamping should be delayed for the initial 60 seconds, unless there are concerns regarding the cord's integrity or the infant's heart rate.

- It is advised that the cord be clamped within 5 minutes, although women should be supported if they prefer a greater delay.

- Postnatal placental transfusion delivers an extra 80–100 mL of blood for a term infant.

- The blood volume per kilogram of body weight in the fetus is comparable to that of an adult, approximately 65–75 mL/kg.

- At birth, this increases to around 90 mL/kg; however, the increase is diminished by 20–35% if the umbilical cord is clamped quickly.

- Prompt cord clamping diminishes placental transfusion and may deprive a term infant of 20–30 mg/kg of iron, adequate for the requirements of a newborn for around 3 months.

- The physiology of placental transfusion in preterm infants and ill term infants, especially those experiencing intrapartum hypoxia, is inadequately comprehended.

- At birth, umbilical circulation diminishes and pulmonary vascular resistance decreases, resulting in a fast augmentation of pulmonary blood flow.

- This marks the initiation of the transition from fetal to neonatal circulation.

DOI: 10.1201/9781003650355-10

- The sustained circulation in the umbilical vein and arteries at birth may contribute to the physiological processes aiding the infant during this transition.

- Prompt cord clamping may hinder the infant's capacity to manage the shift from fetal to neonatal circulation.

- Although the majority of healthy term infants adjust without significant issues, preterm infants or those with pre-existing cardiorespiratory impairments may experience adverse clinical outcomes.

- A slight postponement in cord clamping will augment the infant's blood volume.

- A prolonged delay may yield further benefits, including improved cardiorespiratory transition and more stable blood pressure, potentially occurring without any further alteration in net blood volume.

- The primary factors influencing placental transfusion include the degree of uterine compression on the placenta post-delivery, the vertical positioning of the infant relative to the placenta during this interval, and the duration prior to umbilical cord clamping.

- The administration of a preventive uterotonic agent during the third stage significantly diminishes the likelihood of postpartum hemorrhage. While these medicines seemingly do not affect the ultimate volume of placental transfusion, they do alter the velocity and duration of flow.

- The administration of intramuscular uterotonic agents prior to cord clamping seems improbable to significantly influence placental transfusion.

- Further research is warranted to ascertain the potential clinical significance regarding either duration or net volume.

- The flow of oxygenated blood to the fetus through the umbilical vein is more significantly affected by gravity than the flow in the umbilical artery.

- Elevating the infant above the placenta while the umbilical cord remains intact is anticipated to diminish venous supply to the infant, yet the umbilical artery persists in transporting blood back to the placenta.

- Consequently, elevating the baby may result in blood flow from the newborn to the placenta.

- In contrast, positioning the infant below the placenta enhances blood flow to the infant, although it does not affect the overall volume of placental transfusion.

- In the absence of a uterotonic, gravity significantly impacts placental transfusion when the infant is positioned 20 cm or more above or below the introitus.

- Placental transfusion during a cesarean section seems to be inferior to that during vaginal delivery. This may result from gravity if the infant is elevated prior to cord clamping and diminished uterine tone.

- Cord 'stripping' or 'milking,' conducted either prior to or subsequent to cord clamping, has been evaluated against prompt cord clamping in several recent trials involving preterm and term or near-term infants. The primary focus of interest in this treatment pertains to preterm deliveries.

- Despite the limited scale of the trials, there is evidence indicating enhanced early newborn cardiovascular stability, a diminished requirement for oxygen at 36 weeks of postmenstrual age, and a reduction in blood transfusions.

- The cord blood is swiftly propelled into the fetal circulation through milking, which involves stripping a 20 cm segment of the cord three times, each for around 2 seconds, before clamping.

- Cord milking evidently hinders flow in the umbilical arteries and may have additional effects via endothelial activation. This requires additional randomized trials to assess the potential benefits and unwanted effects.

- No statistically significant differences were seen between the immediate and deferred cord clamping groups regarding postpartum hemorrhage, severe postpartum hemorrhage, or manual placenta removal.

- At 24 to 48 hours of age, infants in the immediate cord clamping cohort exhibited reduced hemoglobin levels compared to those in the deferred clamping cohort.

- By the age of 3 to 6 months, there was no notable difference between the groups.

- Immediate clamping correlated with an elevated risk ratio of iron insufficiency, notwithstanding the presence of heterogeneity among studies.

- Due to less hemolysis linked to rapid clamping, these infants had a decreased relative chance of requiring phototherapy for jaundice.

- The data available are inadequate to draw valid conclusions regarding the comparative effects on other significant short-term outcomes, including symptomatic polycythemia, respiratory issues, hypothermia, infection, and the necessity for special care admission.

- In preterm infants, the timing for immediate cord clamping varied from 5 to 20 seconds, while postponed clamping ranged from 30 to 180 seconds.

- No significant distinction was observed between the groups regarding severe intraventricular hemorrhage or periventricular leukomalacia in preterm infants.

- Delayed cord clamping correlated with a reduction in transfusions for anemia; however, no significant difference was observed in transfusions for hypotension.

- Deferred clamping correlated with elevated mean arterial blood pressures at birth and at 4 hours of age, as well as a reduced necessity for inotropes compared to immediate cord clamping.

- It was also linked to a decreased risk of necrotizing enterocolitis.

- Preterm infants assigned to deferred cord clamping exhibited elevated serum bilirubin levels; however, the three trials reporting this outcome showed no significant difference in jaundice necessitating phototherapy, nor was there a discernible difference in oxygen requirements at 36 weeks of postmenstrual age between the groups.

QUESTIONS

1. What is the meaning of the term 'immediate cord clamping' for a term fetus?

    A. When the cord is clamped within 10 seconds of birth of the baby

    B. When the cord is clamped within 30 seconds of birth of the baby

    C. When the cord is clamped within 60 seconds of birth of the baby

    D. When the cord is clamped within 120 seconds of birth of the baby

2. What is the definition of the term 'deferred cord clamping' for a term fetus?

    A. Not clamping the cord until at least 30 seconds after birth of the baby

    B. Not clamping the cord until at least 60 seconds after birth of the baby

    C. Not clamping the cord until at least 2 minutes after birth of the baby

    D. Not clamping the cord until at least 5 minutes after birth of the baby

3. According to NICE guidelines, what is the recommendation regarding umbilical cord clamping after the birth of the baby in healthy young women?

    A. Not clamping the cord in the first 30 seconds after birth of the baby

    B. Not clamping the cord in the first 60 seconds after birth of the baby

    C. Not clamping the cord in the first 2 minutes after birth of the baby

    D. Not clamping the cord in the first 5 minutes after birth of the baby

4. How much blood does postnatal placental transfusion provide to a term baby?

  A. 60–80 mL

  B. 80–100 mL

  C. 100–140 mL

  D. 140–180 mL

5. What is the blood volume/kilogram of body weight for the growing fetus during pregnancy?

  A. 40–50 mL/kg

  B. 50–65 mL/kg

  C. 65–75 mL/kg

  D. Around 90 mL/kg

6. What is the blood volume/kilogram of body weight for the term fetus at birth?

  A. 40–50 mL/kg

  B. 50–65 mL/kg

  C. 65–75 mL/kg

  D. Around 90 mL/kg

7. How much iron is a term baby deprived of due to 'immediate cord clamping'?

  A. 10–20 mg/kg of iron

  B. 20–30 mg/kg of iron

  C. 60–80 mg/kg of iron

  D. 80–100 mg/kg of iron

8. All of the following factors are important determinants of postnatal placental transfusion, except?

  A. Intensity of uterine contractions compressing the placenta

  B. Elevation of the fetus in relation to the placenta

  C. Timing of umbilical cord clamping

  D. Administration of uterotonic drugs during the third stage of labor

9. What is the definition of 'milking the cord' or 'cord stripping'?

  A. A 20 cm length of cord is stripped three times, each time for about 2 seconds, before clamping the cord.

  B. A 20 cm length of cord is stripped six times, each time for about 3 seconds, before clamping the cord.

  C. A 10 cm length of cord is stripped three times, each time for about 2 seconds, before clamping the cord.

  D. A 10 cm length of cord is stripped six times, each time for about 3 seconds, before clamping the cord.

10. Which of the following neonatal outcomes is increased with immediate cord clamping?

  A. Need for phototherapy for jaundice

  B. Iron deficiency

  C. Need for admission to NICU

  D. Symptomatic polycythemia

11. Which of the following neonatal outcomes is decreased with immediate cord clamping?

    A. Need for phototherapy for jaundice

    B. Iron deficiency

    C. Need for admission to NICU

    D. Symptomatic polycythemia

12. In preterm babies, deferred cord clamping has all of the following neonatal outcomes, except?

    A. Fewer transfusions for anemia

    B. Elevated mean arterial pressure at birth and at 4 hours of birth

    C. Decreased risk of necrotizing enterocolitis

    D. Decreased risk of periventricular leucomalacia

13. In all of the following maternal conditions immediate cord clamping should be considered, except?

    A. Hemodynamic instability of the mother

    B. Placental abruption

    C. Placenta previa or accreta

    D. Multiple pregnancy

14. Immediate cord clamping should be contemplated in all of the below fetal situations, with the exception of which one?

    A. In patients with vasa previa requiring rapid neonatal resuscitation

    B. Fetal growth restriction accompanied by abnormal Doppler findings

    C. Cord avulsion

    D. All preterm newborns, regardless of gestational age at birth

15. At what gestational age is 'milking the cord' contraindicated?

    A. <28 weeks

    B. <30 weeks

    C. <32 weeks

    D. <34 weeks

ANSWERS

1. B	6. D	11. A
2. C	7. B	12. D
3. B	8. D	13. D
4. B	9. A	14. D
5. C	10. B	15. A

11 SIP – Congenital Cytomegalovirus (CMV) Infection

Source: Congenital Cytomegalovirus Infection–Update on Screening, Diagnosis and Treatment Scientific Impact Paper No. 56 April 2018. https://www.rcog.org.uk/guidance/browse-all-guidance/scientific-impact-papers/congenital-cytomegalovirus-infection-update-on-screening-diagnosis-and-treatment-scientific-impact-paper-no-56/

IMPORTANT POINTS FROM THE GUIDELINE

- Cytomegalovirus (CMV) is a double-stranded DNA virus belonging to the human herpesvirus family. It is the predominant cause of viral infection in neonates, affecting 1 in 200 infants in high-income nations and 1 in 71 babies in low- and middle-income countries.

- It is the predominant non-genetic etiology of sensorineural hearing loss (SNHL) and a significant contributor to neurological disability.

- The primary source of infection for pregnant women is the saliva and urine of small children.

- The risk of fetal damage is highest following a primary infection in women during the first trimester and significantly decreases after 12 weeks of gestation.

- The UK National Screening Committee does not endorse routine universal prenatal and newborn screening for CMV infection.

- The presence of immunoglobulin IgM is frequently indicative of a recent primary infection in other viral illnesses. Nonetheless, this does not apply to CMV for various reasons:
  - IgM may be detectable for several months following the first CMV infection.
  - IgM can be identified in cases of non-primary infection.
  - Cross-reactivity with IgM may occur due to an alternative viral infection.
  - IgM may be identified due to nonspecific polyclonal activation of the immune system.

- IgG avidity testing is frequently employed to more accurately ascertain the timing of infection.

- Avidity levels are measured by the avidity index, which indicates the ratio of IgG bound to the antigen after exposure to denaturing agents.
  - A high avidity score (>60%) indicates a likely prior infection (>3 months ago).
  - A low avidity index (<30%) indicates a recent primary infection (within the last 3 months).
  - The avidity index (30–60%) represents a gray zone, indicating that maternal primary CMV infection cannot be definitively excluded.

- The diagnosis of primary CMV infection during pregnancy can be established by one of the following methods:
  - The emergence of CMV-specific IgG in a woman who was previously seronegative.
  - The identification of CMV IgM antibodies with low IgG avidity, signifying a recent primary infection.

- After maternal primary CMV infection during the first trimester, oral valaciclovir treatment may be taken promptly to decrease the risk of transplacental transmission.

- Upon confirmation of fetal CMV infection via amniocentesis, serial ultrasound evaluations of the fetus should be conducted every 2–3 weeks until delivery.

- Even when maternal CMV infection is present without definite fetal infection, repeated ultrasound examinations of the fetus should be conducted every 2–3 weeks until delivery.

- Cerebral MRI is recommended for infected fetuses at 28–32 weeks of gestation (with potential repetition after 3–4 weeks) utilizing T1, T2, and diffusion sequences.

DOI: 10.1201/9781003650355-11

- Infected fetuses are classified into three categories:
  - Asymptomatic: The prognosis for these fetuses is highly favorable, albeit with a residual chance of hearing impairment. Continuous observation is advised for signs of progression of the impairment.
  - Mild-to-moderately symptomatic fetuses have an ambiguous prognosis, and additional follow-up with ultrasound and potentially MRI may assist in refining the prognosis. Antiviral therapy and other therapeutic alternatives are currently under evaluation, however their application remains confined to research purposes only. Oral valaciclovir treatment may be contemplated on a case-by-case basis following a thorough conversation with the parents. The possibility of pregnancy termination should also be addressed.
  - Severely symptomatic fetuses: The prognosis is unfavorable, and counseling regarding the option of pregnancy termination should be conducted.
- All newborns born to mothers with proven or suspected CMV infection must undergo testing for congenital CMV using urine or saliva samples within the initial 21 days of life.
- A birth plan must be recorded in the maternal notes, specifying the necessity for clinical assessment and investigation.

QUESTIONS

1. Which of the following is the most common cause of viral infection in newborns?
   A. Herpes simplex virus
   B. Parvovirus
   C. CMV
   D. Varicella zoster

2. What is the incidence of CMV infection in newborns in high-income countries?
   A. 1 in 70
   B. 1 in 100
   C. 1 in 200
   D. 1 in 1000

3. What is the incidence of CMV infection in newborns in low- and middle-income countries?
   A. 1 in 70
   B. 1 in 100
   C. 1 in 200
   D. 1 in 1000

4. What is the most common source of CMV infection in pregnant women?
   A. Respiratory droplets
   B. Transfusion of blood products
   C. Saliva and urine of young children
   D. Skin-to-skin contact

5. How many babies born with CMV infection show symptoms of the infection at birth?
   A. 1 in 2
   B. 1 in 4
   C. 1 in 6
   D. 1 in 8

6. How long should babies born with CMV infection be followed after birth to check their hearing and brain development?

   A. 3 months

   B. 6 months

   C. 12 months

   D. 24 months

7. A 32-year-old primigravida patient, who works as a primary school teacher, presents to your OPD with flu-like symptoms during the last few days. She has been complaining of joint aches, fever, malaise for 1 week. Her GP has referred her to you as on examination there is significant cervical lymphadenopathy. She is currently 14 weeks into her pregnancy. Her routine blood investigations and combined screen test were normal. Her latest liver function test performed by the GP is suggestive of markedly elevated transaminases. What will be your working diagnosis in her case?

   A. Rubella infection

   B. Acute viral hepatitis

   C. CMV infection

   D. Toxoplasmosis infection

8. A 28-year-old primigravida patient, who works as a primary school teacher, presents to your outpatient department (OPD) with flu-like symptoms during the last few days. She has been complaining of joint aches, fever, and malaise for 1 week. Her GP has referred her to you as on examination there is significant cervical lymphadenopathy. She is currently 10 weeks into her pregnancy. Her routine blood investigations were normal. Her latest liver function test performed by the GP is suggestive of markedly elevated transaminases. Considering her working diagnosis of CMV infection, what is your recommended drug of choice in her case?

   A. Acyclovir

   B. Valacyclovir

   C. Oseltamivir

   D. Ribavarin

9. Which of the following is the leading non-genetic cause of SNHL in newborns?

   A. Rubella

   B. CMV

   C. Syphillis

   D. Toxoplasmosis

10. What percentage of babies born will be symptomatic in cases of women with primary CMV infection during their first trimester?

    A. 1–2%

    B. 3.9–5.2%

    C. 8%

    D. 20%

11. What is the risk of congenital infection in women with non-primary CMV infection during their pregnancy?

    A. 1–2%

    C. 8%

    B. 3.9–5.2%

    D. 20%

12. In cases of CMV infection, which of the following statements regarding the IgM antibodies is NOT true?

   A. IgM can be detectable for several months following the first infection.

   B. IgM is undetectable during non-primary infections.

   C. There may be cross-reactivity with other viral infections.

   D. IgM may be identified as a result of non-specific polyclonal activation of the immune system.

13. A 29-year-old primigravida patient, who is a primary school teacher, presents to your OPD with a history of fever, flu-like symptoms, and joint aches. On examination, there is significant cervical lymphadenopathy. A working diagnosis of CMV infection is made. Which of the following tests will best determine the timing of the infection?

   A. CMV-specific IgM levels

   B. CMV polymerase chain reaction (CMV-PCR) on maternal blood

   C. CMV-PCR on maternal urine

   D. IgG avidity testing

14. A 29-year-old primigravida patient, who is a primary school teacher, presents to your OPD with a history of fever, flu-like symptoms, and joint aches. On examination, there is significant cervical lymphadenopathy. A working diagnosis of CMV infection is made. On IgG avidity testing, there is a low avidity index of less than 30%. According to her test results, what is the timing of her CMV infection?

   A. Past infection > 3 months before

   B. Non-primary infection

   C. Recent primary infection within last 3 months

   D. Reactivation of CMV infection

15. Which of the following is the mainstay for diagnosis of fetal CMV infection?

   A. Amniocentesis for real-time PCR for CMV viral genome

   B. Level 2 scan showing echogenic bowel, ventriculomegaly

   C. IgG avidity index testing

   D. CMV-specific IgM testing

16. Sensorineural hearing loss and neurological impairment is maximum in fetuses affected during which of the following phases of pregnancy?

   A. Periconception period

   B. First trimester

   C. Second trimester

   D. Third trimester

17. The transmission rate of CMV infection is maximum during which phase of pregnancy?

   A. Periconception period

   B. First trimester

   C. Second trimester

   D. Third trimester

18. Which of the following statements regarding amniocentesis for diagnosis of fetal infection with CMV is true?

    A. It should be conducted no sooner than 17 weeks once fetal urination is established.

    B. It should ideally be conducted after 20 weeks of gestation.

    C. It should be conducted 6–8 weeks post-maternal infection to prevent false-negative outcomes.

    D. All of the above.

    E. A and B.

19. Women with primary CMV infection during pregnancy are at how much of a higher risk of congenital CMV infection and its sequelae, respectively, when compared to the general population?

    A. 8-fold and 2-fold, respectively

    B. 16-fold and 4-fold, respectively

    C. 24-fold and 6-fold, respectively

    D. 30-fold and 10-fold, respectively

20. Which of the following tests should be done to confirm congenital CMV infection in the neonate at birth?

    A. Saliva and urine swab CMV-PCR with 3 weeks of birth

    B. Saliva and urine swab CMV-PCR with 6 weeks of birth

    C. Saliva and urine swab CMV-PCR with 3 months of birth

    D. Saliva and urine swab CMV-PCR with 6 months of birth

21. Which of the following is the recommended treatment for symptomatic neonates with congenital CMV infection at birth?

    A. Acyclovir should be started within 4 weeks of birth

    B. Valganciclovir/Ganciclovir should be started within 4 weeks of birth

    C. Oseltamivir should be started within 8 weeks of birth

    D. Valganciclovir/Ganciclovir should be started within 8 weeks of birth

22. What percentage of neonates with symptomatic congenital CMV infection at birth can be prevented from progression of SNHL?

    A. Up to 34%   C. Up to 84%

    B. Up to 54%   D. Up to 94%

23. A 28-year-old primigravida patient, who works as a primary school teacher, presents to your OPD with flu-like symptoms for the last few days. She has been complaining of joint aches, fever, and malaise for 1 week. Her GP has referred her to you as on examination there is significant cervical lymphadenopathy. She is currently 15 weeks into her pregnancy. Her routine blood investigations were normal. Her latest liver function test performed by the GP is suggestive of markedly elevated transaminases. Considering her working diagnosis of CMV infection, how would you follow-up the patient during pregnancy?

    A. Offer amniocentesis for CMV-PCR after 20 weeks

    B. Offer detailed targeted ultrasound every 2–4 weeks

    C. Offer a fetal brain MRI at 28–32 weeks of pregnancy and repeat 3–4 weeks later if required

    D. All of the above

    E. A and B

24. Which of the following tests on a fetal blood sample is an independent prognostic indicator of neonatal outcome?

    A. Beta-2 microglobulin

    B. Platelet count

    C. Fetal IgM levels

    D. CMV-PCR of fetal blood

25. A 32-year-old primigravida patient, who works at a child welfare center, presents to your antenatal OPD to discuss her anomaly scan report. Her GP has referred her to you due to concerning features in her scan report, suggestive of vetriculomegaly (>15 mm), ascites and pleural effusion, early-onset fetal growth restriction, hyperechogenic bowel, and significant placentomegaly. Upon retrospective history taking the patient confirms a history of fever with malaise and joint aches about 6 weeks previously. What will be your diagnostic suspicion in her case?

    A. Congenital rubella syndrome

    B. Congenital CMV infection

    C. Congenital varicella syndrome

    D. Congenital syphilis infection

26. On MRI of a fetus with congenital CMV infection, which of the following brain lesions is the most commonly seen finding?

    A. Subependymal cysts

    B. White matter lesions

    C. Ventricular dilatation

    D. Polymicrogyria

27. On MRI findings of a fetus with suspicion of congenital CMV infection, involvement of white matter of which of the following lobes is associated with the worst prognosis?

    A. Frontal lobe

    B. Parietal lobe

    C. Temporal lobe

    D. Occipital lobe

28. Which of the following is not included in the classic triad of symptoms in symptomatic fetuses affected by congenital CMV infection?

    A. Jaundice

    B. Petechiae

    C. Chorioretinitis

    D. Hepatosplenomegaly

29. In terms of signs of clinical presentation which of the following is not typically seen in congenital CMV infection?

    A. Periventricular calcifications

    B. Ventriculomegaly

    C. Scattered calcifications in the brain

    D. SNHL

ANSWERS

1. C	11. A	21. B
2. C	12. B	22. C
3. A	13. D	23. D
4. C	14. C	24. B
5. D	15. A	25. B
6. D	16. B	26. B
7. C	17. D	27. C
8. B	18. D	28. C
9. B	19. C	29. C
10. B	20. A	

12 SIP – Congenital Uterine Anomalies (CUA)

Source: Reproductive Implications and Management of Congenital Uterine Anomalies (2024 Second Edition) Scientific Impact Paper No. 62 February 2025. https://www.rcog.org.uk/guidance/browse-all -guidance/scientific-impact-papers/reproductive-implications-and-management-of-congenital-uterine -anomalies-2024-second-edition-scientific-impact-paper-no-62/

IMPORTANT POINTS FROM THE GUIDELINE (SIP)

- Congenital uterine anomalies (CUAs) are anatomical aberrations arising from the embryological maldevelopment of the Müllerian ducts.

- The general prevalence of CUAs is 5.5% in an unselected population, 8.0% in women with infertility, 13.3% in those with a history of miscarriage, and 24.5% in those experiencing both miscarriage and infertility.

- The development of Müllerian ducts occurs in three phases, and any malfunction during these periods leads to the formation of CUAs.

  - Organogenesis (formation of both Müllerian ducts) – deficiencies in Müllerian duct development result in agenesis or hypoplasia (e.g. aplastic/hypoplastic uterus and unicornuate uterus).

  - The fusion of both Müllerian ducts results in the development of a uterus and the upper vagina.

    - Horizontal fusion or unification of the lower segments of the paired Müllerian ducts results in the formation of the uterus, cervix, and upper vagina. Defects in this process can lead to varying degrees of fusion or unification anomalies, such as a bicornuate uterus (partial fault) or uterine didelphys (full defect).

    - Vertical fusion of the descending Müllerian duct and ascending urogenital sinus to create the vaginal canal – deficiencies result in an imperforate hymen or a transverse vaginal septum.

  - Septal resorption or canalization entails the absorption of the horizontally fused Müllerian ducts, resulting in the formation of the uterine cavity. Inadequate resorption or canalization, contingent upon the severity of the defect, results in complete septate uterus, partial septate uterus, or arcuate uterus.

- The European Society of Human Reproduction and Embryology (ESHRE) and European Society of Gastrointestinal Endoscopy (ESGE) classification encompasses descriptions for all female genital tract abnormalities, not limited to the uterus, akin to the VCUAM (Vagina Cervix Uterus Adnex–associated Malformation) classification (uterine U0–U6, cervical C0–C4, and vaginal V0–V4).

  - U0: Typical uterus.

  - U1: Dysmorphic uterus (mostly infantile and T-shaped).

  - U2: Septate uterus–uterine cavity is divided by a fibromuscular septum, while maintaining a normal exterior contour/shape.

  - U3: Bicorporeal uterus (partial and complete – bicornuate and uterus didelphys according to AFS) – the uterus manifests as two distinct uterine horns, a double uterus with or without two separate cervices, and infrequently a double vagina. Each uterine horn is connected to a single fallopian tube and ovary.

  - U4: Hemi-uterus (unicornuate) – only one uterine horn is present, connected to a single fallopian tube and ovary, while the other uterine horn is either missing or rudimentary.

  - U5 Aplastic uterus (uterus missing).

  - U6: Designated for cases that remain unclassified.

  - Cervical: C0–C4 (C0, normal cervix; C1, septate cervix; C2, double cervix; C3, unilateral cervical aplasia; C4, cervical aplasia).

- Vaginal: V0–V4 (V0, normal vagina; V1, longitudinal non-obstructive vaginal septum; V2, longitudinal obstructive vaginal septum; V3, transverse vaginal septum and/or imperforate hymen; V4, vaginal aplasia).

■ The 2016 ARSM paper, 'Uterine Septum: A Guideline,' indicated that an arcuate uterus is not clinically significant, providing distinct criteria for the diagnosis of septate and bicornuate uteri, differing from those suggested by ESHRE/ESGE.

- Normal/arcuate: Depth from interstitial to apex of indentation exceeds 1 cm, and the angle of indentation surpasses 90°.

- Sepate: Depth of the interstitial to the apex exceeds 1.5 cm, and the angle of indentation is less than 90°.

- Bicornuate: External fundal indentation exceeding 1 cm.

- This creates an ambiguous category between normal/arcuate and septate, wherein certain women may not fulfill the requirements for either diagnosis.

■ The Congenital Uterine Malformation Experts (CUME) group established a straightforward and replicable criterion for identifying septate uterus, defined as an interior indentation exceeding 10 mm.

- The CUME group presented diagnostic criteria for T-shaped uterus in 2020, based on 3D ultrasound assessment, which includes a lateral indentation angle <130°, a lateral indentation depth >7 mm, and a T-angle ≤40°, demonstrating good diagnostic accuracy and moderate reliability.

■ In 2021, the American Society for Reproductive Medicine (ASRM) revised and broadened the traditional American Fertility Society (AFS) classification, integrating cervical, vaginal, and all complex anomalies into nine distinct categories: Müllerian agenesis, cervical agenesis, unicornuate uterus, didelphys, bicornuate uterus, septate uterus, longitudinal vaginal septum, transverse vaginal septum, and complex anomalies.

- The ASRM has established diagnostic criteria for septate, arcuate, and bicornuate uteri.

  – The septate uterus is characterized by a septal length over 1 cm and a septal angle of less than 90°.

  – The arcuate uterus is identified when the septal indentation is 1 cm or less and the angle is 90° or greater.

  – A bicornuate uterus is identified when the exterior indentation exceeds 1 cm.

■ Three-dimensional transvaginal sonography (TVS) is now regarded as the gold standard for evaluating congenital uterine defects due to its minimally invasive nature and its ability to accurately diagnose different forms of uterine malformations.

■ An MRI of the pelvis is both sensitive and specific for diagnosing CUAs and is effective in outlining the endometrium, identifying uterine horns, and clarifying aberrant gonadal positioning or renal architecture. It is also less invasive than the combination of laparoscopy and hysteroscopy.

■ Although MRI is not generally advised for all individuals with a suspected CUA, it is beneficial for those with an unconfirmed diagnosis via 3D ultrasound and for those with suspected complicated abnormalities.

■ CUAs may be linked to congenital renal malformations, with unilateral renal agenesis being the most prevalent, due to their closely related embryonic origin.

■ The incidence of renal abnormalities was 18.8%, with unilateral renal agenesis identified as the predominant defect.

■ Upon evaluation of various subtypes according to the ESHRE/ESGE criteria, the prevalence of renal abnormalities was found to be 5% in normal (U0), 0% in dysmorphic (U1), 15.6% in septate (U2), 24.7% in bicorporeal (U3), 29.5% in hemi uterus (U4), and 11.7% in aplastic (U5) cases, respectively.

- An ultrasound, MRI, or intravenous pyelogram should be advised for all women diagnosed with a CUA, selecting the most suitable option based on the clinical presentation.

- Although a link exists between canalization abnormalities and diminished reproductive performance, the precise etiology and pathophysiological mechanisms behind infertility, miscarriage, and other negative reproductive outcomes, including fetal growth limitation, remain ambiguous.

- Multiple hypotheses have been proposed, including the abnormal endometrium overlying the septum, which may create a suboptimal implantation site; disordered and diminished blood supply inadequate for placentation and embryonic development; and uncoordinated uterine contractions or reduced uterine capacity.

- Although hysteroscopic septal division is generally a safe technique when performed by skilled practitioners, it is not devoid of dangers. The TRUST trial indicated a complication rate of 4.6%.

- The objectives of CUA management are to address anatomical distortions linked to obstructive anomalies to alleviate symptoms such as pain, thus enhancing quality of life, and to prevent long-term health and reproductive complications.

- For non-obstructive anomalies, the goal is to enhance reproductive outcomes in infertile women or those who have suffered recurrent miscarriages.

- The primary objective is to enhance the incidence of term live births while concurrently decreasing long-term infant morbidity and mortality.

- A universally accepted and flawless classification method for CUAs is currently unavailable.

- The ESHRE/ESGE (2013), ASRM (2016), CUME (2018), and ASRM (2021) standards endeavor to scientifically delineate CUAs utilizing 3D ultrasound data.

- Precise 3D ultrasound measurements of exterior and internal fundal indentation must be conducted and documented in each instance to establish a suitably extensive database.

- It is advisable to document septal measurements, specifics of surgical septal excision, and related reproductive results. The reported categories could thereafter be assessed and improved based on observed reproductive outcomes.

- Although 2D pelvic TVS and hysterosalpingography (HSG) serve as effective screening modalities for low-risk women, 3D pelvic ultrasonography is advised for the precise diagnosis and classification of CUAs in individuals with suspicious screening results or those experiencing recurrent miscarriages.

- MRI or a combination of laparoscopy and hysteroscopy should be utilized exclusively for the diagnosis of intricate CUAs.

- The majority of women with a CUA achieve a normal reproductive outcome.

- It is essential to inform women with a CUA, based on its kind and severity, of the heightened risks associated with first- or second-trimester miscarriages, premature labor, fetal malpresentation, as well as fetal growth issues and pre-eclampsia.

- Women with a significant fusion or unification defect exhibit unilateral placental implantation, perhaps resulting in the functional exclusion of one uterine artery from the uteroplacental circulation. This is associated with placental insufficiency, fetal growth complications, and stillbirth.

- Hysteroscopic resection of a uterine septum may be considered on an individualized basis by qualified doctors for women with recurrent miscarriage due to its potential benefits.

- The management of inadvertently identified septum in infertile women is contentious and requires additional research.

- Women should be well apprised of the scant data on the efficacy of surgery, as well as the intraoperative and postoperative dangers involved, if a surgical procedure is contemplated.

- The unit responsible for managing CUAs must establish suitable systems for clinical governance and auditing.

- Multicentered randomized controlled trials, sufficiently powered to evaluate reproductive outcomes following hysteroscopic resection of uterine septum in women experiencing recurrent miscarriages and/or recurrent implantation failure after assisted reproduction, are necessary to establish evidence-based recommendations.

- Presently, abdominal or laparoscopic metroplasty for fusion or unification deficits is typically contraindicated due to its potential for considerable intraoperative and postoperative morbidity, as well as insufficient evidence to demonstrate enhanced reproductive outcomes.

- Due to the correlation between CUAs and renal tract anomalies, doctors should contemplate imaging the renal tract in individuals with CUAs.

- All women with CUAs (e.g. unicornuate, bicornuate, didelphys, or septate uterus, contingent on severity) and those who have undergone hysteroscopic resection of a uterine septum should be monitored within 12 weeks utilizing a suitable preterm birth care protocol as delineated in the UK Preterm Birth Clinical Network Guidance.

- The guidance indicates that all acute maternity units must implement fundamental measures to identify and manage women at elevated risk of preterm birth (Level 1).

- More specialized care may be offered by advanced centers within or near each Local Maternity System, which can deliver additional services such as high vaginal or transabdominal cerclage.

QUESTIONS

1. What is the overall prevalence of CUAs in the general population?

   A. 5.5%

   B. 8%

   C. 13.3%

   D. 24%

2. What is the prevalence of CUAs in women with infertility?

   A. 5.5%

   B. 8%

   C. 13.3%

   D. 24%

3. What is the prevalence of CUAs in women with a history of miscarriage?

   A. 5.5%

   B. 8%

   C. 13.3%

   D. 24%

4. What is the prevalence of CUAs in women with a history of miscarriage and infertility?

   A. 5.5%

   B. 8%

   C. 13.3%

   D. 24%

5. Which of the following investigations is the gold standard for assessment of CUA?

   A. Routine transvaginal 2D scan

   B. MRI pelvis

   C. 3D transvaginal ultrasound

   D. CECT pelvis

6. Which of the following CUAs develops due to a horizontal fusion defect of Müllerian duct development?

   A. Unicornuate uterus

   B. Bicornuate uterus

   C. Septate uterus

   D. Arcuate uterus

7. Which of the following CUAs develops due to a defect in resorption or canalization during the Müllerian duct development?

   A. Uterus didelphys

   B. Transverse vaginal septum

   C. Imperforate hymen

   D. Septate uterus

8. Which of the following CUAs develops due to a vertical fusion defect of Müllerian duct development?

   A. Bicornuate uterus

   B. Transverse vaginal septum

   C. Septate uterus

   D. Arcuate uterus

9. All of the following CUAs are due to the defect in organogenesis/development of Müllerian ducts, except?

   A. Mayer–Rokitansky–Küster–Hauser (MRKH) syndrome

   B. Hypoplastic uterus

   C. Unicornuate uterus

   D. Bicornuate uterus

10. According to the ESHRE/ESGE classification of CUAs, an internal indentation at the fundal midline exceeding 50% of the uterine wall thickness has been used to diagnose which of the following CUAs?

    A. Arcuate uterus

    B. Septate uterus

    C. Bicorporeal uterus

    D. Unicornuate uterus

11. According to the ESHRE/ESGE classification of CUAs, an external indentation at the fundal midline exceeding 50% of the uterine wall thickness has been used to diagnose which of the following CUAs?

    A. Arcuate uterus

    B. Septate uterus

    C. Bicorporeal uterus

    D. Unicornuate uterus

12. Which of the following is not included in U0–U6 according to the ESHRE/ESGE classification of CUAs?

    A. Arcuate uterus

    B. Septate uterus

    C. Bicorporeal uterus

    D. Unicornuate uterus

13. According to the ESHRE/ESGE classification of U0–U6, which of the following is incorrectly matched?

    A. U0 – Normal uterus

    B. U2 – Septate uterus

    C. U4 – Bicorporeal uterus

    D. U6 – Unclassified

14. According to the CUME group, how is a septate uterus defined?

    A. Internal indentation of more than 5 mm

    B. Internal indentation of more than 10 mm

    C. Internal indentation of more than 15 mm

    D. Internal indentation of more than 20 mm

15. According to the CUME group, what is the diagnostic criteria for a T-shaped uterus depending upon the 3D ultrasound assessment?

    A. Lateral indentation angle ≤130°

    B. Lateral indentation depth ≥7 mm

    C. T-angle ≤40°

    D. All of the above

    E. A and B

16. Which of the following statements regarding the ASRM classification of CUAs is NOT true?

    A. It has six different groups – including uterine, cervical, vaginal, and all complex anomalies.

    B. Septate uterus is defined as septal length of >1 cm and septal angle of <90°.

    C. Arcuate uterus is diagnosed when septal indentation is ≤1 cm and angle of ≥90°.

    D. Bicornuate uterus is diagnosed when the external indentation is >1 cm.

17. What is the estimated risk of congenital renal anomalies in patients with a CUA?

    A. 5%

    B. 10%

    C. 18%

    D. 30%

18. Which of the following is the most common congenital renal anomaly noted in patients with a CUA?

    A. Duplex kidney

    B. Unilateral renal agenesis

    C. Ectopic kidney

    D. Horseshoe kidney

19. According to the ESHRE/ESGE classification, which of the following has the highest risk of congenital renal anomaly?

   A. U1 – Dysmorphic uterus

   B. U2 – Septate uterus

   C. U3 – Bicorporeal uterus

   D. U4 – Unicornuate uterus

20. Which of the following CUAs has the poorest reproductive outcomes and reduced conception rate?

   A. Bicornuate uterus

   B. Uterus didelphys

   C. Septate uterus (partial/complete)

   D. Unicornuate uterus

21. Which of the following causes a dysmorphic T-shaped uterus?

   A. Intrauterine diethylstilbesterol (DES) exposure

   B. Tuberculosis infection

   C. Marginal intrauterine adhesions (IUAs)

   D. All of the above

   E. A and B

22. According to the TRUST trial, what is the estimated complication rate after hysteroscopic septal division?

   A. 0.1%

   B. 1%

   C. 4–5%

   D. 10%

23. OHVIRA syndrome includes a triad of all of the following, except?

   A. Uterus didelphys

   B. Obstructed hemi-vagina

   C. Hypoplasia of urinary bladder

   D. Ipsilateral renal anomaly

24. Which of the following anomalies is not linked to intrauterine DES exposure?

   A. T-shaped uterus

   B. Cervical incompetence

   C. Hypoplastic uterus

   D. Oblique transverse vaginal septum obstructing the vagina

25. MURCS association does not include which of the following?

   A. Duplex ureter

   B. Aplasia of the Müllerian duct

   C. Renal agenesis

   D. Cervicothoracic somite dysplasia causing abnormalities in vertebrae development

26. In patients with persistent Müllerian duct syndrome (PMDS), which of the following phenotype/genotype combinations is correctly matched?

   A. Phenotype Female/Genotype is 46 XX

   B. Phenotype Female/Genotype is 46 XY

   C. Phenotype Male/Genotype is 46 XYY

   D. Phenotype Male/Genotype is 46 XY

27. A 17-year-old girl is accompanied by her mother to your gynecology outpatient department (OPD) with primary amenorrhoea. On examination her breasts are well developed (Tanner Stage 4), her pubic and axillary hair are normal. On per vaginum examination, there is a dimple noted through the vaginal introitus. Her karyotyping is done which is 46 XX. Her pelvis MRI is suggestive of hypoplastic uterus and agenesis of the upper part of her vagina. What is your working diagnosis in this case?

   A. MRKH syndrome

   B. MURCS association

   C. Herlyn–Werner–Wunderlich syndrome (HWWS)

   D. PMDS

28. A young couple has been trying to conceive for the last 5 years. All investigations of the female partner are normal. The male partner has a low sperm count for which an ultrasound of the scrotum is advised, which is suggestive of undescended testes. The karyotype of the male partner is 46 XY. His ultrasound of the abdomen is suggestive of Müllerian elements noted in his groin area. Considering the above findings, what is your working diagnosis in this case?

   A. MRKH syndrome

   B. MURCS association

   C. HWWS

   D. PMDS

29. A 18-year-old female presents to your gynecology OPD with primary amenorrhoea and cyclical lower abdomen pain. Her examination is suggestive of well-developed breasts and normal pubic and axillary hair. Her karyotype is 46 XX. Her pelvis MRI is suggestive of a didelphys uterus, associated with a large pelvic mass of about 10 cm with ground-glass appearance with left-sided endometrioma, with an oblique septum obstructing the left side of her vagina, and left renal agenesis. What is your working diagnosis in her case?

   A. MRKH syndrome

   B. MURCS association

   C. HWWS

   D. PMDS

30. All of the following are true about PMDS, except?

   A. Phenotype is male

   B. Karyotype is 46 XXY

   C. Arises from a genetic defect in the production of anti-Müllerian hormone

   D. The persistent Müllerian components present an elevated risk of cancer

31. A 34-year-old patient presents to your gynecology OPD with her hysterosalpingogram (HSG) report. She has been married for 5 years and the couple has been trying to conceive since marriage. She has regular ovulatory cycles and her hormonal profile is normal. Her husband has normal semen analysis. They want to opt for intrauterine insemination, prior to which you had offered her an HSG. Her HSG report is suggestive of a small, curved, 'banana-shaped' uterine cavity located off-midline. What is your working diagnosis in her case?

   A. Arcuate uterus

   B. Complete septate uterus

   C. Partial septate uterus

   D. Unicornuate uterus

32. A 19-year-old patient presents to your gynecology OPD with complaints of primary amenorrhoea. She is referred to you by her GP with her MRI report. Her MRI report is suggestive of absent uterus, but there are fibrous linear structures seen just above the bladder dome. Both her ovaries are noted to be normal. There is presence of an ectopic right kidney (noted in the pelvis), and renal agenesis on the left side. On general examination, the patient is noted to have significant thoracic scoliosis. What is your working diagnosis in her case?

   A. Type 1 MRKH

   B. Type 2 MRKH

   C. HWWS

   D. PMDS

33. A 18-year-old patient presents to your gynecology OPD with primary amenorrhoea. She is referred to you by her GP with her MRI report. Her MRI report is suggestive of hematometro-colpos, right-sided hematosalpinx with both ovaries normally placed. Her uterus, cervix, and vagina are noted to be anatomically normal but distended with heterogeneously echogenic fluid. Both her kidneys are noted to be normal. Her karyotype is 46 XX. On local examination, there is a 'bluish bulge' noted at the vaginal opening. What is your working diagnosis in her case?

   A. MRKH syndrome

   B. Low-transverse vaginal septum

   C. Imperforate hymen

   D. HWWS

ANSWERS

1. A	12. A	23. C
2. B	13. C	24. D
3. C	14. B	25. A
4. D	15. D	26. D
5. C	16. A	27. A
6. B	17. C	28. D
7. D	18. B	29. C
8. B	19. D	30. B
9. D	20. C	31. D
10. B	21. D	32. B
11. C	22. C	33. C

13 SIP – Elective Egg Freezing

Source: Elective Egg Freezing for Non-Medical Reasons Scientific Impact Paper No. 63 February 2020. https://www.rcog.org.uk/guidance/browse-all-guidance/scientific-impact-papers/elective-egg-freezing-for-non-medical-reasons-scientific-impact-paper-no-63/

IMPORTANT POINTS FROM THE GUIDELINE (SIP)

- Elective egg freezing offers women, who are not ready to initiate family planning, a means to counteract the inevitable decrease in fertility associated with advancing age.

- Although sometimes regarded (and marketed) as a type of insurance, it is crucial for women considering egg freezing to possess a comprehensive awareness of the probabilities of success, along with the associated expenses and risks.

- It is imperative that women are thoroughly informed about the probable success rates of egg freezing, especially as it is exclusively offered by the commercial sector, raising concerns over financial implications and misleading marketing practices.

- The success of egg freezing is significantly influenced by the woman's age at the time of the procedure, with markedly greater success rates for those aged 35 and under.

- Younger women face disadvantages due to the current statutory limit of 10 years for storage, which should ideally be revised.

- An age-based upper limit for storage and usage may be more rational for medical, biological, and social reasons; nonetheless, due to the challenge of establishing a universally applicable age, such a limit in basic law should be eliminated.

- The substantial expenses related to the operation and subsequent egg preservation hinder many women from considering it, hence raising concerns regarding equitable access.

- As the NHS and similar state insurance systems in other nations do not cover elective egg freezing, this practice is exclusively available in the private sector, resulting in unavoidable financial ramifications.

- The future will undoubtedly witness a rise in the number of women opting to store their eggs, primarily due to the absence of a stable partnership.

- Societal changes are necessary to enable women to pursue family life at a biologically optimal age, should they choose, without jeopardizing their career opportunities, and to ensure sufficient childcare provisions that do not disadvantage women or families facing financial hardships.

- The growing acknowledgment of the necessity to enhance public education on age-related alterations in female fertility should underscore the significance of men's understanding alongside that of women.

QUESTIONS

1. Egg-freezing cycles account for what percentage of the IVF cycles?

    A. <1%

    B. 2%

    C. 5%

    D. 10%

2. Which of the following factors is a key determinant of a woman's fertility?

    A. Anti-Müllerian hormone levels

    B. Age of the woman

    C. Antral follicle count

    D. Body mass index (BMI) of the woman

DOI: 10.1201/9781003650355-13

3. In the absence of any medical indication, what is the timeframe that UK legislation allows for egg freezing after which the eggs are discarded?

   A. 10 years

   B. 15 years

   C. 20 years

   D. 25 years

4. After egg freezing, the likelihood of future live birth depends upon which of the following factors?

   A. Anti-Müllerian hormone levels

   B. Age of the woman and number of oocytes stored

   C. Antral follicle count

   D. BMI of the woman

5. All of the following are methods to determine the ovarian reserve of a woman planned for egg freezing, except?

   A. Anti-Müllerian hormone levels

   B. Antral follicle count measurements

   C. Follicle-stimulating hormone levels

   D. Luteinizing hormone levels

6. Which of the following is the most common reason for elective egg freezing to postpone child-bearing in women of reproductive age group?

   A. Absence of a reliable partner/relationship

   B. Awaiting financial stability

   C. Anticipating improved job opportunities and stability

   D. Escalating expenses associated with childrearing

7. Which of the following age groups of young women have high-cumulative live birth rates?

   A. <35 years

   B. 36–40 years

   C. 40–45 years

   D. None of the above

8. What is the reported cumulative live birth rate in women who have undergone elective egg freezing at the age of 35 years and under?

   A. 60%

   B. 70%

   C. 80%

   D. 90%

9. In clinical practice, which of the following techniques is not routinely available for elective egg freezing in women of reproductive age group for non-medical reasons?

   A. Elective freezing of embryos

   B. Elective freezing of eggs

   C. Elective freezing of ovarian tissue

   D. B and C

10. All of the following are obstetric risks associated with planning pregnancy at a later age after egg freezing, except?

   A. Pre-eclampsia

   B. Gestational diabetes mellitus

   C. Preterm birth causing cerebral palsy

   D. Intrahepatic cholestasis of pregnancy

11. Which of the following methods best reduces the risk of ovarian hyperstimulation syndrome in women undergoing egg freezing?

   A. GnRH antagonist trigger

   B. GnRH agonist trigger

   C. Coasting

   D. Using low-dose aspirin

12. Which of the following European countries funds 'elective egg freezing'?

   A. Germany

   B. Belgium

   C. Denmark

   D. B and C

   E. None of the above

13. Among the factors affecting the likelihood of a successful live birth using cryopreserved oocytes, which of the following is deemed the most significant?

   A. BMI of the patient

   B. Type of protocol used for ovarian stimulation

   C. Number of cycles performed of controlled ovarian stimulation

   D. The number of mature oocytes retrieved

14. According to research, what is the minimum number of mature oocytes that should retrieved to achieve a pregnancy?

   A. 5–7 oocytes

   B. 8–10 oocytes

   C. 15–20 oocytes

   D. >25 oocytes

15. Which of the following mediums is used for storage of cryopreserved oocytes?

   A. Ethylene glycol

   B. Sucrose

   C. Dimethyl sulfoxide

   D. Liquid nitrogen

16. Which of the following is considered the most common reason for women not utilizing their stored oocytes?

    A. Not wanting to be a single parent

    B. Preferring to conceive naturally

    C. Not wanting to use a sperm donor

    D. All of the above

    E. B and C

17. Long-term cryopreservation of oocytes in liquid nitrogen affects which of the following factors in in vitro fertilization?

    A. Euploidy rate

    B. IVF success outcomes

    C. Both of the above

    D. None of the above

ANSWERS

1. B	7. A	13. D
2. B	8. D	14. B
3. A	9. C	15. D
4. B	10. D	16. D
5. D	11. A	17. D
6. A	12. E	

14 SIP – Endometrial Cancer in Obese Women

Source: Endometrial Cancer in Obese Women Scientific Impact Paper No. 32 May 2012. https://www
.rcog.org.uk/guidance/browse-all-guidance/scientific-impact-papers/endometrial-cancer-in-obese
-women-scientific-impact-paper-no-32/

IMPORTANT POINTS FROM THE GUIDELINE (SIP)

- The 2007 Foresight report, commissioned by the UK government, projected that without intervention, 60% of men, 50% of women, and 25% of children will be obese by 2050.

- Excess body weight is linked to a heightened risk of numerous malignancies, with a particularly strong correlation between obesity and endometrial cancer risk.

- Obesity is more linked to type 1 (endometrioid) endometrial cancers rather than type 2 (non-endometrioid kinds such as serous or carcinosarcoma) endometrial cancer; yet, both subtypes are elevated with obesity.

- The risk of endometrial cancer is elevated in women with a body mass index (BMI) exceeding 30 kg/m², and this risk escalates linearly with rising BMI.

- In the United Kingdom, over 50% of endometrial malignancies are linked to obesity.

- The preoperative evaluation of endometrial cancer can be challenging in obese women.

- Magnetic resonance imaging (MRI) is frequently employed to evaluate endometrial cancer; however, several scanners include weight restrictions that prevent the examination of severely obese individuals.

- A BMI exceeding 30 kg/m² signifies obesity and correlates with an elevated risk of perioperative complications, but a BMI surpassing 40 kg/m² is classified as morbid obesity and is linked to heightened complication rates.

- Obesity is linked to various illnesses, particularly diabetes, hypertension, and cardiovascular disease.

- In morbidly obese women, perioperative problems including obstructive sleep apnea, arrhythmias, acute cardiac events, and venous thromboembolic events are more prevalent.

- Obese and morbidly obese women are likely to necessitate a more comprehensive preoperative evaluation to mitigate the consequences of concurrent morbidity and require more rigorous postoperative management.

- The conventional management for endometrial cancer involves surgical intervention, typically total hysterectomy and bilateral salpingo-oophorectomy, entailing the excision of the uterus, cervix, fallopian tubes, and ovaries, with or without lymphadenectomy, supplemented by adjuvant therapies such as radiotherapy and/or chemotherapy as warranted.

- Laparoscopic hysterectomy and bilateral salpingo-oophorectomy have been established as the preferred surgical method for women with endometrial cancer in three extensive randomized controlled trials.

- Laparoscopic hysterectomy offers advantages such as decreased hospital stay, lower analgesic needs, enhanced quality of life metrics, and quicker return to daily activities.

- The projected risk of conversion from laparoscopy to laparotomy escalates with BMI, with a significant increase in women with a BMI over 35 kg/m².

- The complication rate in women with a BMI exceeding 35 kg/m² undergoing laparoscopic surgery was comparable to that of open surgery (25%).

- The conclusion is that laparoscopic hysterectomy is not cost-effective for women with high BMI.

- Laparoscopic hysterectomy has shown to enhance patient-reported outcomes relative to open surgery in the near term; however, there is no significant difference, save from body image, at 6 months.

DOI: 10.1201/9781003650355-14

- Vaginal hysterectomy and bilateral salpingo-oophorectomy conducted under regional anesthesia may serve as an alternate surgical approach for obese women unsuitable for general anesthesia.

- This approach does not permit direct visualization of the peritoneal surfaces and may pose difficulties in severely obese postmenopausal women.

- In obese patients, surgical time is markedly extended.

- Moreover, abdominal hysterectomy in obese women is associated with elevated morbidity, including a marked rise in wound infections, wound dehiscence, and re-hospitalization compared to non-obese patients.

- A key benefit of laparoscopic hysterectomy in obese women is the reduced incidence of wound infection relative to laparotomy.

- A significant controversy in the management of endometrial cancer is regarding the use of lymph node dissection (pelvic and maybe para-aortic) during surgical intervention.

- Lymph node dissection may be employed for precise staging of endometrial cancer or may serve a therapeutic purpose.

- Endometrial cancer exhibits radiosensitivity, allowing radiotherapy to serve as a singular therapeutic option.

- Radiotherapy is delivered either as a combination of external beam radiotherapy and brachytherapy or solely as brachytherapy.

- Radiotherapy is regarded as a primary treatment for endometrial cancer only in exceptional circumstances; a recent retrospective research has found recurrence rates of up to 18% in these individuals.

- Numerous clinicians confronted with the challenge of low-grade endometrial cancer in women with morbid obesity and comorbidities are inclined to utilize progestogens, especially via intrauterine system (IUS), as a conservative approach to disease management.

- Nonetheless, there are no substantial case series documenting the results of this medical therapy as a primary treatment, and the long-term outcomes of such administration remain ambiguous.

- Research in a recurrent context (regardless of the patient's weight) utilizing high-dose oral progestogens indicates an objective response rate ranging from 11% to 25%.

- The correlation between obesity, the consequent metabolic alterations, and endometrial cancer is widely documented.

- The combined contraceptive pill is linked to a decreased incidence of endometrial cancer; nevertheless, its safety in obese women is questionable (UKMEC).

- The Mirena IUS, weight reduction, physical activity, and the administration of oral hypoglycemic agents (e.g. metformin) have all been proposed as strategies for the prevention of endometrial cancer in obese women.

- Bariatric surgery leading to sustained weight loss has been associated with a decreased risk of cancer development, particularly in women.

- Obesity is linked to non-cancerous comorbidities, including diabetes, cardiovascular disease, hypertension, and pulmonary disease, which may adversely affect morbidity and survival.

- Data indicates that obesity adversely affects both cancer-related outcomes and women's overall wellness.

- Elevated conversion rates in morbidly obese patients in certain randomized controlled trials of laparoscopic hysterectomy demonstrate that the selection of surgical approach must be meticulously evaluated based on local knowledge.

- Laparoscopic or open surgery in morbidly obese women imposes significant demands on the local healthcare economy: preoperative assessments may be extensive, surgical duration can be extended, patients frequently necessitate high-dependency postoperative care, surgical wards require specialized equipment for these patients, and hospitalization may be prolonged.

- Apronectomy resulted in a 4-fold decrease in wound morbidity relative to the conventional laparotomy method.

- The surgical duration for hysterectomy combined with apronectomy in obese women is markedly extended compared to hysterectomy performed in isolation.

- The combination of hysterectomy and apronectomy has been demonstrated to lead to extended hospitalization.

QUESTIONS

1. What is the overall 5-year survival of patients with endometrial cancer?

    A. 57%   C. 77%

    B. 67%   D. 87%

2. What is the 5-year survival of patients with stage I endometrial cancer?

    A. 60–70%   C. 80–85%

    B. 70–80%   D. >90%

3. All of the following statements regarding stage I endometrial cancer according to the latest FIGO staging (2023) are true, except?

    A. Stage I (IA1): Non-aggressive histological type of endometrial carcinoma limited to a polyp or confined to the endometrium.

    B. Stage I (IA2): Non-aggressive histological types of endometrium involving less than 50% of the myometrium with no or focal lymphovascular space invasion (LVSI) as defined by WHO criteria.

    C. Stage I (IA3): Low-grade endometrioid carcinomas limited to the uterus with simultaneous low-grade endometrioid ovarian involvement.

    D. Stage I (IB): Aggressive histological types such as serous, high-grade endometrioid, clear cell, carcinosarcomas, undifferentiated, mixed, and other unusual types without any myometrial invasion.

4. According to the molecular profiling of high-grade endometroid endometrial cancer (ECC) patients with which of the following have excellent prognosis?

    A. Pathogenic POLE mutation (POLEmut)

    B. Mismatch repair deficiency (MMRd)

    C. Microsatellite instability and no specific molecular profile (NSMP)

    D. P53 abnormal (p53abn)

5. According to the molecular profiling of high-grade ECC patients having which of the following have poor prognosis?

    A. Pathogenic POLEmut

    B. MMRd

    C. Microsatellite instability and NSMP

    D. p53abn

6. According to the WHO definition, substantial/extensive LVSI involves how many vessels?

    A. ≥2 vessels   C. ≥4 vessels

    B. ≥3 vessels   D. ≥5 vessels

7. Which of the following factors is not considered for staging of endometrial cancer?

    A. Histological type and grade of endometrial cancer

    B. LVSI

    C. Cervical stromal invasion

    D. Cervical glandular extension

8. Which of the following monoclonal antibodies has been recently approved for the treatment of endometrial cancer?

    A. Transtuzumab

    B. Pembrolizumab

    C. Certolizumab

    D. Ibritumomab

9. What is the time period during which maximum recurrences of endometrial cancer occur after primary surgical treatment?

    A. First 3 months

    B. First 6 months

    C. First 1 year

    D. First 2 years

10. Regarding women with BMI >35 kg/m² undergoing surgical management of endometrial cancer, which of the following statements is incorrect?

    A. The rate of major complications associated with laparoscopy in these women is comparable to that of open surgery.

    B. Elevated BMI does not increase the likelihood of conversion from laparoscopy to laparotomy.

    C. Laparoscopic surgery is not cost-effective for women with high BMI.

    D. All patient-reported outcome markers improved after laparoscopic surgery in women with BMIs under 35 kg/m².

11. Regarding the use of apronectomy in obese women during surgical management of endometrial cancer, which of the following statements is true?

    A. It has the benefit of not prolonging the duration of surgery.

    B. It results in a 4-fold reduction in wound morbidity among obese women.

    C. It does not prolong hospitalization for obese women.

    D. Hysterectomy in conjunction with apronectomy is the optimal surgical intervention for all women with a BMI exceeding 30 kg/m².

12. The principal characteristics of Muir–Torre syndrome include all of the following, with the exception of?

    A. The predominant characteristic is the presence of sebaceous adenomas

    B. It has an autosomal recessive inheritance pattern

    C. It possesses mutations in genes implicated in DNA mismatch repair, including MLH1, MSH2, and MSH6

    D. It includes visceral malignancies such as colorectal and endometrial tumors

13. Which of the following describes an aggressive endometrial cancer histological subtype?

   A. Grade 1 endometroid carcinoma

   B. Grade 2 endometroid carcinoma

   C. Grade 3 endometroid carcinoma

   D. B and C

14. Which of the following is the tumor type that gains the most from using molecular classification and is heterogeneous in terms of prognosis, clinical presentation, and molecular makeup?

   A. Grade 2 endometroid carcinoma

   B. Grade 3 endometroid carcinoma

   C. Serous carcinoma

   D. Mucinous carcinoma

15. Which of the following statements about high-grade (grade 3) endometroid carcinoma is incorrect?

   A. In high-grade (grade 3) endometroid cancer, molecular profiling is especially crucial and strongly advised.

   B. High-grade endometroid carcinomas are classified with the aggressive histological categories if the molecular categorization is unclear.

   C. High-grade endometroid carcinomas that belong to the non-specific molecular profile (NSMP) group have a favorable prognosis, particularly when they are estrogen receptor (ER)-negative.

   D. The prognosis for high-grade endometroid carcinomas with POLEmut is very good.

16. Nuclear atypia observed in low-grade endometrioid carcinoma is a significant criterion to exclude which aggressive kind of endometrial cancer?

   A. Mucinous carcinoma

   B. Serous carcinoma

   C. Carcinosarcoma

   D. Clear cell carcinoma

17. Which of the following statements regarding grading of EEC is true?

   A. Grade 1 low-grade endometroid carcinoma has up to 10% non-glandular solid growth.

   B. Grade 3 high-grade endometroid carcinoma has >50% solid component.

   C. Grading is not significant in NSMP endometrioid tumors.

   D. The binary grading method exhibits inadequate reproducibility and hence lacks clinical significance.

ANSWERS

1. C	7. D	13. C
2. D	8. B	14. B
3. D	9. D	15. C
4. A	10. B	16. C
5. D	11. B	17. B
6. D	12. B	

15 SIP – Endometrial Scratch

Source: Local Endometrial Trauma (Endometrial Scratch): A Treatment Strategy to Improve Implantation Rates Scientific Impact Paper No. 54 December 2016. https://www.rcog.org.uk/guidance/browse-all-guidance/scientific-impact-papers/local-endometrial-trauma-endometrial-scratch-a-treatment-strategy-to-improve-implantation-rates-scientific-impact-paper-no-54/

IMPORTANT POINTS FROM THE GUIDELINE (SIP)

- Implantation remains a critical factor in the efficacy of assisted reproductive technologies.

- For implantation to happen, a blastocyst must adhere to the endometrium under the influence of estrogen and progesterone.

- Numerous factors can influence an embryo's implantation potential, including the quality of sperm, oocyte, and embryo, as well as iatrogenic factors such laboratory settings and embryo transfer techniques.

- Moreover, many conditions of the uterine cavity may affect the embryo's capacity for implantation, including submucosal fibroids, intrauterine adhesions, and endometrial polyps.

- Numerous studies have investigated the effects of endometrial injury during the luteal phase prior to an in vitro fertilization (IVF) cycle in women experiencing recurrent implantation failure (RIF), which seem to offer compelling evidence supporting the efficacy of superficial endometrial injury (or scratch) in enhancing the implantation rate in this population.

- Although a globally agreed definition for RIF has not been established, it is considered the inability to attain a clinical pregnancy following the transfer of at least four high-quality embryos throughout a minimum of three fresh or frozen cycles in women under 40 years of age.

- Two systematic reviews and meta-analyses have demonstrated a positive impact of local endometrial damage in RIF, but they recommended that additional randomized trials are necessary.

- An inclination toward enhancement in clinical pregnancy rates and live birth rates was noted following endometrial damage after four implantation failures.

- The process via which endometrial injury may enhance IVF results in women with RIF is not well understood.

- Successful implantation necessitates the simultaneous development of the endometrium and the embryo.

- It has been proposed that recurrent IVF failure may be associated with a temporal mismatch between the endometrium and the embryo stage, indicating that endometrial development in IVF cycles may be 2–4 days more advanced than in natural cycles.

- It is hypothesized that localized endometrial injury during stimulated cycles postpones endometrial maturation due to the wound healing process, thereby rectifying the asynchrony between the endometrial and embryonic stages.

- Embryo implantation in natural cycles occurs during the endometrial 'window of implantation,' marked by the expression of several components by endometrial epithelial cells, including adhesion molecules, cytokines, growth factors, and enzymes.

- Numerous researchers hypothesize that the repair process after localized injury correlates with heightened synthesis of different growth factors that facilitate implantation.

- The repair process following tissue injury is somewhat facilitated by immunological components, some of which also play a role in embryo implantation.

- A potential explanation for enhanced embryo implantation following endometrial scratching is the generation of immune factors induced by the trauma.

- There is heightened expression of tumor necrosis factor alpha (TNF-α), interleukin (IL)-15, and other immune mediators in the endometrium of women who previously underwent a biopsy during the proliferative phase of the same cycle.

- TNF is a pivotal proinflammatory cytokine that enhances the synthesis of various other cytokines, including leukemia inhibitory factor, IL-11, IL-6, and granulocyte-macrophage colony-stimulating factor, all of which are hypothesized to contribute to the implantation process.

- Endometrial damage during the proliferative phase of the cycle elevated the numbers of uterine natural killer (uNK) cells that had diminished due to ovarian stimulation.

- IL-15 is crucial for regulating uNK cells, and variations in uNK cell quantities may correlate with alterations observed after IL-15 treatment.

- uNK cells, a specialized subset of NK cells, constitute the predominant lymphocytes in the uterus, particularly during early pregnancy and the secretory phase of the menstrual cycle, and are essential for placental development and the success of early pregnancy.

- They facilitate the development of immunological tolerance at the maternal-fetal interface, inhibiting the maternal immune system from targeting the fetus.

- Altered uNK cell function or quantity has been associated with reproductive failure, including recurrent miscarriage (RM) and RIF.

- A further mechanism for the sustained impact of tissue damage on endometrial function may entail the recruitment and activation of endometrial stem cells.

- It is recommended that endometrial scratching be performed roughly 7 days before the onset of menstruation, just prior to the initiation of ovarian stimulation for IVF treatment.

- All couples should be informed about the significance of protected intercourse during the month of the endometrial scratch, as doing the procedure in the luteal phase of the cycle poses the danger of occurring in the presence of an early pregnancy.

- Endometrial damage or scratch is typically done utilizing an endometrial biopsy sampler (pipelle).

- The sampler is inserted into the endometrial cavity, and the inner shaft is subsequently retracted to generate negative pressure.

- The sampler is then systematically rotated while being moved vertically within the endometrial cavity multiple times to facilitate the 'scratching' process.

- Current information indicates that endometrial trauma may be advantageous for women with RIF.

- Evidence suggests a possible advantage of endometrial biopsy in women with RIF when conducted in the cycle prior to the IVF treatment cycle.

- Existing evidence about the efficacy of the technique for women initiating their first IVF cycle is insufficient.

QUESTIONS

1. What is the recommended ideal timing for performing the 'endometrial scratch'?

    A. During the early follicular phase of the cycle preceding the IVF cycle

    B. During the late follicular phase of the cycle preceding the IVF cycle

    C. During the luteal phase of the cycle preceding the IVF cycle (about 7 days prior to the expected period)

    D. During the week immediately after the embryo transfer

2. Which of the following is an important proinflammatory cytokine that plays a crucial role in implantation?

    A. IL-10

    B. IL-4

    C. TNF-α

    D. TGF-β

3. TNF-α is an important proinflammatory cytokine that stimulates production of all of the following cytokines to play a role in the embryo implantation process, except?

   A. IL-6

   B. IL-10

   C. IL-11

   D. Granulocyte colony-stimulating factor (G-CSF)

4. Which of the following cytokines has a crucial role in the regulation of uNK cells?

   A. IL-10

   B. IL-4

   C. IL-13

   D. IL-15

5. Which of the following are important functions of uNK cells?

   A. They are crucial for the transformation of spiral arteries.

   B. They are crucial in trophoblastic invasion and the initial stages of placental development.

   C. They induce immunological tolerance to prevent the maternal immune system from attacking the fetus.

   D. All of the above.

   E. B and C.

6. Abnormal uNK cell function is implicated in all of the following conditions, except?

   A. RIF

   B. RM

   C. Pre-eclampsia

   D. Gestational diabetes

7. Regarding RIF, which of the following components of the definition is incorrect?

   A. Failure to achieve pregnancy after transfer of at least four good-quality embryos

   B. In three or more fresh/frozen embryo transfers

   C. In women above 40 years of age

   D. During a time span of 1 year

8. According to evidence, all of the following are proven advantages of endometrial scratching, except?

   A. Improved live birth rates

   B. Better implantation rates

   C. Increased clinical pregnancy rates

   D. Reduced rates of RMs

9. What is the suggested threshold for the cumulative predicted probability of implantation to identify RIF for the purpose of commencing further workup/investigation of the cause of RIF?

   A. >30%

   B. >40%

   C. >60%

   D. >80%

10. Endometrial scratch is performed using which of the following instruments?

    A. Uterine sound

    B. Pipelle catheter

    C. Blunt uterine curette

    D. Ovum forceps

11. According to European Society of Human Reproduction and Embryology (ESHRE) guidelines, all of the following are recommended investigations in a couple suspected of RIF, except?

    A. Reassess lifestyle factors

    B. Reassess endometrial thickness

    C. Test for antiphospholipid antibody syndrome

    D. Test for sperm DNA fragmentation and uNK cells

12. Which of the following assertions concerning 'endometrial scratching' is inaccurate?

    A. It is a safe and well-accepted process.

    B. It markedly enhances live birth rates in women with RIF.

    C. It should be conducted during the luteal phase of the cycle.

    D. It may normalize endometrial receptivity, hence enhancing implantation rates.

ANSWERS

1. C	5. D	9. C
2. C	6. D	10. B
3. B	7. D	11. D
4. D	8. D	12. B

16 SIP – Enhanced Recovery in Gynecology

Source: Enhanced Recovery in Gynaecology Scientific Impact Paper No. 36 February 2013. https://www
.rcog.org.uk/guidance/browse-all-guidance/scientific-impact-papers/enhanced-recovery-in-gynaecol-
ogy-scientific-impact-paper-no-36/

IMPORTANT POINTS FROM THE GUIDELINE (SIP)

- Enhanced recovery (ER) is often referred to as 'fast track,' 'rapid,' or 'accelerated recovery.'

- The ER model for elective surgery integrates various care components to create a pathway that mitigates physiological stress responses and organ dysfunction associated with surgical procedures.

- This facilitates expedited recovery for patients.

- The objective of ER is to mitigate the physical and psychological effects of elective gynecological surgery on patients, hence promoting expedited recovery, decreased hospital stay, and a swift return to normal activities.

- The rates of complications and readmissions are equivalent to, or superior to, those observed in the UK after standard recovery.

- Engaging the patient at each stage of the process, from decision-making to discharge, is a crucial aspect of ER care.

- Informed decision-making equips women with comprehensive information regarding treatment alternatives, including surgical possibilities.

- A formal preoperative risk assessment of the patient's health and fitness for surgery should be conducted in a timely manner to facilitate the optimization of any recognized issues, potentially reducing intra- and postoperative complications and mortality.

- The procedure should initiate within the community before referral and persist in preadmission clinics, maybe necessitating specialized assistance from anesthetics or medical specialties.

- The ideal location for early postoperative recovery must be identified and arranged, potentially necessitating elective admission to intensive or high-dependency care facilities.

- Preoperative patient education might diminish the necessity for analgesics and enhance patients' hospital admission experience.

- Procedure-specific information and consent significantly enhance the information dissemination phase of the preadmission process.

- Patients ought to engage in discussions regarding their surgical procedures and pain management with gynecologists and anesthetists, respectively.

- The pivotal role of professional nurses in this process is undeniable.

- The admission of patients on the day of surgery has become routine practice in units following the successful implementation of ER protocols, resulting in substantial cost savings.

- Preoperative discharge planning is a crucial component of ER.

- On the day of surgery, dehydration is mitigated by limiting the fasting duration to 2 hours for clear fluids before anesthesia.

- Complex carbohydrate beverages have demonstrated advantages in non-diabetic patients undergoing colorectal surgery, alleviating preoperative thirst, hunger, and anxiety, as well as mitigating postoperative insulin resistance.

- This decreases the duration of hospitalization and enhances patient satisfaction.

- Mechanical bowel preparation entails temporal and financial ramifications and is discomforting for patients.

- It is linked to morbidity, and there is no evidence that it enhances outcomes for colorectal patients undergoing elective rectal surgery, where bowel continuity is reestablished.

DOI: 10.1201/9781003650355-16

- Refraining from long-acting sedative premedication facilitates postoperative mobilization.

- All care routes must be suitably evidence-based, necessitating the inclusion of antibiotic administration prior to incision and thromboprophylaxis.

- The utilization of minimal access surgical approaches is highly endorsed.

- An abdominal incision should be minimized to facilitate safe surgical procedures.

- The routine use of nasogastric, abdominal, and vaginal drains offers minimal benefit and should be avoided, as they elevate morbidity and extend hospital stays.

- The use of vaginal packs should be avoided due to their discomfort and tendency to impede mobilization.

- Preventing intraoperative hypothermia diminishes postoperative problems.

- Goal-directed fluid therapy during surgery, utilizing stroke volume to steer fluid management, has been shown to decrease surgical mortality and shorten hospital stay.

- Minimizing variability in anesthetic techniques enhances patient outcomes and fosters patient safety.

- Postoperative pain must be preemptively managed and addressed, as it exacerbates the surgical stress response and extends recovery time.

- Spinal, epidural, and regional analgesic techniques diminish opioid consumption, enhance patient satisfaction, and correlate with a quicker return to work.

- Prompt initiation of meals and the reduction of standard intravenous fluid infusion volume are recommended.

- This method is secure and correlates with less nausea, decreased duration of hospitalization, and enhanced patient satisfaction.

- Early mobilization is essential to ER.

- It mitigates the adverse consequences of bed rest, including muscular atrophy and debilitation, compromised pulmonary function and tissue oxygenation, heightened insulin resistance, and an elevated risk of thrombosis.

- Mobilization is promoted by appropriate multimodal analgesia protocols that minimize the use of systemic opioids because of their potential side effects, which may encompass regional blocks.

- Regimens incorporate antiemetics to address postoperative nausea and vomiting, as well as laxatives if necessary to alleviate constipation.

- Catheters, drains, vaginal packs, and intravenous drips impede mobilization and should be removed promptly.

- Furthermore, the early removal of foreign bodies diminishes the likelihood of related illnesses.

- Women are susceptible to experiencing transient voiding difficulties after pelvic surgery.

- Consequently, the assessment of voiding and post-void residuals should be conducted after catheter removal.

- This should prevent the long-term irreversible voiding issues linked to bladder overdistension.

- Discharge for ER patients is dependent on specific criteria/protocols.

- Patients are discharged when they can mobilize, manage their discomfort with oral analgesics, pass flatus, and consume food and beverages.

- Women may be administered a mild laxative for home use until their initial bowel movement.

- Re-catheterization should not impede discharge, as women may be discharged with an indwelling catheter and return later for a trial without a catheter.

- Patients must receive written discharge information that encompasses emergency contact details, practical recovery guidance, and the anticipated duration for resuming normal function.

- Generally, there is no rise in readmissions or postoperative responsibilities for primary care.

- Minimal net investment is necessary for the effective implementation of ER.

- The ER allocates beds for enhanced operational capacity or cost reduction.

- The length of stay, accessible through Hospital Episode Statistics (HES) data for interhospital comparison, serves as a proxy indicator of care quality, as shorter durations imply reduced complications and adherence to ER protocols.

- A further indicator of quality is patient satisfaction.

- The NHS inpatient survey, questionnaires, and patient diaries gather these measures; patient feedback reinforces ER.

- Implementing ER may pose challenges to established customary practices.

- Successful implementation necessitates the involvement, participation, and commitment of all stakeholders in primary, secondary, and social care, including senior clinical and management teams, to ensure the sustainability of the transformation.

- A core team of stakeholders, referred to as 'ER champions,' should be designated to spearhead this transition.

- This typically involves a multidisciplinary team comprising a surgeon, anesthesiologist, specialized nurses, and managerial personnel.

- Education is crucial for the effective implementation of ER protocols.

- The implementation of locally established pathways and protocols derived from the ER pathway documentation can substantially facilitate change and empower all staff to enhance their knowledge.

- The primary components of ER provide secure, high-quality perioperative care and should be established as standard practice for all women undergoing elective gynecological surgery.

- This technique provides advantages for both patients and the NHS by generating savings from diminished complications and shortened hospital stays.

- These advantages are seen as:

  - Enhancing the patient's physical and psychological condition through preoperative evaluation, facilitating their planning and preparation prior to admission.

  - Preoperative discharge planning to address socio-domestic variables that may hinder early release.

  - Minimizing physiological stress during the operation by adopting a laparoscopic technique for hysterectomy to decrease length of stay and short-term postoperative mortality.

  - Implementing a systematic strategy for perioperative management by minimizing treatment variability using ER protocols within a department to decrease the utilization of high-dependency beds, complications, and duration of hospital stay.

  - Facilitating patient engagement across the entire process, from decision-making to discharge, enhances their sense of being informed, involved, motivated, and contributes to an overall improved experience.

QUESTIONS

1. Which of the following are proven advantages of the 'ER program'?

   A. Enables quicker recovery of patients

   B. Reduces physical and psychological stress of the surgical procedure

   C. Reduces length of stay at the hospital and hence the cost implications on the healthcare system

   D. All of the above

2. Which of the following are considered surrogate markers for quality of patient care after successful implementation of an ER program?

   A. HES data

   B. Patient satisfaction – collected by surveys and questionnaires

   C. Admission prediction dataset

   D. A and B

   E. All of the above

3. According to the latest guidelines, how much time prior to a gynecology surgical procedure, should estrogen-containing contraceptives and hormone replacement therapy be stopped to reduce the risk of venous thromboembolism?

   A. 2 weeks   C. 6 weeks

   B. 4 weeks   D. 12 weeks

4. According to latest guidelines, how much time prior to a gynecology surgical procedure, should smoking tobacco and alcohol be stopped?

   A. 2 weeks   C. 6 weeks

   B. 4 weeks   D. 12 weeks

5. For patients who are known cases of diabetes mellitus on treatment, what is the optimal level of HbA1c that should be ensured preoperatively before an elective gynecological procedure?

   A. <6.5%   C. <7.5%

   B. <7%   D. <8.5%

6. According to the recommendations, which of the following medications should be withheld on the day of surgery?

   A. Metformin

   B. Angiotensin inhibitors

   C. Beta-blockers

   D. A and B

   E. All of the above

7. According to latest evidence regarding fasting preoperatively, how many hours prior to a gynecological surgery should solid food intake be restricted?

   A. Up to 2 hours preoperatively

   B. Up to 4 hours preoperatively

   C. Up to 6 hours preoperatively

   D. Up to 8 hours preoperatively

8. According to latest evidence regarding fasting preoperatively, how many hours prior to a gynecological surgery should clear fluid intake be restricted?

   A. Up to 2 hours preoperatively

   B. Up to 4 hours preoperatively

   C. Up to 6 hours preoperatively

   D. Up to 8 hours preoperatively

9. Regarding mechanical bowel preparation prior to a surgery, which of the following statements is correct?

   A. Mechanical bowel preparation (e.g. bisacodyl, sodium picosulfate) should not be routinely administered prior to surgery.

   B. Bowel preparation is deemed to enhance intraoperative visualization, bowel manipulation, or surgical convenience.

   C. It does not exacerbate patient distress or dehydration.

   D. It diminishes the surgical time intraoperatively.

10. For patients on oral warfarin, how many days prior to a laparoscopic procedure should it be stopped?

    A. No need to stop warfarin

    B. To be stopped 5 days preoperatively

    C. To be stopped 7 days preoperatively

    D. To be stopped 10 days preoperatively

11. For patients on clopidogrel, how many days prior to a laparoscopic procedure should it be stopped?

    A. No need to stop warfarin

    B. To be stopped 5 days preoperatively

    C. To be stopped 7 days preoperatively

    D. To be stopped 10 days preoperatively

12. Regarding prevention of surgical site infections (SSIs), which of the following recommendations regarding antibiotic administration preoperatively/intraoperatively is not true?

    A. Prophylactic broad-spectrum antibiotics should be given during the hour prior to skin incision.

    B. Antibiotics should be repeated if surgical time is more than 3 hours.

    C. Antibiotics should be repeated if blood loss is greater than 500 mL.

    D. 1.5 gm cefuroxime and 500 mg metronidazole is the preferred prophylactic antibiotic combination of choice prior to skin incision for a patient planned for hysterectomy.

13. Patients undergoing which of the following surgical procedures do not require a 'trial of void' according to latest evidence?

    A. Diagnostic laparoscopy

    B. Laparoscopic ovarian cystectomy or surgery for minimal/mild endometriosis

    C. Patients who have undergone surgery for prolapse

    D. A and B

    E. All of the above

14. According to latest recommendations regarding 'trial of void' in patients during the postoperative period, which of the following statements is not true?

  A. Patients who have undergone a minor operation do not require a 'trial of void.'

  B. Patients who have undergone surgery for prolapse require a voiding trial after 4 hours or upon experiencing a strong urge to void.

  C. The success of the 'trial of void' is determined by a post-void residual volume of less than 100 mL or if at least two-thirds of the bladder volume has been passed by the patient.

  D. If the initial trial is unsuccessful, the patient should be catheterized and discharged with an indwelling catheter.

ANSWERS

1. D	6. D	11. C
2. D	7. C	12. C
3. B	8. A	13. D
4. B	9. A	14. D
5. D	10. B	

17 SIP – Evaluating Misoprostol/Mechanical Methods of Induction of Labor (IOL)

Source: Evaluating Misoprostol and Mechanical Methods for Induction of Labour Scientific Impact Paper No. 68 April 2022. https://www.rcog.org.uk/guidance/browse-all-guidance/scientific-impact-papers/evaluating-misoprostol-and-mechanical-methods-for-induction-of-labour-scientific-impact-paper-no-68/

IMPORTANT POINTS FROM THE GUIDELINE (SIP)

- Induction of labor (IOL) is the artificial initiation of labor, generally involving cervical ripening with pharmacological agents, artificial rupture of membranes, and continuous uterine stimulation as necessary, utilizing oxytocin infusion.

- Historically, mechanical methods were employed for IOL; however, they have mostly been supplanted by dinoprostone (prostaglandin E2 [PGE2]) and synthetic oxytocin.

- Recently, focus has shifted to misoprostol and the transcervical balloon catheter as simple and perhaps safer alternatives for cervical ripening. These are permissible, secure, and efficacious.

- The National Institute for Health and Care Excellence (NICE) advocates using vaginal PGE2, low-dose oral misoprostol, or balloon catheter for cervical ripening and IOL.

- This aligns with the recommendations from the World Health Organization (WHO), but NICE also advocates for low-dose vaginal misoprostol.

- NICE additionally endorses outpatient cervical ripening for women with a 'low-risk' pregnancy, with hospital admission occurring with the onset of contractions or membrane rupture.

- Misoprostol is an orally active E1 prostaglandin commonly utilized off-label during pregnancy.

- The advised dosages range from 25 to 800 μg, contingent upon gestation and indication, with the necessary dose markedly decreasing as gestation progresses and uterine sensitivity increases.

- The oral and sublingual routes exhibit quick absorption, reaching peak levels in around 30 minutes, compared to 70–80 minutes for buccal or vaginal administration. Oral misoprostol possesses a half-life of 20–40 minutes, leading to a shorter duration of effect of 2 hours, in contrast to approximately 4 hours for vaginal administration and 3 hours for sublingual administration.

- High-dose vaginal misoprostol (50 μg or more), dinoprostone, and low-dose oral misoprostol solution (less than 50 μg) resulted in the highest number of vaginal deliveries within 24 hours.

- In comparison to other prostaglandins, low-dose oral misoprostol solution is linked to reduced incidences of cesarean delivery due to fetal heart rate abnormalities and labor progression.

- All techniques were generally safe; however, the incidence of uterine hyperstimulation was greatest with high-dose vaginal misoprostol and least in women induced with a double-balloon catheter (two fluid-filled balloons positioned on either side of the cervix).

- Titrated (low-dose) oral misoprostol solution provided the greatest advantages for women and infants, whereas buccal/sublingual misoprostol incurred the least expense.

- The oral regimen offers possible logistical benefits, including oral route of administration, cost-effectiveness, and thermal stability.

- Participants administered oral misoprostol exhibited a markedly reduced cesarean delivery rate and significantly less hyperstimulation in comparison to dinoprostone.

- The objective of mechanical interventions is to apply direct pressure on the internal cervical os, hence enhancing local secretion of prostaglandins and oxytocin to facilitate cervical ripening and dilation.

- Single balloon catheters (normal 16F Foley catheter), are commonly utilized after being inflated above the cervix with 30 mL of saline instilled into the balloon.

DOI: 10.1201/9781003650355-17

- A commercial double-balloon catheter, which compresses the cervix from both superior and inferior positions, is also available.

- Laminaria tents and osmotic dilators can be put into the cervical canal to have a same effect; however, research regarding their efficacy is lacking.

- The utilization of balloon catheters does not elevate the incidence of infection or the likelihood of preterm birth in subsequent pregnancies.

- Women induced with oral misoprostol had a greater likelihood of vaginal delivery compared to those induced with the Foley catheter; no other outcome differences were observed.

- The use of the Foley catheter (30 mL single balloon) or cervical ripening balloons for induction is efficacious and associated with reduced rates of hyperstimulation and neonatal morbidity compared to dinoprostone.

- A Foley catheter may induce less maternal discomfort compared to a double-balloon catheter.

- Oral misoprostol (25 μg every 2 hours) is currently approved for induction in the UK and seems to yield decreased rates of cesarean delivery and hyperstimulation compared to dinoprostone. It is possibly appealing for self-administration or for individuals seeking to circumvent frequent vaginal inspections.

- Vaginal misoprostol (25 μg every 4 to 6 hours) yields effects comparable to those of dinoprostone.

- In individuals with a history of cesarean delivery requiring cervical ripening, balloon catheter induction may present a reduced incidence of uterine rupture compared to dinoprostone.

- In women receiving outpatient induction, balloon catheterization or long-acting dinoprostone are appropriate techniques with minimal adverse effects.

- The balloon has the benefit of reduced hyperstimulation rates; however, there is an increased requirement for oxytocin augmentation.

QUESTIONS

1. What is the incidence of induced births in the UK?

   A. 10%   C. 30%

   B. 20%   D. 40%

2. What is misoprostol?

   A. E1 prostaglandin (PGE1)

   B. E2 prostaglandin (PGE2)

   C. D2 prostaglandin (PGD2)

   D. F2-alpha prostaglandin (PGF2-alpha)

3. What is dinoprostone?

   A. PGE1

   B. PGE2

   C. PGD2

   D. PGF2-alpha

4. For IOL, misoprostol can be administered by all of the following routes, except?

   A. Oral

   B. Sublingual

   C. Buccal

   D. Per-rectal

5. The main complication of uterine hyperstimulation is lowest with which of the following methods of IOL?

   A. High-dose vaginal misoprostol (50 μg or more)

   B. Dinoprostone

   C. Low-dose oral misoprostol solution (less than 50 μg)

   D. Transcervical double-balloon catheter

6. Comparing dinoprostone and low-dose oral misoprostol as labo-inducing agents, all of the following statements are true, except?

   A. Oral misoprostol is inexpensive.

   B. Oral misoprostol exhibits thermal stability.

   C. Oral misoprostol is easy to administer.

   D. Oral misoprostol is associated with a markedly elevated cesarean delivery rate and a dramatically increased incidence of uterine hyperstimulation.

7. Compared to dinoprostone, by what percentage does induction by balloon catheter reduce the risk of uterine hyperstimulation with abnormalities in fetal heart rates?

   A. 25%

   B. 45%

   C. 65%

   D. 85%

8. Compared to dinoprostone, by what percentage does induction by balloon catheter reduce serious neonatal morbidity and perinatal mortality?

   A. 22%

   B. 32%

   C. 42%

   D. 52%

9. Pain associated with induction is least with which of the following methods?

   A. Double-balloon catheter

   B. Single-balloon catheter

   C. Dinoprostone (PGE2)

   D. Misoprostol (PGE1)

10. What is the recommended dosage of oral misoprostol licensed in the UK for IOL?

    A. 25 μg half-hourly

    B. 25 μg hourly

    C. 25 μg 2 hourly

    D. 25 μg 4–6 hourly

11. Which of the following routes for administration of misoprostol has the highest peak levels and highest bioavailability due to bypassing the first-pass metabolism by the liver?

    A. Oral

    B. Vaginal

    C. Sublingual

    D. Per-rectal

12. Comparing oral and vaginal routes of misoprostol administration, which of the following characteristics is not correctly described?

   A. Oral route has higher peak levels

   B. Oral route has higher sustained blood levels

   C. Oral route has rapid absorption

   D. Vaginal route has higher bioavailability

13. During IOL with misoprostol, to ensure good uterine contractions which of the following pharmacokinetic characteristics is considered to be the most important?

   A. Higher peak levels

   B. Rapid absorption

   C. Higher sustained levels in blood

   D. Higher bioavailability

14. Which of the following routes of misoprostol administration has the quickest onset of action?

   A. Sublingual

   B. Oral

   C. Vaginal

   D. Rectal

15. Which of the following routes of misoprostol administration has the longest duration of action?

   A. Sublingual

   B. Oral

   C. Vaginal

   D. Rectal

16. Which of the following routes of misoprostol administration has the most delayed peak of desired action?

   A. Sublingual

   B. Oral

   C. Vaginal

   D. Rectal

ANSWERS

1. C	7. C	13. C
2. A	8. D	14. B
3. B	9. B	15. D
4. D	10. C	16. D
5. D	11. C	
6. D	12. B	

18 SIP – Expanded Carrier Screening

Source: The Use of Expanded Carrier Screening in Reproductive Medicine Scientific Impact Paper No. 74 June 2024. https://www.rcog.org.uk/guidance/browse-all-guidance/scientific-impact-papers/the-use-of-expanded-carrier-screening-in-reproductive-medicine/

IMPORTANT POINTS FROM THE GUIDELINE (SIP)

- Expanded carrier screening (ECS) is a comprehensive blood test for numerous genetically linked disorders.

- This check can identify whether an individual unknowingly possesses gene variations linked to prevalent genetic disorders, such as cystic fibrosis, which may be transmitted to their offspring.

- This procedure is commonly used in reproductive medicine for individuals contemplating family planning, whether through natural means or fertility treatments.

- Numerous sperm and egg banks, especially in the United States and Europe, do comprehensive ECS testing on all potential donors.

- ECS is not already standard practice in the UK; nonetheless, an increasing number of patients are seeking it prior to therapy.

- ECS may evaluate for over 100 genetic disorders.

- A panel refers to the list of conditions that are checked for.

- Standard panels consist of 250 or 600 genes.

- Not all extended carrier screening tests analyze the same genes.

- Some individuals may screen for genes that may not precipitate significant illnesses or that manifest later in life, while others may search for genes associated with severe pediatric problems.

- There is no consensus regarding the specific panel of genes that should be assessed in an ECS.

- Commercial enterprises providing direct-to-consumer genetic and genomic testing, including ECS, have intensified their online marketing efforts both domestically and internationally, specifically targeting healthy individuals.

- The NHS England (NHSE) National Genomic Test Directory stipulates that carrier testing for partners of carriers should be provided only when the carrier frequency exceeds 1 in 70 in pertinent populations, when the gene is appropriate for carrier testing (pseudogenes and/or elevated rates of benign variants complicating the process), and/or when identifying an affected fetus would significantly influence reproductive decisions.

- While the Human Fertilisation and Embryology Authority (HFEA) offers recommendations to UK reproductive clinics regarding donor screening, there is presently no national directive in the UK specifically addressing ECS, nor are there any mandates for UK fertility clinics to implement ECS or for gamete donors.

- Moreover, the majority of donors would not satisfy the testing standards established in the NHSE National Genomic Test Directory.

- Emerging research suggests that ECS may be beneficial for consanguineous couples, with reports indicating that between 12–28% of such couples may possess probable harmful or pathogenic mutations previously unknown to them.

- More extensive investigations including additional populations are necessary.

- Prospective parents pursuing assisted reproductive technology, particularly those already engaged in preimplantation genetic testing for monogenic disorders, may find ECS appealing.

- Their principal goal is to prevent the transfer of a genetic disorder to their progeny, and hence, they may seek to broaden their screening alternatives.

- All individuals are carriers of many autosomal recessive diseases.

DOI: 10.1201/9781003650355-18

- This often has little bearing on the individual's health, and there is only a risk to progeny if they procreate with someone who is a carrier of the same gene variant.

- Presently, ECS panels encompass a minimum of 41 conditions and a maximum of 1556.

- A minimal number of the 500–600 genes evaluated in the predominant ECS panels in the United States meet the standards set out by the NHSE National Genomic Test Directory.

- A carrier rate of 1 in 70 indicates a prevalence of the condition/disease of approximately 1 in 20,000.

- An individual choosing a gamete donor identified as a carrier of a disorder with a carrier frequency of 1 in 70, will themselves have a 1 in 70 probability of being a carrier for that condition, and if they are a carrier, there is a 1 in 4 (25%) likelihood of producing an affected offspring.

- In the absence of carrier testing for the receiver, the probability of a child being impacted by the disease is 1 in 280 (0.36%).

- Although carrier rates vary by ethnicity, the advantage of utilizing ECS is its superior accuracy compared to self-reported ethnicity and ethnicity-based panels.

- Providers of ECS differ significantly, with some offering testing for diseases characterized by low prevalence, variable expressivity, inadequate penetrance, late onset, or moderate phenotype.

- Certain providers lack standardized best practices or regulatory supervision.

- The precision of ECS data is often ambiguous concerning the classification of variants (pathogenic, probable pathogenic, or of unknown importance) and their reliability level.

- Variant reports must be regarded with caution and assessed independently.

- ECS facilitates informed decision-making regarding preconception; yet, its responsible implementation presents technical, legal, ethical, and societal challenges.

- Since all individuals possess variants responsible for autosomal recessive disorders, the utilization of a broader panel (usually comprising either 250 or 600 genes) increases the likelihood of identifying a recessive gene variant.

- It is beneficial if the prospective parents are carriers of variants of the same gene; however, certain situations are more severe than others.

- The utilization of ECS is increasing among individuals pursuing reproductive treatment with both autologous and donor gametes.

- Comprehension of ECS is thus essential for all doctors engaged in fertility and reproductive medicine.

- All people possess several autosomal recessive disorders; nevertheless, there is inadequate data to advocate for routine prenatal testing of all couples, as the likelihood of having an affected child is minimal.

- Preconception targeted carrier screening is suitable for potential parents at elevated risk of possessing a gene associated with severe disease, based on personal or familial history, or population/ethnic predominance.

- There is an absence of standardization among commercially available ECS panels, and comprehension of the utilized panel is crucial prior to interpreting any results.

- While selecting a larger panel may be advantageous due to its broader gene coverage, it is advisable to utilize panels with identical gene coverage for both people, donors, and couples to facilitate direct comparison.

- The interpretation of ECS data must be conducted with prudence by qualified healthcare practitioners possessing adequate expertise in clinical genetics.

- Additional research is required to identify the suitable genes for inclusion in ECS panels, taking into account variances in population and ethnicity, while weighing the advantages for patients and their prospective progeny against the risks of superfluous screening, anxiety, and counseling.

QUESTIONS

1. What is the cut-off value of carrier frequency, above which it is recommended to offer carrier testing for certain genetic conditions?

    A. 1 in 10

    B. 1 in 25

    C. 1 in 70

    D. 1 in 100

2. According to the NHSE National Genomic Test Directory, which of the following is not an indication for performing carrier testing?

    A. The carrier frequency of the genetic disorder must exceed 1 in 70.

    B. The gene in question must be appropriate for conducting carrier testing.

    C. There should be a significantly high incidence of benign variants of the genetic condition.

    D. In instances where an aberrant fetus is diagnosed, there are solutions available to facilitate informed decisions that promote improved reproductive outcomes.

3. What percentage of consanguineous couples may have pathogenic variants in which ECS could be of benefit?

    A. 10%

    B. 12–28%

    C. 40%

    D. 50–65%

4. All of the following are examples of autosomal recessive genetic conditions, except?

    A. Sickle cell anemia

    B. Cystic fibrosis

    C. Gaucher disease

    D. Huntington's disease

5. All of the following are examples of autosomal dominant genetic conditions, except?

    A. Marfan's syndrome

    B. Achondroplasia

    C. Leigh syndrome

    D. Familial hypercholesterolemia

6. All of the following are examples of mitochondrial inheritance disorders, except?

    A. Leigh syndrome

    B. Duchenne muscular dystrophy

    C. Leber's hereditary optic neuropathy

    D. NARP (Neuropathy, Ataxia, and Retinitis Pigmentosa) syndrome

7. All of the following are examples of single-gene disorders, except?

    A. Huntington's disease

    B. Duchenne muscular dystrophy

    C. Tay–Sachs disease

    D. Silver–Russell syndrome

8. A couple is planned for in vitro fertilization with oocyte donation. The husband is 46 years old and the wife is 43 years old. The oocyte donor is a known carrier of autosomal recessive polycystic kidney disease, which has a carrier rate of 1 in 70. In this situation, if the couple carrier status is unknown, what is the probability of the child being affected by the disease?

A. 1 in 70

B. 1 in 280

C. 1 in 490

D. 1 in 4

9. How many genes are being studied in a commonly used panel while performing ECS?

A. <50

B. 120–250

C. 250–600

D. >1000

10. Regarding recommendations for ECS in the UK, which of the following statements is incorrect?

A. ECS can assess for more than 100 genetic diseases.

B. A panel denotes the enumeration of genetic conditions that are evaluated.

C. Standard panels comprise 250 or 600 genes.

D. ECS is well recognized as a standard procedure in the UK.

ANSWERS

1. C	5. C	9. C
2. C	6. B	10. D
3. B	7. D	
4. D	8. B	

19 SIP – Fertility-Sparing Surgeries for Gynecological Cancers

Source: Fertility Sparing Treatments in Gynaecological Cancers Scientific Impact Paper No. 35 February 2013. https://www.rcog.org.uk/guidance/browse-all-guidance/scientific-impact-papers/fertility-sparing-treatments-in-gynaecological-cancers-scientific-impact-paper-no-35/

IMPORTANT POINTS FROM THE GUIDELINE (SIP)

- The advancement of information regarding gynecological cancers has facilitated the provision of fertility-sparing surgery for women who want to maintain their reproductive capacity.

- This must consistently be addressed with the patient in relevant situations.

- The management of these women is intricate and necessitates contributions from a multidisciplinary team, comprising specialists with expertise in handling such cases.

- The work of specialized gynecological oncology nurses is crucial in assisting patients with their decision-making processes.

- Collaboration and dialogue with fertility specialists are crucial for women to maximize their likelihood of attaining a successful pregnancy.

- The objective of radical vaginal trachelectomy (RVT) is to excise the cervix, upper vagina, and para-cervical tissue via the vaginal route, to laparoscopically resect the regional lymph nodes, while preserving the body and fundus of the uterus to facilitate conception.

- A cerclage is positioned in the neocervix to reduce the occurrence of mid- and late-pregnancy loss.

- In the aggregated series, 10–12% of patients necessitated supplementary treatment due to positive margins, positive lymph nodes, or unfavorable prognostic characteristics.

- The recurrence rate ranged from 4.2% to 5.6%, with a 5-year survival rate of 96.8% to 97.5%.

- The tumor's location, rather than its histological classification, is paramount; thus, RVT is a viable option for individuals with early stage cervical adenocarcinoma.

- A notably elevated recurrence rate has been documented in tumors over 2 cm in diameter; it is thus advocated to limit the application of RVT to patients with smaller tumors.

- This procedure is unsuitable for those with metastatic illness.

- The rates of intraoperative and postoperative complications seem satisfactory and comparable to those of radical hysterectomy.

- Approximately 15% of RVT patients experience cervical stenosis, which may result in dysmenorrhea or infection.

- The miscarriage rate in the first trimester was comparable to the general population at 16–20%, but the risk of miscarriage in the second trimester increased to 8–10%.

- Only 70–75% of pregnancies culminated in term delivery (>37 weeks of gestation), while the incidence of substantial prematurity was under 12%.

- While most available data pertains to the application of RVT, there is a growing number of publications regarding the application of radical abdominal trachelectomy (RAT).

- This procedure is executed similarly to a radical hysterectomy, meticulously dissecting the parametrium in a manner familiar to gynecological oncologists, thereby replicating the excision of the identical paracervical tissue as in a radical hysterectomy.

- The dissection may be conducted via a laparotomy incision or laparoscopically.

- While RVT is recommended just for tumors measuring less than 2 cm in diameter, this procedure may prove particularly advantageous for tumors over 2 cm that would typically warrant a major hysterectomy.

- To diminish morbidity and the extent of surgical intervention, certain researchers have advocated for the administration of preoperative chemotherapy, succeeded by a straightforward cone biopsy and pelvic lymphadenectomy.

- This option warrants further investigation and may enable the treatment of tumors over 2 cm in a manner that ensures a favorable prognosis.

- Nonetheless, chemotherapy will adversely impact ovarian function.

- The extent of fertility impact will depend on the woman's pre-existing fertility status, the chemotherapy type, and the dosage administered.

- In microscopic tumors (stage 1A1), the occurrence of metastatic nodal or parametrial illness is minimal; hence, a simple cone biopsy has been employed for treatment for many years. Lymphadenectomy is unnecessary, and fertility outcomes are outstanding.

- If pelvic irradiation is deemed necessary in the treatment of cervical cancer, such as in cases of pelvic nodal metastases or parametrial invasion, ovarian translocation may be contemplated.

- The ovaries can be elevated and sutured to the lateral abdominal wall while maintaining their vascular supply.

- They must be positioned well above the pelvic brim to be excluded from the radiation field.

- This treatment may avert early menopause, allowing for the future utilization of ovaries for egg retrieval, in vitro fertilization (IVF), and obtaining conception via surrogacy if deemed suitable.

- Nonetheless, there is a significant chance of ovarian failure; so, oocyte retrieval should be contemplated prior to the initiation of radiotherapy.

- The application of progestogen in managing stage IA endometrioid endometrial cancer without myometrial invasion is now firmly established, although the number of patients seeking this treatment remains limited.

- A significant percentage of early endometrial malignancies in young women are well-differentiated and localized to the endometrium, with many patients also having polycystic ovarian syndrome.

- Endometrial cancer is often diagnosed in reproductive clinics.

- A significant issue is that endometrial cancer is staged histopathologically during hysterectomy, and in the absence of uterine removal, alternative methods must be employed to ascertain whether the tumor has infiltrated the myometrium.

- MRI exhibits a 90% accuracy rate and is employed in most instances.

- Multiple progestogenic regimens have been employed, with the most prevalent being Medroxyprogesterone acetate at 400–800 mg in divided daily dosages or megestrol at 160 mg daily. The response rate was 75% and the recurrence rate was 23%.

- The levonorgestrel-containing intrauterine device has been utilized in recent studies and may be beneficial for maintenance therapy.

- There is no agreement on the suitable length of treatment.

- It is supported by most studies that the endometrial samples can be taken at three-monthly intervals, with response times ranging from 3 to 12 months across all studies.

- There is a lack of consensus regarding long-term treatment.

- A hysterectomy post-childbearing may reduce the risk of long-term disease, whereas hormone maintenance by the IUS, progestogen-only pill, or combined oral contraceptive has been employed to postpone the hysterectomy.

- Young women diagnosed with epithelial ovarian cancer exhibit greater heterogeneity compared to those with cervical or endometrial cancer.

- Despite numerous documented series, it remains uncertain if histological subtype, breast cancer (BRCA) gene status, or other factors affect the prognosis of patients with early stage illness undergoing conservative treatment.

- To comprehensively stage a patient with ovarian cancer, it is acknowledged that a hysterectomy, bilateral oophorectomy, omentectomy, excision of pelvic and para-aortic lymph nodes, collection of peritoneal washings, and several random peritoneal biopsies are necessary.

- No further advantage is seen in performing a biopsy on a macroscopically normal contralateral ovary.

- Individuals diagnosed with stage I illness exhibit a favorable prognosis.

- However, if the uterus and the contralateral ovary are retained, there is likely a danger that microscopic metastatic illness may be unrecognized, resulting in an elevated risk of recurrence.

- Stage IA grade 1 and maybe grade 2 tumors of mucinous, endometrioid, or serous forms are appropriate for fertility-sparing surgery. Grade 1 stage IC may also be regarded.

- Borderline ovarian tumors are more prevalent in younger women and are often managed with conservative surgical approaches.

- The survival rates range from 95% to 97% at 5 years; however, recurrences sometimes manifest later, perhaps creating a misleading sense of security.

- Most gynecological oncologists would likely recommend conservative surgery for stage 1A disease; however, concerns arise when the disease has metastasized.

- The 5-year survival rates for stage II or III disease range from 65% to 85%, and due to the indolent nature of these tumors, a greater number of patients will ultimately succumb to the disease during an extended follow-up period.

- Radical surgery does not enhance the prognosis in germ cell tumors, which are typically highly responsive to chemotherapy. Survival rates in advanced disease exceed 90%, and most individuals will regain normal menstrual function after treatment. These cases predominantly arise in extremely young adults and children and are rare, hence necessitating referral to specialized centers.

- In instances where fertility-sparing surgery is unsuitable, ovarian tissue harvest and cryopreservation, ovarian stimulation with oocyte retrieval, and/or IVF with embryo cryopreservation may be viable alternatives.

- Surrogacy will be necessary to attain conception if the uterus is excised.

- Oocyte cryopreservation is technically demanding and necessitates ovarian stimulation, which may consequently postpone cancer treatment. It may be contraindicated if the tumor is considered hormone-sensitive, although there is no scientific evidence to support this.

- Oocyte vitrification may provide higher success rates than slow freezing but is constrained by the quantity of oocytes that can be harvested.

- This method has been endorsed by NICE fertility but only offers a 3–5% probability of achieving a successful pregnancy per frozen egg.

QUESTIONS

1. A 30-year-old patient presents to your outpatient department (OPD) with her cervical biopsy report. Her report is suggestive of squamous cell carcinoma of the cervix which is staged as stage 1B1. The patient is very keen to start a family soon and has been trying for 1 year. She wants to experience pregnancy and childbirth and is very concerned and depressed due to the current situation. Which of the following fertility-sparing treatment options can be offered to her?

   A. RAT

   B. RVT

   C. Neoadjuvant chemotherapy and cone biopsy

   D. Large loop excision of the transformation zone (LLETZ)

2. What is the tumor size below which a fertility-sparing surgery such as RVT can be performed?

   A. <2 cm

   B. 2–4 cm

   C. Cancer involving the lower third of the vagina

   D. Cancer involving the upper third of the vagina

3. Which of the following is not an indication for RVT in women requiring fertility-sparing surgery for cervical cancer?

   A. Early stage cervical cancer (FIGO stage IA2–IB1)

   B. Tumors larger than 2 cm

   C. No evidence of lymph node involvement

   D. No upper endocervical canal involvement

4. What is the 5-year survival rate of patients managed with RVT for early stage cervical cancer?

   A. 67%

   B. 77%

   C. 87%

   D. 97%

5. What is the recurrence rate in patients managed with RVT for early stage cervical cancer?

   A. 4–6%

   B. 10%

   C. 15%

   D. 20%

6. What is the incidence of cervical stenosis in patients managed with RVT for early stage cervical cancer?

   A. 4–6%

   B. 10%

   C. 15%

   D. 25%

7. What is the risk of second-trimester miscarriage in women managed with RVT for early stage cervical cancer?

   A. 4–6%

   B. 8–10%

   C. 15%

   D. 25%

8. All of the following are indications for RAT, except?

   A. FIGO stage IA1 with lymphovascular space invasion

   B. FIGO stage IA2

   C. FIGO stage IB1 and IB2 tumors with a size ≤2 cm

   D. Evidence of involvement of upper endocervical canal on preoperative MRI

9. A 34-year-old patient, who has a known case of polycystic ovarian disease, presents to your OPD with her endometrial biopsy report. She has a history of heavy and prolonged periods, for which her GP offered her an endometrial biopsy. The report is suggestive of stage 1A endometroid adenocarcinoma. The patient is very keen to start a family. Regarding fertility-sparing management of early stage endometrial cancer, which of the following statements is true?

A. Staging of endometrial cancer is clinical rather than histopathological.

B. MRI of the pelvis is not accurate in detecting the extent of invasion of the cancer into the myometrium.

C. MIRENA (LNG-IUS) is the recommended first-line treatment option.

D. The most common progesterone regimen used is medroxyprogesterone acetate 400–800 mg in daily divided doses.

10. What is the response rate to oral medroxyprogesterone acetate (400–800 mg daily divided doses) used in treatment of early stage endometrial cancer in women opting for fertility preservation?

A. 30%

B. 50%

C. 75%

D. 85%

11. What is the recurrence rate after oral medroxyprogesterone acetate (400–800 mg daily divided doses) used in treatment of early stage endometrial cancer in women opting for fertility preservation?

A. 10%

B. 23%

C. 40%

D. 75%

ANSWERS

1. B	5. A	9. D
2. A	6. C	10. C
3. B	7. B	11. B
4. D	8. D	

20 SIP – Induction of Labor (IOL) in Older Mothers

Source: Induction of Labour at Term in Older Mothers Scientific Impact Paper No. 34 February 2013. https://www.rcog.org.uk/guidance/browse-all-guidance/scientific-impact-papers/induction-of-labour-at-term-in-older-mothers-scientific-impact-paper-no-34/

IMPORTANT POINTS FROM THE GUIDELINE (SIP)

- The average age of childbirth is significantly increasing in Western nations.

- In the United Kingdom (UK), the percentage of births to women aged 35 years or older has significantly risen over the past few decades.

- Advanced maternal age presents a continuum of risk for both the mother and the fetus, with numerous research documenting various bad outcomes linked to this demographic factor.

- The prevalence of stillbirth during 39–40 weeks of gestation is 2 in 1000 for women aged 40 and older, in contrast to 1 in 1000 for women under 35 years old.

- Obstetric problems such as placental abruption, placenta previa, malpresentation, low birth weight, post-term delivery, and postpartum hemorrhage are more prevalent in older women.

- As fertility diminishes with age, the utilization of assisted reproductive techniques (ARTs) escalates, hence heightening the likelihood of multiple pregnancies. This may independently negatively impact the reported risks.

- Existing maternal medical problems, including hypertension, obesity, and diabetes, escalate with growing maternal age, as do pregnancy-related complications such as pre-eclampsia and gestational diabetes.

- These medical comorbidities can all affect fetal health and are likely to exacerbate the impact of age on the risk of pregnancy in an older mother.

- Nonetheless, despite adjusting for these comorbidities, advanced maternal age remains independently correlated with an elevated risk of prenatal and intrapartum stillbirth. It is also linked to a rise in neonatal mortality.

- Epidemiological studies indicate that women aged 40 years or older have a stillbirth risk at 39 weeks of gestation comparable to that of 25–29 year olds at 41 weeks of gestation.

- Unexplained stillbirths rise with advancing maternal age and gestational age in both nulliparous and multiparous women.

- When evaluating the risks of stillbirth at term, it is essential to determine the stillbirth risk as a fraction of ongoing pregnancies at a specific gestational age.

- The perinatal mortality rate at a specific gestational age is an imprecise indicator of antepartum stillbirth, as the at-risk population for continuing the pregnancy includes all current pregnancies, not solely the infants delivered that week.

- While the perinatal mortality rate is minimal at 41 weeks of gestation, the gestational age linked to the lowest cumulative risk of perinatal death is 38 weeks of gestation.

- Afro-Caribbean women exhibit stillbirth rates exceeding double (1.8%) across nearly all maternal age categories compared to Caucasian and Asian women (0.47% and 0.63%, respectively), even after adjusting for parity and medical comorbidities.

- Nulliparous women have a greater incidence of stillbirth compared to multiparous women across all maternal age categories.

- The influence of maternal age remained significant even after controlling for medical conditions, parity, race, and ethnicity.

- Women classified as nulliparous, aged >40 years and at term, exhibit a heightened incidence of intrapartum stillbirth attributable to intrapartum anoxia, with an adjusted risk ratio relative to younger women.

DOI: 10.1201/9781003650355-20

- The etiology of the increased stillbirth risk in women of advanced maternal age, following the removal of congenital anomalies, remains unidentified.

- Data indicate that fetal growth restriction (FGR) escalates with advancing maternal age.

- Scientific and clinical evidence indicates that aging diminishes myometrial function, with numerous extensive population studies documenting elevated incidence of cesarean sections due to dystocia and assisted deliveries among older moms experiencing both spontaneous and induced labor.

- Research indicates a linear correlation between maternal age and assisted delivery, intrapartum cesarean section, and labor duration in nulliparous women.

- Women aged 35 years and older necessitate elevated doses and prolonged administration of oxytocin to attain a successful vaginal birth.

- Neonatal mortality fluctuates with maternal age, with elevated rates among younger mothers (<25 years old) and older mothers (≥40 years old) compared to the overall maternity population.

- A Cochrane analysis indicates that induction at 41 weeks of gestation enhances perinatal outcomes without elevating the cesarean section rate.

- The statistics have resulted in a National Institute for Health and Care Excellence (NICE) guideline in the UK that women exceeding 41 weeks of gestation should have labor induction to prevent stillbirth associated with post-maturity.

- Growing research indicates that labor induction at 37 weeks of gestation enhances perinatal outcomes without elevating cesarean section rates.

- This contradicts the prevailing notion that labor induction results in elevated cesarean section rates.

- A recent comprehensive evaluation of research employing this technology identified only three randomized controlled trials (RCTs) that included women induced before 41 weeks of gestation. They did not identify a statistically significant elevation in the risk of cesarean section.

- The Hypertension and Pre-eclampsia Trial (HYPITAT) was a randomized controlled trial published subsequent to this systematic review, indicating that for women with gestational hypertension and mild pre-eclampsia at or beyond 37 weeks of gestation, labor induction did not result in a higher cesarean section rate compared to expectant management.

- Women aged 40 and older have a comparable risk of stillbirth at 39 weeks of gestation to that of women in their mid-20s at 41 weeks of gestation, at which point it is generally agreed that labor induction should be proposed to mitigate the risk of late stillbirth.

- Consequently, there is a rationale for providing induction of labor at 39–40 weeks of gestation to women aged 40 years or older.

- The research indicates that this strategy would decrease late antenatal stillbirths and mitigate maternal risks associated with a continued pregnancy, including pre-eclampsia.

- The reasoning is more compelling in the presence of concurrent medical comorbidities, nulliparity, or Afro-Caribbean heritage, all of which are associated with elevated stillbirth rates.

- Increasing research suggests that such a protocol would not elevate the incidence of operational vaginal births or emergency cesarean sections. Such matters should be addressed with older pregnant women.

- It is anticipated that older women, particularly those who are nulliparous, will opt for elective cesarean section as a preferred method of delivery instead of labor induction.

- In these conditions, it is crucial to discuss the risks and benefits of labor induction compared to elective cesarean section.

QUESTIONS

1. Which of the following risk factors is independently strongly linked to antenatal and intrapartum stillbirth and neonatal mortality?

    A. Pre-existing medical conditions such as hypertension and diabetes

    B. Obesity with BMI >30 kg/m²

    C. Advanced maternal age

    D. ARTs

2. By definition, what does vAMA (very advanced maternal age) mean?

    A. Women who are 35 years or more at the time of delivery

    B. Women who are 40 years or more at the time of delivery

    C. Women who are 42 years or more at the time of delivery

    D. Women who are 45 years or more at the time of delivery

3. At what gestation during pregnancy is the perinatal mortality rate the lowest?

    A. 38 weeks

    B. 39 weeks

    C. 40 weeks

    D. 41 weeks

4. At what gestation during pregnancy is the cumulative risk of perinatal death the lowest?

    A. 38 weeks

    B. 39 weeks

    C. 40 weeks

    D. 41 weeks

5. What is the overall incidence of stillbirth in the UK?

    A. 1 in 100

    B. 1 in 250

    C. 1 in 500

    D. 1 in 1000

6. What percentage of stillbirths are unexplained?

    A. 10%

    B. 25%

    C. 40%

    D. About 60%

7. A 43-year-old primigravida presents to your outpatient department (OPD) at 37 weeks of gestation. She has recently read a patient information leaflet on the risk of stillbirth in older women. Her pregnancy has been uncomplicated so far. She is very concerned about the same and has come to discuss her further management and delivery options. In terms of planned induction of labor (IOL) at 39–40 weeks of gestation in women ≥40 years of age, which of the following statements is incorrect?

    A. IOL at 39–40 weeks reduces the risk of late antenatal stillbirths in older women.

    B. It reduces the maternal risks such as pre-eclampsia.

    C. It increases the risk of need for emergency cesarean sections.

    D. It does not increase the risk of operative vaginal births.

8. By how many folds is the risk of stillbirth increased in the current pregnancy, in a patient with history of stillbirth in previous pregnancy compared to women who had a live birth in their previous pregnancy?

   A. 2-fold

   B. 5-fold

   C. 10-fold

   D. 15-fold

9. Regarding chronic histiocytic intervillositis (CHI) as a cause of stillbirth, which of the following statements is correct?

   A. It is an obstructive placental lesion.

   B. It does not recur in future pregnancies.

   C. Placentomegaly is observed upon examination of the placenta.

   D. The combination of aspirin, low-molecular-weight heparin, prednisolone, and hydroxychloroquine has demonstrated superior pregnancy outcomes compared to the use of aspirin alone.

10. In women of vAMA, which of the following statements regarding their risk of complications is correct?

    A. They are three times more predisposed to placenta previa and placental abruption.

    B. Postpartum hemorrhage impacts 25% of women of advanced maternal age.

    C. They exhibit a heightened incidence of cesarean delivery, particularly if primiparous.

    D. All of the above.

    E. A and C.

11. According to latest evidence by the American College of Obstetrics and Gynecology, at what gestation should elderly pregnant women (≥40 years) be offered planned delivery due to the risk of stillbirth?

    A. 37–37^{+6} weeks

    B. 38–38^{+6} weeks

    C. 39–39^{+6} weeks

    D. 40–40^{+6} weeks

12. The growing fetus in elderly pregnant women (≥40 years) is at increased risk of which of the following neonatal outcomes?

    A. Large-for-gestational-age babies

    B. Small-for-gestational-age babies

    C. Risk of stillbirth

    D. All of the above

    E. B and C

13. According to the evidence, which of the following chromosomal abnormalities does not increase significantly with maternal age?

    A. Trisomy 13

    B. Sex chromosome aneuploidy (XXX, XYY, 45XO)

    C. Microarray or rare chromosomal abnormalities

    D. B and C

    E. All of the above

14. What is the estimated risk of stillbirth between 37 to 41 weeks of gestation in women ≥40 years of age?

   A. 1 in 150

   B. 1 in 267

   C. 1 in 382

   D. 1 in 1000

ANSWERS

1. C	6. D	11. C
2. D	7. C	12. D
3. D	8. B	13. D
4. A	9. D	14. B
5. B	10. D	

21 SIP – Laser Treatment for Genitourinary Syndrome of Menopause (GSM)

Source: Laser Treatment for Genitourinary Syndrome of Menopause Scientific Impact Paper No. 72 July 2022. https://www.rcog.org.uk/guidance/browse-all-guidance/scientific-impact-papers/laser-treatment-for-genitourinary-syndrome-of-menopause-scientific-impact-paper-no-72/

IMPORTANT POINTS FROM THE GUIDELINE (SIP)

- Genitourinary syndrome of menopause (GSM) is a condition characterized by vulvovaginal symptoms such as vaginal pain, dyspareunia, vaginal dryness, itching, tissue friability, and sexual dysfunction, along with urological symptoms including urinary frequency, urgency, incontinence, hematuria, and recurrent urinary tract infections.

- Indicators of GSM encompass atrophic alterations of the external and internal female genitalia, characterized by regression and thinning of the labia minora, retraction of the introitus, and prominence of the urethral meatus.

- Histological alterations include the thinning of the stratified squamous epithelium, diminished glycogen reserves in the epithelial cells, and a reduction in vascularity and dermal papillae.

- The symptoms of GSM might adversely affect sexual function and quality of life in postmenopausal women.

- Traditionally, they have been managed with either non-hormonal or hormonal therapy.

- Non-hormonal therapy encompass water- or silicone-based vaginal lubricants, vaginal moisturizers, and herbal medicines.

- Hormonal therapies: Low-dose vaginal estrogens are regarded as the optimal treatment and are both safe and well tolerated.

- Potential options comprise vaginal dehydroepiandrosterone and an oral selective estrogen receptor modulator (ospemifene).

- Laser therapy functions by activating processes that facilitate tissue repair, growth, and healing, leading to enhanced capillary density and remodeling of connective tissue.

- In gynecology, tissue remodeling primarily utilizes two sorts of lasers based on the medium employed to produce the laser energy: the CO_2 laser and the erbium YAG (Er:YAG) laser.

- Lasers induce collagen remodeling in the subepithelial connective tissue; however, the mechanism of action varies based on whether the laser effects are ablative or non-ablative.

- Ablative lasers generate short pulses of high-peak power, delivering concentrated microablation to the epithelium and subepithelial tissue by forming microscopic columns of thermal injury in deeper layers, while preserving superficial tissue. This process subsequently stimulates fibroblast activation and collagen synthesis without inducing fibrosis.

- Various lasers, regardless of the material employed for energy generation, exhibit distinct tissue penetration capabilities and can induce varying degrees of collateral heat damage and tissue fibrosis.

- The CO_2 laser MonaLisa Touch (DEKA, Italy) features a proprietary system that can produce unique pulse modes to selectively target mucosal or cutaneous tissue. The specialized D-Pulse exerts a pronounced impact on the vaginal epithelium and lamina propria through an initial high-peak phase that vaporizes the epithelium, followed by a low-peak, prolonged tail that disperses laser energy into the connective tissue. Repetitive pulses can enhance these effects to be suitable for any vaginal tissue. These technological attributes promote vaginal tissue regeneration devoid of fibrosis.

- The Er:YAG laser SMOOTH (Fotona, Slovenia) features a patented 'smooth mode' that produces a non-ablative impact on tissues, inducing a gradual thermal effect that leads to controlled heating of the subepithelial connective tissue, abundant in water, thereby facilitating the disruption of collagen cross-linkages and the contraction of collagen fibers. Following the contraction of collagen fibrils, following thermomechanical interactions with the underlying tissues result in

DOI: 10.1201/9781003650355-21

tissue shrinkage and retraction, ultimately leading to the creation of new collagen fibers over time.

- Laser treatments are often conducted in an outpatient environment, with or without prior application of topical analgesics.

- Treatment sessions typically endure for 15 to 20 minutes and are scheduled 4 to 6 weeks apart, necessitating a total of three to five treatments.

- No standardized protocols exist for laser therapy.

- Adverse effects also seem to be moderate and temporary.

- The prevalent adverse effects include: Vaginal discharge (4%), edema (3.4%), discomfort, occurring solely during therapy (1.4%), and pinpoint bleeding (1.2%). Symptoms are transient and diminish within 2 weeks.

- Vaginal estrogens remain the definitive treatment for alleviating symptoms of GSM.

- Patients must undergo thorough investigation and receive guidance on the substantial safety and efficacy of vaginal estrogens, as well as be informed about non-hormonal treatments prior to contemplating vaginal laser therapy for GSM.

- The existing research, however limited, indicates that laser therapy may serve as an effective non-hormonal treatment for managing GSM, demonstrating comparable efficacy in alleviating symptoms to vaginal estrogen.

- Additional research and randomized controlled trials are needed to assess and confirm the long-term efficacy and safety of this technology prior to its endorsement for the management of GSM.

- Evidence indicates that the longevity of the effects of laser therapy diminishes over time, with symptom scores reverting to baseline levels by 18 months.

- Recommendations from international consensus groups and the National Institute for Health and Care Excellence (NICE) indicate that laser therapy should be confined to research environments until substantial data are accessible.

- Clinicians utilizing energy-based devices must possess adequate training in both laser use and the specific conditions being treated (e.g. GSM, SUI, etc.).

QUESTIONS

1. A 65-year-old postmenopausal woman presents to your outpatient department (OPD) with complaints of vaginal dryness and itching, associated with dyspareunia and increased urinary frequency and urgency. A working diagnosis of GSM is made. Which of the following is a histological diagnostic feature of GSM?

   A. Atypical basal cell proliferation marked by basal layer involvement, larger nuclei, hyperchromasia, pleomorphic cells, and an elevated number of mitotic figures.

   B. Thinning of the stratified squamous epithelium, reduction of glycogen reserves in the epithelial cells, and depletion of vascularity and dermal papillae.

   C. A band-like lymphocytic infiltrate obscuring the dermal–epidermal junction, accompanied by hyperkeratosis, hypergranulosis, sawtoothed rete ridges, and Civatte bodies.

   D. Atrophic epidermis exhibiting loss of rete ridges, accompanied by a subepidermal band of sclerosis (homogenized collagen) and a lichenoid inflammatory infiltration of lymphocytes situated beneath that band.

2. Which of the following is the gold standard treatment for GSM?

   A. Vaginal lubricants

   B. Vaginal estrogens

   C. Dehydroepiandrosterone

   D. Ospemifene

3. Which of the following are indications for laser treatment of GSM?

   A. Women who refuse vaginal estrogens

   B. Women for whom vaginal estrogens have proven ineffective

   C. Women for whom vaginal estrogens, vaginal dehydroepiandrosterone, and ospemifene are contraindicated, such as those undergoing active therapy for breast cancer

   D. All of the above

   E. B and C

4. Mechanisms of action of ablative lasers include all of the following, except?

   A. It generates short pulses with high-peak power

   B. It induces concentrated microablation of the epithelium and subepithelial tissue by forming microscopic columns of thermal damage in the deeper tissues

   C. It results in the destruction of superficial tissue

   D. This is followed by the stimulation of fibroblast activation and collagen synthesis without fibrosis

5. Which of the following statements regarding the mechanism of the CO_2 laser MonaLisa Touch is NOT true?

   A. It produces distinct pulse modes to selectively target mucosal or cutaneous tissues.

   B. The specialized D-Pulse exerts a heightened influence on the vaginal epithelium and lamina propria.

   C. It features an initial high-peak segment (to vaporize the epithelium) followed by a low-peak, extended tail to disperse laser energy into the connective tissue.

   D. It promotes the regeneration of vaginal tissue accompanied by tissue fibrosis.

6. What is the wavelength of the CO_2 laser MonaLisa Touch used for GSM?

   A. 2940 nm

   B. 3600 nm

   C. 1064 nm

   D. 10,600 nm

7. What is the wavelength of the Er:YAG laser used for GSM?

   A. 2940 nm

   B. 3600 nm

   C. 1064 nm

   D. 10,600 nm

8. Regarding the mechanism of action of the Er:YAG laser SMOOTH, all of the following are true, except?

   A. It produces an ablative impact on tissues and generates a significant thermal effect

   B. It induces regulated heating of the subepithelial connective tissue

   C. It facilitates the disruption of collagen cross-linkages and the contraction of collagen fibers

   D. Subsequent thermomechanical interaction with deeper tissues induces tissue shrinking and retraction, followed by the production of new collagen fibers over time

9. Which of the following are validated assessment scores for vaginal health in women with GSM?

    A. Visual analog scale (VAS)

    B. Vaginal health index score (VHIS)

    C. DIVA (day-to-day impact of vaginal aging) questionnaire

    D. All of the above

    E. B and C

10. What is the most common side effect of vaginal laser therapy done for GSM?

    A. Pinpoint bleeding

    B. Pain

    C. Vaginal discharge

    D. Edema

11. How long do the beneficial effects of laser therapy persist, after which symptom scores return to baseline levels?

    A. 3 months

    B. 6 months

    C. 9 months

    D. 18 months

ANSWERS

1. B	5. D	9. D
2. B	6. D	10. C
3. D	7. A	11. D
4. C	8. A	

22 SIP – Magnesium Sulfate

Source: Magnesium Sulphate to Prevent Cerebral Palsy Following Preterm Birth Scientific Impact Paper No. 29 August 2011. https://www.rcog.org.uk/guidance/browse-all-guidance/scientific-impact-papers/magnesium-sulphate-to-prevent-cerebral-palsy-following-preterm-birth-scientific-impact-paper-no-29/

IMPORTANT POINTS FROM THE GUIDELINE (SIP)

- The incidence of preterm birth is rising.

- Although the survival rates of preterm infants have increased, the incidence of cerebral palsy has also escalated.

- The prevalence of cerebral palsy markedly diminishes with advancing gestational age: 14.6% at 22–27 weeks, 6.2% at 28–31 weeks, 0.7% at 32–36 weeks, and 0.1% in term newborns.

- Twenty-five percent of cerebral palsy instances occur in infants delivered before 34 weeks of gestation.

- The percentage of infants born preterm with cerebral palsy attributed to a perinatal etiology (49%) exceeds that of children born at term (35%).

- Research on infants born to mothers administered magnesium sulfate for the prevention of eclamptic convulsions or as tocolysis indicated a decrease in the incidence of cystic periventricular leucomalacia (PVL) and cerebral palsy.

- The predominant pathological lesion linked to cerebral palsy in preterm newborns is periventricular white matter damage.

- Oligodendrocytes represent a significant glial population within the white matter.

- N-methyl-D-aspartic acid (NMDA) receptors on oligodendrocytes are believed to play a significant role in the process of glial damage.

- NMDA receptor antagonists serve as effective neuroprotective medicines in several animal models of prenatal brain injury.

- Magnesium sulfate may mitigate the detrimental consequences of hypoxic/ischemic brain injury by inhibiting NMDA receptors, functioning as a calcium antagonist, and decreasing calcium influx into the cells.

- Magnesium sulfate is involved in tissue protection against free radicals, functions as a vasodilator, diminishes vascular instability, minimizes hypoxic injury, mitigates cytokine or excitatory amino acid-induced cellular damage, and exhibits anti-apoptotic properties.

- The MAGPIE trial was primarily intended to assess the maternal neurological effects of magnesium while simultaneously documenting newborn outcomes.

- The study encompassed women delivering at all gestational stages, with 80% of participants sourced from underdeveloped nations.

- Pediatric follow-up indicated a reduced incidence of mortality or cerebral palsy in children at 2 years of age when mothers received magnesium sulfate instead of a placebo.

- The magnesium sulfate group shown no rise in mortality or sensory impairment, thereby assuring long-term safety for children born following maternal magnesium sulfate administration.

- The Cochrane review of studies determined that antenatal magnesium sulfate therapy administered to mothers at risk of preterm birth significantly decreased the likelihood of cerebral palsy in their offspring, with a relative risk of 0.68.

- A notable decrease in the incidence of considerable gross motor impairment was observed.

- The advised dosage is an intravenous loading dose of 4 g administered over 20–30 minutes, followed by a maintenance regimen of 1 g/hr for 24 hours or until delivery, whichever occurs first.

- The Australian guideline recommends that infusion should preferably begin at least 4 hours before birth but acknowledges that there may still be advantages if administered less than 4 hours before delivery.

- Magnesium sulfate administered exclusively for the prevention of cerebral palsy is stopped post-delivery.

- Intravenous magnesium sulfate can cause maternal adverse effects, including face flushing, and may seldom lead to muscle weakening and paralysis in those with neuromuscular diseases.

- The concomitant administration of calcium channel antagonists may amplify cardiovascular and neuromuscular effects.

- No evidence was found regarding an impact on maternal mortality, cardiac respiratory arrest, pulmonary edema, respiratory depression, severe postpartum hemorrhage, or cesarean section rates.

- A 50% rise in hypotension and tachycardia was noted.

- Seventy percent reported adverse symptoms including flushing, nausea, vomiting, sweating, and complications at the injection site.

QUESTIONS

1. What is the incidence of cerebral palsy in infants born at term?

    A. 25%
    B. 15%
    C. 5%
    D. 0.1%

2. Of all cases of infants born with cerebral palsy, what percentage of infants are born at less than 34 weeks?

    A. 10%
    B. 15%
    C. 25%
    D. 35%

3. What is the most common pathological associated with cerebral palsy in preterm infants?

    A. Intraventricular hemorrhage
    B. Periventricular white matter injury
    C. Demyelination
    D. Cerebellar hemorrhage

4. Magnesium sulfate acts on which of the following receptors to maintain a neuroprotective effect?

    A. It blocks NMDA receptors
    B. It stimulates GABA receptors
    C. It stimulates glutamate receptors
    D. It blocks dopamine receptors

5. Mechanisms of action of magnesium sulfate in neuroprotection include all of the following, except?

    A. It acts as a calcium antagonist
    B. It is a vasoconstrictor
    C. It has anti-apoptotic action
    D. It reduces cytokine or excitatory amino acid-induced cell damage

6. According to the Cochrane review of trials, what is the reported relative risk reduction in cerebral palsy in children born to mothers at risk of preterm birth, who have received magnesium sulfate antenatally?

   A. About 50–60%

   B. About 30–40%

   C. About 20–25%

   D. About 10–15%

7. What is the recommended dosage of magnesium sulfate for neuroprotection in patients at risk of preterm birth?

   A. Administered via intravenous route a loading dosage of 4 g should be administered over 20–30 minutes, followed by a maintenance regimen of 1 g/hr for 12 hours or until delivery, whichever occurs later.

   B. Administered via intravenous route a loading dosage of 6 g should be administered over 20–30 minutes, followed by a maintenance regimen of 1 g/hr for 12 hours or until delivery, whichever occurs later.

   C. Administered via intravenous route a loading dosage of 4 g should be administered over 20–30 minutes, followed by a maintenance regimen of 1 g/hr for 24 hours or until delivery, whichever occurs first.

   D. Administered via intravenous route a loading dosage of 6 g should be administered over 20–30 minutes, followed by a maintenance regimen of 1 g/hr for 24 hours or until delivery, whichever occurs first.

8. While patients are on intravenous magnesium sulfate regimen, all of the following maternal parameters need to be monitored, except?

   A. Deep tendon reflexes

   B. Respiratory rate, pulse rate, blood pressure

   C. Urine output

   D. Temperature

9. What is the normal range of magnesium in blood?

   A. 1.7–2.2 mg/dL

   B. 2.3–2.8 mg/dL

   C. 2.9–3.4 mg/dL

   D. 3.5–4.0 mg/dL

10. A primigravida patient with IVF conception presents to the emergency department with preterm labor at 30 weeks. She is offered steroid cover and intravenous magnesium sulfate for neuroprotection. During her treatment she develops flushing, nausea, and vomiting. Her respiratory rate is 12/minute, blood pressure is 90/60 mmHg, and she has muscle paralysis. You suspect magnesium toxicity and send for serum magnesium level, which is 3.5 mg/dL. What is your recommended management in her case?

    A. Intravenous calcium carbonate

    B. Intravenous calcium citrate

    C. Intravenous calcium gluconate

    D. Intravenous calcium phosphate

ANSWERS

1. D	5. B	9. A
2. C	6. B	10. C
3. B	7. C	
4. A	8. D	

23 SIP – Metformin Therapy in Polycystic Ovary Syndrome (PCOS)

Source: Metformin Therapy for the Management of Infertility in Women with Polycystic Ovary Syndrome Scientific Impact Paper No. 13 August 2017. https://www.rcog.org.uk/guidance/browse-all -guidance/scientific-impact-papers/metformin-therapy-for-the-management-of-infertility-in-women -with-polycystic-ovary-syndrome-scientific-impact-paper-no-13/

IMPORTANT POINTS FROM THE GUIDELINE (SIP)

- While several individuals with polycystic ovaries may not exhibit polycystic ovary syndrome (PCOS), it remains a prevalent endocrine illness impacting 4–12% of women.

- The diagnostic criteria for PCOS are widely recognized, necessitating the presence of two of the following:

  - Oligo-ovulation and/or anovulation (menstrual irregularity and/or anovulatory infertility), i.e., menstrual disruption.

  - Clinical and/or biochemical indicators of hyperandrogenism (hirsutism, acne, baldness).

  - Ultrasound examination reveals polycystic ovaries.

- The World Health Organization (WHO) categorizes normal weight for adults as a body mass index (BMI) of 18.5–24.99 kg/m², overweight as a BMI of 25 kg/m² or above, and obesity as a BMI of 30 kg/m² or greater.

- The established definition of PCOS acknowledges obesity as a correlation rather than a diagnostic criterion, given that only 40–50% of women with PCOS are classified as overweight.

- Other etiologies of menstrual irregularities and hyperandrogenism must be ruled out with suitable endocrine evaluations.

- Ovarian hyperandrogenism is predominantly influenced by luteinizing hormone in women of normal weight.

- In individuals with excess weight, insulin may enhance the effects of luteinizing hormone by increasing androgen release from the ovaries.

- Insulin inhibits the liver's release of sex hormone-binding globulin, resulting in elevated amounts of free circulating testosterone.

- Individuals with PCOS have greater insulin resistance (IR) compared to weight-matched individuals without the disease.

- IR occurs in roughly 10–15% of lean and 20–40% of obese women with PCOS.

- Women with PCOS face an elevated risk of developing type II diabetes.

- As an individual's weight increases, the severity of IR also escalates.

- Maternal weight significantly impacts both natural and assisted conception, affecting the probability of achieving pregnancy and the chances of a healthy pregnancy.

- Research has shown elevated incidences of preterm birth, miscarriages, and low birth weight in infants born to obese mothers compared to those of normal weight with PCOS.

- IR is characterized by a diminished glucose response to a certain quantity of insulin, typically arising from defects in the insulin receptor and post-receptor signaling pathways.

- Consequently, circulating insulin concentrations increase.

- Elevated circulating insulin levels in the ovary are believed to facilitate excessive androgen production and anovulation.

- The yearly incidence of diabetes in women with PCOS and pre-existing IR was 10.4%.

- IR is a prevalent characteristic irrespective of weight; however, not all women with PCOS have elevated IR.

- Given that IR is affected by age and ethnicity, establishing a globally accepted cut-off level for IR can be challenging.

- Consequently, the assessment of IR is not incorporated into the diagnostic criteria for PCOS.

- IR can be assessed using various costly tests; but, in clinical practice, it is more crucial to evaluate for impaired glucose tolerance (IGT).

- Basic screening assessments encompass evaluating BMI, waist circumference, and monitoring fasting blood glucose levels.

- If the fasting blood glucose is below 5.2 mmol/L, the risk of IGT is minimal.

- The 2-hour 75 g oral glucose tolerance test (OGTT) is the definitive diagnostic test and may be administered to individuals at elevated risk (BMI exceeding 30 kg/m² in Caucasian women or surpassing 25 kg/m² in women from specific ethnic groups, such as South Asians, who exhibit a heightened susceptibility to IR at lower body weights).

- Women with impaired fasting glucose (fasting plasma glucose level 6.1–6.9 mmol/L) or IGT (plasma glucose 7.8 mmol/L or greater, but less than 11.1 mmol/L following a 2-hour 75 g OGTT) should have an annual OGTT.

- An evaluation of glycosylated hemoglobin (HbA1c) may be conducted if women cannot complete an OGTT and can be utilized for annual screening.

- Metformin suppresses hepatic glucose production, diminishes lipid synthesis, enhances fatty acid oxidation, and inhibits gluconeogenesis, leading to reduced circulating insulin and glucose levels.

- Metformin improves insulin sensitivity at the cellular level and seems to exert direct effects on the ovary.

- No consensus existed on the dosage and duration of metformin therapy.

- Although many research indicate that metformin medication may facilitate weight loss, the majority of extensive randomized controlled trials have not substantiated this claim.

- A recent subgroup study in a systematic review suggested that metformin medication, when paired with lifestyle adjustment, had a modest effect on obese women with PCOS.

- Moreover, metformin alone did not enhance weight loss relative to placebo or no intervention.

- Consequently, enhancing lifestyle and assisting women through personalized assessment, goal planning, and a combination of nutrition and exercise continues to be the primary strategy.

- Clomiphene citrate demonstrated higher rates of ovulation and clinical pregnancy compared to metformin, a finding that remained consistent when analyzed by BMI.

- It was established that metformin alone is much less successful than clomiphene citrate alone as a first-line therapy for treating anovulatory and infertile women with PCOS.

- Moreover, metformin does not improve metabolic markers, including fasting insulin, glucose, testosterone, and lipid profiles.

- Metformin is generally considered safe during pregnancy; nonetheless, the standard recommendation is to discontinue its use after conception, except for individuals with diabetes.

- A meta-analysis comparing metformin to clomiphene in women with a BMI below 32 kg/m² indicated no significant differences in ovulation, pregnancy, live birth, miscarriage, and multiple pregnancy rates between the two treatments.

- Metformin usage is consistently linked to a higher incidence of side effects compared to clomiphene citrate or placebo, notably nausea, vomiting, and other gastrointestinal disturbances.

- The utilization of long-acting formulations may mitigate gastrointestinal side effects.

- The ideal metformin regimen remains undetermined, with dosages ranging from 500 mg/day to 3000 mg/day utilized.

- The predominant regimens are 500 mg administered three times daily or 850 mg administered twice daily.

- The necessity of adjusting the dose based on body weight or other variables remains ambiguous.

- Women with PCOS unresponsive to clomiphene citrate may be presented with one of the following second-line therapies:

  - Laparoscopic ovarian drilling

  - Clomiphene citrate and metformin, provided these have not been administered as initial therapy

  - Gonadotrophins

- Co-treatment with metformin may enhance the efficacy of exogenous gonadotrophins or the results of assisted reproduction.

- Metformin reduced the risk of OHSS in patients undergoing in vitro fertilization, likely by modifying the ovarian response to stimulation.

- Currently, the short GnRH antagonist protocol is advised for women at risk of OHSS, but the function of metformin remains ambiguous.

- Women with PCOS face heightened risks of pregnancy-related problems, such as gestational diabetes, pregnancy-induced hypertension, pre-eclampsia, and newborn morbidity.

- Given the beneficial benefits of metformin on metabolic, cardiovascular, and thrombotic events in the diabetic population, it appears plausible that outcomes in PCOS pregnancies could be enhanced with metformin.

- A substantial Norwegian multicenter randomized controlled trial revealed no enhancement in these problems with the sustained administration of metformin during pregnancy.

- Metformin exhibits a favorable safety profile during pregnancy, with no evidence of teratogenic effects.

- Insufficient data exists to endorse the use of other insulin sensitizers, such as thiazolidinediones (glitazones), D-chiro-inositol, and myo-inositol, for the management of anovulatory PCOS.

- Recent insulin-sensitizing drugs, including glucagon-like peptide 1 (GLP-1) analogs such as exenatide and liraglutide, are presently being studied.

- Metformin seems to have a restricted impact on enhancing reproductive outcomes in women with PCOS, although it may be advantageous for particular patient subsets, such as obese women when used in conjunction with clomiphene citrate, those exhibiting resistance to clomiphene citrate, and individuals diagnosed with either IGT or type II diabetes.

- The administration of Metformin may result in undesirable side effects, including nausea, vomiting, stomach discomfort, diarrhea, disorientation, and atypical fatigue.

- Moreover, although there is data indicating a decrease in diabetes onset among high-risk women without PCOS, the efficacy of prolonged metformin usage in enhancing metabolic parameters remains uncertain.

- Consequently, lifestyle recommendations emphasizing nutrition and exercise continue to be fundamental for young women with PCOS.

QUESTIONS

1. According to the WHO, what is the normal body mass index?

    A. Less than 18.5 kg/m²

    B. Between 18.5–24.99 kg/m²

    C. Between 25–29.99 kg/m²

    D. More than 30 kg/m²

2. According to the WHO, which body mass index represents the overweight category?

   A. Less than 18.5 kg/m²

   B. Between 18.5–24.99 kg/m²

   C. Between 25–29.99 kg/m²

   D. More than 30 kg/m²

3. According to the WHO, which body mass index represents the obese category?

   A. Less than 18.5 kg/m²

   B. Between 18.5–24.99 kg/m²

   C. Between 25–29.99 kg/m²

   D. More than 30 kg/m²

4. What percentage of patients with PCOS are overweight?

   A. 10–20%   C. 30–40%

   B. 20–30%   D. 40–50%

5. In women with PCOS, who are within normal weight BMI range, which of the following hormones are responsible for driving ovarian hyperandrogenism?

   A. Follicle-stimulating hormone (FSH)

   B. Luteinizing hormone (LH)

   C. Insulin

   D. Testosterone

6. In overweight PCOS women, which of the following statements regarding hormonal effects is NOT true?

   A. Insulin enhances the effects of LH.

   B. Insulin enhances the secretion of androgens by the ovaries.

   C. Insulin elevates sex hormone-binding globulin (SHBG) levels.

   D. There is an elevated concentration of free-circulating testosterone.

7. What percentage of slim women with PCOS are insulin resistant?

   A. <10%

   B. 10–15%

   C. 20–40%

   D. 40–50%

8. What percentage of obese women with PCOS are insulin resistant?

   A. <10%   C. 20–40%

   B. 10–15%   D. 40–50%

9. Which of the following effects on pregnancy are increased in obese women with PCOS, in comparison to normal weight women?

   A. Preterm birth

   B. Low birth weight babies

   C. Spontaneous miscarriages

   D. All of the above

10. All of the following statements regarding IR are true, except?

    A. It manifests exclusively in overweight and obese women diagnosed with PCOS.

    B. It is affected by age and race.

    C. IR arises from a diminished glucose response to a specific amount of insulin.

    D. It typically arises from a malfunction in the insulin receptor and post-receptor signaling pathways.

11. What is the annual rate of developing diabetes in women with PCOS who have IR?

    A. 5%

    B. 10%

    C. 15%

    D. 20%

12. Which of the following are simple screening tests for IR for checking the IGT?

    A. BMI

    B. Waist circumference

    C. Fasting blood glucose

    D. All of the above

    E. B and C

13. Which of the following is the gold standard investigation to diagnose IGT?

    A. BMI

    B. Waist circumference

    C. Fasting blood glucose

    D. 2-hour 75 gm OGTT

14. All of the following are high-risk groups that should be offered 2-hour OGTT, except?

    A. BMI greater than 30 kg/m^2 in Caucasian women

    B. BMI greater than 25 kg/m^2 in South Asian women

    C. BMI greater than 30 kg/m^2 in Black women

    D. In women with IGT – fasting glucose between 7.8–11.1 mmol/L (offer annual OGTT)

15. Regarding the mechanism of action of metformin, which of the following statements is not true?

    A. Metformin suppresses hepatic glucose production.

    B. It reduces lipid synthesis and enhances fatty acid oxidation.

    C. It stimulates gluconeogenesis at the cellular level.

    D. It improves insulin sensitivity at the cellular level.

16. Which of the following is considered the mainstay treatment for young women with PCOS?

    A. Lifestyle modification with diet and exercise for weight reduction

    B. Metformin 850 mg twice daily

    C. Offer myo-inositol and di-chiro inositol

    D. Offer thiazolidinediones

17. Metformin has been proven to be advantageous in all of the following patient categories, except?

   A. Utilized independently in young individuals with PCOS

   B. Employed in obese women when combined with clomiphene citrate

   C. In women demonstrating resistance to clomiphene citrate

   D. In patients diagnosed with reduced glucose tolerance or type II diabetes

18. Regarding the homeostasis model assessment (HOMA)-IR, which of the following statements is incorrect?

   A. It signifies the HOMA-IR.

   B. The calculation involves multiplying fasting insulin and glucose levels, then dividing the product by a factor of 22.5.

   C. A high HOMA-IR score indicates elevated insulin sensitivity.

   D. It assists in assessing the risk of acquiring type II diabetes mellitus.

19. Regarding the impact of metformin on hyperandrogenism in women with PCOS, which of the following statements is inaccurate?

   A. Metformin reduces testosterone levels.

   B. Metformin does not enhance the free androgen index (FAI) in non-obese women.

   C. Metformin improves insulin sensitivity.

   D. Metformin improves biochemical hyperandrogenism.

20. Which of the following effects of metformin in patients with PCOS is incorrect?

   A. It improves ovulation by mitigating hyperandrogenism and hyperinsulinemia

   B. It improves the regularity of menstrual cycles

   C. It improves reproductive outcomes

   D. It is acknowledged for improving lipid profiles primarily in women with a BMI of 25 kg/m² or lower

ANSWERS

1. B	8. C	15. C
2. C	9. D	16. A
3. D	10. A	17. A
4. D	11. B	18. C
5. B	12. D	19. B
6. C	13. D	20. D
7. B	14. C	

24 SIP – Management of Malignant Ovarian Germ Cell Tumors (MOGCT)

Source: Management of Female Malignant Ovarian Germ Cell Tumours Scientific Impact Paper No. 52 November 2016. https://www.rcog.org.uk/guidance/browse-all-guidance/scientific-impact-papers/management-of-female-malignant-ovarian-germ-cell-tumours-scientific-impact-paper-no52/

IMPORTANT POINTS FROM THE GUIDELINE (SIP)

- Malignant ovarian germ cell tumors (MOGCTs) in females are uncommon.

- Prompt detection and multiagent treatment correlate with elevated cure rates of 85.6% (ranging from 81.2% to 90.0%).

- MOGCTs, encompassing dysgerminomas, immature teratomas, embryonal tumors, and endodermal sinus (yolk sac) tumors, represented merely 1.5% of ovarian malignancies in a EUROCARE study on ovarian cancer survival in Europe.

- Roughly one-third of these instances are dysgerminomas, another one-third are immature teratomas, and the other one-third comprises embryonal tumors, endodermal sinus tumors, choriocarcinoma, and mixed-cell types.

- MOGCTs predominantly manifest during the initial two decades of life; however, they can arise at any age, with 82.3% of all MOGCTs occurring between the ages of 14 and 54 years.

- The manifestation of MOGCTs is diverse, potentially encompassing acute and subacute pelvic pain, menstrual irregularities, and the presence of a pelvic or abdominal mass.

- The preliminary assessment should encompass a pelvic ultrasound.

- If imaging indicates MOGCT, blood levels of alpha-fetoprotein (AFP) and human chorionic gonadotropin (hCG) should be assessed to assist in identifying women with germ cell tumors (GCTs).

- The existing Royal College of Obstetricians and Gynaecologists Green-top Guideline for ovarian masses in premenopausal women advises the assessment of serum lactic dehydrogenase (LDH), AFP, and hCG in all women under 40 years of age.

- This guideline advises measuring AFP and hCG levels anytime there is a suspicion of GCT, especially in women under 40 years or in older women when imaging suggests a GCT.

- The elevation of AFP and hCG corresponds with the stage and survival in MOGCT, with increased levels of both markers linked to a more advanced disease stage and diminished survival, independent of stage.

- The detection of a solid mass on ultrasonography in younger women may suggest a MOGCT.

- If there is a strong suspicion of a MOGCT, further imaging of the abdomen, pelvis, and chest by contrast-enhanced computed tomography (CT) should be conducted.

- Magnetic resonance imaging (MRI) may yield supplementary insights compared to CT imaging of the ovaries.

- The surgical approach for young women wishing to preserve future fertility should be conservative, aimed at achieving a tissue diagnosis and assessing the disease's extent.

- MOGCTs are often unilateral; however, 10–15% of pure dysgerminomas are bilateral.

- When indicated, surgery should consist of unilateral oophorectomy, peritoneal washing, omental biopsy, and selective excision of enlarged lymph nodes.

- A biopsy of the normal contralateral ovary is unwarranted.

- The surgical approach should be open to facilitate the evacuation of the afflicted ovary along with its tumor intact, rather than fragmented or ruptured.

- Lymph node metastases did not negatively impact long-term outcomes.

DOI: 10.1201/9781003650355-24

- Moreover, women who received routine lymphadenectomy did not experience improved outcomes; hence, systematic lymphadenectomy has little relevance in MOGCT.

- If nodes are enlarged, the excision of only the afflicted nodes is warranted.

- For women diagnosed with advanced disease (stage Ic/IIa and beyond), neoadjuvant chemotherapy should be contemplated to facilitate fertility preservation and simplify later surgical procedures.

- In women who have finished childbearing, a bilateral salpingo-oophorectomy and hysterectomy may be contemplated, especially in the presence of other gynecological comorbidities.

- Most MOGCTs (60–70%) are diagnosed with illness localized to the ovaries or pelvis.

- In stage I testicular GCTs localized to the testis, surveillance without adjuvant radiation (for seminomas) or chemotherapy (for both seminomas and non-seminomatous GCTs) is currently the standard of care in the UK.

- Research indicates that women who had adjuvant radiation following the resection of early-stage dysgerminomas (stage IA) later experienced infertility due to the dysfunction of the remaining ovary and the emergence of additional malignancies in later life.

- As a result, radiation is no longer advised for resected early-stage dysgerminomas.

- Adjuvant carboplatin or bleomycin–etoposide–cisplatin (BEP) treatment may be contemplated; nevertheless, this subjects women to potentially superfluous toxicity.

- A burgeoning body of evidence supports a 'surveillance only' strategy following resection in women with stage IA/B dysgerminomas.

- Relapse rates during surveillance are approximately 20% for women with resected stage IA dysgerminomas, and nearly all of these cases are eventually treated successfully with chemotherapy.

- Stage IA/B non-dysgerminomatous MOGCT and all grades of immature MOGCT are likely manageable with surveillance following the removal of the ovarian tumor.

- The relapse rates for the non-dysgerminomatous group may be marginally elevated at approximately 25–35%; however, nearly all will achieve remission with treatment upon recurrence.

- Currently, there is inadequate evidence to endorse surgery followed by surveillance alone for women with stage IC illness.

- Women with immature grade I or II teratomas may be eligible for surveillance.

- The safety of treatment for women with stage Ic grade III illness, which should be regarded as a malignant tumor that has not been fully removed, remains uncertain.

- In the UK, all women with stage IA MOGCT are provided with surveillance, irrespective of histological subtype. Operative details, comprehensive pathology assessment, tumor markers, and whole-body imaging are essential to confirming accurate staging.

- Post-surgery, increased tumor markers should be assessed weekly until they normalize to confirm their decline aligns with the anticipated half-life (AFP, 6–7 days; hCG, 1–2 days).

- Surveillance encompasses routine clinical evaluations, examinations, periodic imaging, and tumor marker assessments (hCG, AFP, CA-125, and LDH).

- The significance of CA-125 and LDH in the surveillance of MOGCTs remains inadequately established and is considerably less specific compared to hCG and AFP.

- The frequency of surveillance through tumor marker monitoring is greatest initially, as current data indicate that the majority of relapses occur within 2 years.

- As risk diminishes, the frequency of surveillance decreases over time, resulting in annual appointments only after 7 years.

- The implementation of cisplatin-based combination chemotherapy for MOGCT has significantly enhanced treatment results in women with advanced or incompletely resected illness.

- The long-term prognosis following chemotherapy and limited surgery, while preserving the contralateral ovary and fallopian tube, is favorable; around 90% of women with early-stage disease and 75–80% with advanced disease can anticipate long-term survival, along with a significant probability of menstrual resumption and subsequent pregnancies.

- The indications for chemotherapy are contingent upon the severity and classification of the disease at the time of diagnosis.

- For advanced disease, stage II or higher, neoadjuvant combination chemotherapy may be a viable choice.

- Surgery should unequivocally be avoided in women with advanced stage IIIC and IV illness; rather, neoadjuvant chemotherapy must be initiated promptly.

- For the past 30 years, chemotherapy regimens including platinum have been the treatment of choice for GCTs.

- The combined BEP regimen is the global standard of treatment, typically delivered for three cycles in cases of fully resected illness and four cycles for macroscopic residual disease.

- Bone marrow growth factors are administered, if necessary, as a decrease in chemotherapy dose intensity may result in inferior outcomes.

- Cisplatin should be substituted with carboplatin alone in women exhibiting substantial renal function impairments, peripheral neuropathy, or ototoxicity.

- Adjuvant carboplatin and etoposide have demonstrated superior treatment results for totally resected dysgerminoma.

- Women diagnosed with MOGCT necessitate prompt assessment and intervention.

- The disease may advance quickly, exhibiting a short tumor doubling time, and metastasize to the peritoneum, lungs, liver, and brain.

- Metastatic illness exhibits an increased likelihood of pharmacological resistance and severe consequences, particularly intratumoral hemorrhage.

- For severely unwell women with extensive disease and/or diminished performance status, a weekly induction regimen of etoposide 100 mg/m^2 and cisplatin 20 mg/m^2 (low-dose induction EP) is advised to achieve an early response and enhance the woman's condition prior to the administration of full-dose chemotherapy.

- Approximately 75% of MOGCT recurrences occur within the initial year; hence, rigorous early follow-up every 4–8 weeks seems warranted and should be evaluated.

- Frequent sites of recurrence include the peritoneal cavity and, less commonly, the retroperitoneal lymph nodes or lungs.

- The aim of follow-up should be to assess therapy response, manage treatment-related problems, and facilitate early detection of chronic or recurring disease.

- The follow-up strategy must incorporate the evaluation of tumor markers during each appointment.

- Chest X-ray bi-monthly for 2 years, followed by every 3 to 6 months for the subsequent 3 years.

- CT imaging of the pelvis, abdomen, and chest (if abnormal at presentation) should be conducted 3 months post-chemotherapy completion and subsequently as clinically warranted.

- Women with persistent disease following chemotherapy should be considered for excision, regardless of normal tumor marker levels.

- This aims to eliminate residual disease or any remaining mature teratoma, which may develop into mature teratoma developing syndrome in up to 30% of instances and, less frequently, may undergo malignant transformation into an incurable tumor type, such as squamous carcinoma, over time.

- The potential for mature teratoma growth syndrome, a disorder characterized by the proliferation of mature teratoma deposits, necessitates consideration, as total surgical removal is required. Imaging reveals mixed cystic and solid components with calcification, consistently accompanied by normal hCG and AFP levels, indicating the presence of mature teratoma developing syndrome.

- In the absence of residual disease, a second-look laparotomy or laparoscopy is unwarranted.

- Women with MOGCT who have relapse after initial chemotherapy demonstrate modest salvage rates (about 10%) with repeated treatments, in contrast to male patients, who typically achieve salvage rates above 50%.

- Women experiencing relapse should undergo a contrast-enhanced MRI of the brain and pelvic, CT scans of the chest and abdomen, Doppler ultrasonography of the pelvis, and fluorodeoxy-glucose positron emission tomography/CT.

- The latter may assist in identifying locations of active disease for surgical resection, however, false-positive and false-negative results may arise.

- A multidisciplinary strategy for the management of MOGCT should be implemented.

- The possible loss of fertility due to chemotherapy is a significant worry, necessitating specialized fertility evaluation.

- The majority of women (87–100%) will restore menstrual function and fertility within 1 year post-chemotherapy, with a mere 3% encountering premature menopause.

QUESTIONS

1. What is the cure rate of MOGCT?

    A. 30–40%

    B. 50–60%

    C. 60–70%

    D. 80–90%

2. MOGCT includes all of the following tumors, except?

    A. Dysgerminomas

    B. Choriocarcinoma

    C. Mature teratomas

    D. Endodermal sinus (yolk sac) tumor

3. Which of the following is the most common GCT?

    A. Dysgerminoma

    B. Immature teratoma

    C. Yolk sac tumor

    D. Mixed-germ cell tumor

4. Which of the following tumor markers is not correctly matched with the respective MOGCT?

    A. Endodermal sinus tumor (yolk sac tumor) – increased levels of AFP

    B. Embryonal carcinoma – increased levels of hCG

    C. Dysgerminomas – increased levels of AFP

    D. Immature teratomas – increased levels of CA19-9

5. Regarding the epidemiology of MOGCT, which of the following statements is NOT true?

    A. One-third of MOGCTs are dysgerminomas, one-third are immature teratomas, and the final third include embryonal tumors, endodermal sinus tumors, choriocarcinoma, and mixed-cell types.

    B. They primarily affect women during the first two decades of their lives.

    C. Their cure rates are suboptimal, varying from 30% to 50% with surgical intervention and chemotherapy.

    D. Over 80% of MOGCT cases occur between the ages of 14 and 54 years.

6. What is the preferred initial investigation in women suspected of having MOGCT?

    A. CT scan

    B. Pelvis MRI

    C. Pelvic ultrasound

    D. PET Scan

7. A 20-year-old young woman presents to your emergency department with acute pain in the lower abdomen for the last 2 days. She has been complaining of irregular and prolonged menses for the last 4 to 6 months. On examination, a firm solid abdominal mass is felt in the lower abdomen, which is confirmed by a pelvic ultrasound. What is your next recommended step in her management?

    A. Offer her serum CA-125 levels

    B. Offer her AFP and beta-hCG levels

    C. Offer her a CECT scan of the chest and pelvis

    D. Offer her a PET scan

8. A 18-year-old young woman presents to your emergency department with acute pain in the lower abdomen for the last 2 days. She has been complaining of irregular and prolonged menses for the last 4 to 6 months. On examination, a firm solid abdominal mass is felt in the lower abdomen. Her scan is suggestive of a right-sided solid ovarian mass of about 8 cm. Her AFP levels are 900 ng/mL. A working diagnosis of yolk sac tumor is made. What is your next recommended step in her management?

    A. Offer her serum CA-125 levels

    B. Offer her PET scan

    C. Offer her conservative surgical management aiming for tissue diagnosis and staging the spread of the disease

    D. Intraoperatively biopsy of the contralateral ovary is recommended.

9. All of the following surgical steps are included in the conservative surgery performed for unilateral MOGCT, except?

    A. Unilateral oophorectomy

    B. Peritoneal washings

    C. Omental biopsy and selective removal of enlarged lymph nodes

    D. Biopsy of a normal contralateral ovary

10. What percentage of pure dysgerminomas are bilateral?

    A. 5%

    B. 10–15%

    C. 20%

    D. 30%

11. What percentage of patients with MOGCT are diagnosed with disease confined to the ovaries or pelvis?

    A. 30–40%

    B. 40–50%

    C. 60–70%

    D. >90%

12. All of the following patients with MOGCT can be followed up by 'surveillance-only' strategy after initial surgical resection, except?

    A. Stage IA/IB dysgerminomas

    B. Immature teratomas grade I/II

    C. Stage IA/IB non-dysgerminomatous MOGCT

    D. Stage IC dysgerminomas or non-dysgerminomatous MOGCT

13. What is the relapse rate in early stage (IA) dysgerminomas which are followed up by 'surveillance-only' strategy after initial resection surgery?

    A. <5%   C. 20%

    B. 10%   D. 50%

14. If tumor markers are elevated preoperatively, how frequently should they be monitored after surgery?

    A. Twice weekly until negative

    B. Weekly until negative

    C. Biweekly until negative

    D. Monthly until negative

15. What is the half-life of the tumor marker AFP?

    A. 12 hours   C. 3–4 days

    B. 1–2 days   D. 6–7 days

16. What is the half-life of the tumor marker beta-hCG?

    A. 12 hours   C. 3–4 days

    B. 1–2 days   D. 6–7 days

17. With regard to MOGCT, within what time period do most of the relapses occur?

    A. 6 months   C. 2 years

    B. 1 year   D. 3 years

18. Regarding surveillance in patients with MOGCT, all of the following are recommended at every visit, except?

    A. Clinical review

    B. Clinical examination

    C. Tumor markers (hCG, AFP, CA-125, and LDH)

    D. A CXR and CECT of the abdomen and pelvis at each visit

19. What is the recommended standard of care in terms of chemotherapy for a completely resected disease in patients with MOGCT?

    A. BEP regimen (bleomycin, etoposide, cisplatin) for 3 cycles

    B. BEP regimen (bleomycin, etoposide, cisplatin) for 4 cycles

    C. VAC regimen (vincristine, actinomycin D, cyclophosphamide) for 3 cycles

    D. VAC regimen (vincristine, actinomycin D, cyclophosphamide) for 4 cycles

20. What is the recommended standard of care in terms of chemotherapy for a macroscopic residual disease after surgery in patients with MOGCT?

    A. BEP regimen (bleomycin, etoposide, cisplatin) for 3 cycles

    B. BEP regimen (bleomycin, etoposide, cisplatin) for 4 cycles

    C. VAC regimen (vincristine, actinomycin D, cyclophosphamide) for 3 cycles

    D. VAC regimen (vincristine, actinomycin D, cyclophosphamide) for 4 cycles

21. For how long after management of MOGCT, are women advised against planning pregnancy?

    A. 6 months

    B. 1 year

    C. 2 years

    D. 5 years

22. All of the following are features of mature teratoma growth syndrome, except?

    A. It is a condition marked by the proliferation of adult teratoma deposits

    B. Imaging demonstrates a combination of cystic and solid components accompanied with calcification

    C. Tumor markers, including beta-hCG and AFP, consistently remain within normal ranges

    D. It is usually recognized at the metastatic phase and has a poor prognosis

23. What is the incidence of premature menopause in women with MOGCT treated with chemotherapy?

    A. 1 in 1000

    B. 1%

    C. 3%

    D. 7%

24. Which of the following statements about dysgerminomas is inaccurate?

    A. Lactate dehydrogenase is increased in around 95% of instances.

    B. Bilateral ovarian involvement is observed in 10–15% of cases.

    C. It has a negligible incidence of extraovarian spreading.

    D. Hypercalcemia may present as a paraneoplastic syndrome due to tumor production of 1,25-dihydroxyvitamin D3, the active form of vitamin D.

25. Dysgerminomas are positive for which of the following markers?

    A. D2-40

    B. CD117

    C. Placental alkaline phosphatase

    D. All of the above

26. Which of the following assertions about yolk sac tumor is incorrectly described?

    A. Predominantly unilateral

    B. Frequently painless

    C. The pre-pubertal variant exhibits more aggressiveness and a less favorable prognosis

    D. The post-pubertal form is predominantly associated with germ cell neoplasia in situ (GCNIS) and typically occurs as part of a mixed tumor

27. A 34-year-old patient presents to your gynecology outpatient department (OPD) with complaints of pain in the lower abdomen and awareness of a mass in the lower abdomen for the last 3–4 months. On detailed history, the patient reveals that she was treated for malignant ovarian immature teratoma about 10 years ago. She was told that the treatment was completed successfully at that time. She then again developed recurrence about 4 years ago for which she was again successfully treated. Now she presents for the third time with recurrence and is very concerned and depressed about the situation. Considering the working diagnosis of ovarian growing teratoma syndrome (GTS), which of the following is false about the nature of GTS?

    A. The tumor can typically stay dormant for extended durations.

    B. The tumor exhibits potential for progressive growth, perhaps enlarging significantly, with recurrence possibly occurring multiple times over a span of 10 to 20 years.

    C. Chemotherapy and radiotherapy constitute the principal treatment for both initial and recurring tumors.

    D. The condition exhibits benign biological behavior and, when appropriately treated, has a favorable prognosis

ANSWERS

1. D	10. B	19. A
2. C	11. C	20. B
3. A	12. D	21. C
4. C	13. C	22. D
5. C	14. B	23. C
6. C	15. D	24. C
7. B	16. B	25. D
8. C	17. C	26. C
9. D	18. D	27. C

25 SIP – Multiple Pregnancies after Assisted Reproductive Technology (ART)

Source: Multiple Pregnancies Following Assisted Conception Scientific Impact Paper No. 22 February 2018. https://www.rcog.org.uk/guidance/browse-all-guidance/scientific-impact-papers/multiple-pregnancy-following-assisted-reproduction-scientific-impact-paper-no-22/

IMPORTANT POINTS FROM THE GUIDELINE (SIP)

- Multiple pregnancy, resulting from the transfer >1 embryos into the uterus, is the most prevalent treatment-related adverse consequence of in vitro fertilization (IVF).

- Despite being mostly prevented with the implementation of elective single embryo transfer (eSET) policies, the incidence of multiple pregnancies resulting from IVF remains elevated.

- Data from the UK Human Fertilisation and Embryology Authority (HFEA) indicates that around 19.8% of IVF deliveries in the UK in 2011 resulted in a multiple birth.

- Elevated incidence of multiple births resulting from IVF have been documented throughout Europe and North America.

- Despite being a challenging choice, selective embryo reduction may be contemplated to decrease the incidence of multiple births subsequent to IVF.

- The concerning increase in multiple pregnancies due to assisted reproductive technology (ART) has prompted numerous papers emphasizing the considerable maternal, fetal, and neonatal dangers linked to these pregnancies.

- Maternal problems encompass an elevated risk of pregnancy-induced hypertension, gestational diabetes, peripartum hemorrhage, surgical delivery, postpartum depression, anxiety, and parental stress.

- Multiple pregnancies are linked to a 6-fold elevation in the risk of preterm birth, a primary contributor to infant mortality and enduring mental and physical problems, such as cerebral palsy, learning impairments, and chronic lung disease.

- A study indicates that the projected neonatal expense for a twin in the UK's National Health Service (NHS) is 16 times greater than that for a singleton infant.

- Multiple pregnancies of higher order, arising from cross-border reproductive care or 'fertility tourism,' are exacerbating the issues confronting NHS maternity and neonatal services.

- Both patients and healthcare providers frequently perceive that the success rate of IVF treatment is enhanced with the transfer of two embryos compared to one, hence diminishing safety apprehensions associated with twin pregnancies.

- This perception contradicts the published literature, which has unequivocally shown that, in women with favorable prognoses, the cumulative live birth rate following eSET, succeeded by the transfer of a thawed embryo in a subsequent frozen embryo transfer cycle, is comparable to that after double embryo transfer (DET), albeit with a markedly reduced risk of multiple pregnancies.

- To promote eSET, various techniques have been investigated to ascertain the embryo with the highest implantation potential, including blastocyst culture, preimplantation genetic screening, and time-lapse imaging.

- Additional enhancement of embryo selection techniques is necessary to bridge the disparity in pregnancy rates between eSET and DET, while reducing the danger of multiple gestation.

- The HFEA persists in acknowledging and overseeing the incidence of multiple pregnancies resulting from IVF therapy.

- Following thorough deliberation and collaboration with IVF clinics, professional organizations, patient advocacy groups, and NHS commissioners, the HFEA established a maximum target for multiple birth rates in clinics, commencing at 24% in 2009 and progressively decreasing over 4 years to a cap of 10% of all live births. To attain a decrease in multiple birth rates, IVF clinics were instructed to formulate their own 'multiple birth minimization approach.'

DOI: 10.1201/9781003650355-25

- The UK has had a steady decrease in the multiple pregnancy rate following IVF treatment, declining from 26.6% in 2008 to 15.9% by mid-2014, representing a relative drop of 40%.

- Advancements in clinical and laboratory methodologies have enhanced embryo selection techniques and improved the identification of women most suited for eSET. Consequently, the reduction in multiple pregnancy rates has coincided with a modest yet significant increase in the overall pregnancy rate per cycle, rising from 30% in 2008 to 36.3% in 2014, alleviating concerns that the increased eSET rate might jeopardize the success of IVF treatment.

- The 2013 National Institute for Health and Care Excellence (NICE) guideline on the evaluation and management of fertility issues advocated for governmental financing of three complete IVF cycles, inclusive of associated frozen transfer cycles; yet, today, 60% of IVF cycles in the UK are financed by the patients themselves.

- Rectifying the existing disparities in IVF funding nationwide could substantially enhance the adoption of eSET, thereby maximizing benefits to mother, neonatal, and child health, as well as providing a national economic advantage by decreasing multiple pregnancies following IVF treatment.

- The HFEA has eliminated the 10% maximum multiple birth rate as a licensing requirement for IVF centers. The proposed modifications to the publication of IVF clinic results by the HFEA are expected to encourage eSET by emphasizing the cumulative pregnancy rate following each IVF cycle, which includes both fresh and frozen embryo transfers.

- The HFEA's publication of the live birth rate per embryo transferred is commendable, as it encourages the transfer of fewer embryos.

- Additionally, further advancements in correlating outcomes across fresh and associated frozen cycles are anticipated shortly.

- It is evident that broader use of eSET is necessary, predicated on the ongoing enhancement of laboratory conditions and methodologies to facilitate the selection of a single developmentally competent embryo with greater ease.

- Organizations, including the HFEA, British Fertility Society, Royal College of Obstetricians and Gynaecologists, Association of Clinical Embryologists, Twins and Multiple Births Association, Multiple Births Foundation, and Fertility Network UK, should persist in collaborating with patient groups to promote and disseminate best practices, empower patients through counseling and education, and advocate for the implementation of eSET for all women under 40 with favorable prognoses, who are at the highest risk of multiple pregnancies following DET, as well as for older women who may face elevated risks of multiple pregnancies if multiple embryos are transferred, such as those utilizing donated oocytes.

QUESTIONS

1. What is the most common treatment-related adverse outcome of IVF?

   A. Pre-eclampsia

   B. Placenta previa

   C. Placenta accreta

   D. Multiple pregnancies

2. According to HFEA, what number of IVF deliveries in the UK (in 2011) resulted in multiple births?

   A. 1 in 10 (10%)

   B. 1 in 5 (20%)

   C. 1 in 3 (30%)

   D. 1 in 2 (50%)

3. Which of the following is the recommended method to reduce the number of multiple pregnancies after IVF?

   A. Lower dose of gonadotropin for ovarian stimulation

   B. Single embryo transfer

   C. Fresh embryo transfer

   D. Day 3 embryo transfer

4. What is the increase in likelihood of multiple pregnancies among patients utilizing artificial reproductive procedures compared to those experiencing spontaneous conception?

   A. 2-fold   C. 10-fold

   B. 5-fold   D. 20-fold

5. To what extent does multiple gestation elevate the risk of preterm delivery?

   A. 2-fold   C. 6-fold

   B. 4-fold   D. 10-fold

6. To what extent does the neonatal cost to the NHS increase with twin pregnancies in comparison to singleton pregnancies?

   A. 4-fold   C. 16-fold

   B. 10-fold   D. 20-fold

7. In comparison to DET, which of the following are proven advantages of performing eSET?

   A. Similar cumulative live birth rate

   B. Lower multiple pregnancy rates

   C. Improved overall pregnancy rates per embryo transfer

   D. All of the above

8. Which of the following techniques help to identify embryos with the greatest implantation potential?

   A. Blastocyst culture

   B. Preimplantation genetic screening

   C. Time-lapse imaging

   D. All of the above

9. According to the 2013 NICE guidelines, how many IVF cycles are funded by the government?

   A. Two full cycles

   B. Three full cycles

   C. Four full cycles

   D. Six full cycles

10. Which of the following important factors can increase the acceptance of eSETs among patients and doctors?

    A. Addressing the current differences in IVF funding

    B. Improvising policies of the IVF clinics in terms of eSET

    C. Focusing on cumulative pregnancy rates per embryo transfer

    D. Focusing on live births rates per embryo transfer

11. Which of the following age groups of women undergoing IVF are at greatest risk of multiple pregnancy after DET and hence can benefit from eSET?

   A. <40 years

   B. 40–42 years

   C. 42–45 years

   D. >45 years

ANSWERS

1. D	5. C	9. B
2. B	6. C	10. A
3. B	7. D	11. A
4. D	8. D	

26 SIP – Non-Invasive Prenatal Testing

Source: Non-Invasive Prenatal Testing for Chromosomal Abnormality Using Maternal Plasma DNA Scientific Impact Paper No. 15 March 2014. https://www.rcog.org.uk/guidance/browse-all-guidance/scientific-impact-papers/non-invasive-prenatal-testing-for-chromosomal-abnormality-using-maternal-plasma-dna-scientific-impact-paper-no-15/

IMPORTANT POINTS FROM THE GUIDELINE (SIP)

- Until recently, fetal genetic testing and aneuploidy detection required intrusive sampling methods that posed a minor yet considerable risk of miscarriage.

- In 1997, the detection of cell-free fetal DNA (cffDNA) in maternal circulation was documented.

- Fetal DNA originates from the placenta, may be identified from the initial trimester of gestation, and is swiftly eliminated from the maternal bloodstream post-delivery.

- Maternal blood is hence a dependable source for prenatal diagnostic material.

- Nonetheless, the cffDNA is intermingled with a greater quantity of maternal cell-free DNA, and existing technologies do not facilitate the complete separation of fetal from maternal DNA in vitro.

- Consequently, the initial applications of this phenomenon were on the identification or exclusion of paternally derived fetal DNA sequences absent in the mother, such as Y chromosome sequences in male pregnancies or rhesus D (RhD) sequences in RhD-negative women.

- Recent advancements in DNA sequencing methods provide accurate relative quantification of DNA fragments, facilitating the robust detection of additional material from fetal chromosome trisomy in maternal plasma DNA.

- Fetal RhD typing via cffDNA to ascertain fetal blood group status from maternal blood has been employed since 2000 to guide the management of pregnancies in RhD-negative women sensitized to RhD, who are consequently at risk of hemolytic illness of the fetus and newborn (HDFN).

- In the UK, cffDNA testing has supplanted amniocentesis for fetal blood typing.

- This is significant because if the fetus is RhD positive, amniocentesis for blood typing may elevate the antibody titre, potentially exacerbating moderate disease into severe disease.

- The identification of additional fetal blood groups, including Kell, C, c, and E, with cffDNA has also been documented.

- The application of cffDNA for fetal blood grouping has transitioned from its use in women with antibodies to routine antenatal care for RhD-negative women, thereby enabling the avoidance of antenatal administration of anti-D immunoglobulin (a blood product derived from multiple donors) in 30–40% of RhD-negative women carrying RhD-negative infants.

- The determination of male fetal sex can be achieved through the analysis of cffDNA in maternal plasma by identifying Y chromosomal sequences, such as DYS14 or SRY.

- Numerous studies have documented the precision of non-invasive prenatal sex determination employing various techniques, with real-time polymerase chain reaction (PCR) being the most prevalent.

- In the UK, this method is employed to ascertain fetal sex in women whose fetus is at risk of an X-linked illness, where the early identification of a male fetus necessitates an invasive diagnostic test to confirm the inheritance of the defective X chromosome. An invasive test is unnecessary if the fetus is female.

- In pregnancies susceptible to sex-linked disorders, non-invasive prenatal testing (NIPT) combined with ultrasound has demonstrated a nearly 50% reduction in the utilization of invasive diagnostic procedures.

- This test enables the early discontinuation of dexamethasone medication in pregnancies at risk for congenital adrenal hyperplasia when the fetus is identified as male.

DOI: 10.1201/9781003650355-26

- Intermittent diagnoses of single-gene illnesses have been documented through the identification or exclusion of the paternal allele inherited from a diseased father with an autosomal dominant condition, such as Huntington's disease.

- The UK Genetic Testing Network authorized NIPT for achondroplasia and thanatophoric dysplasia in 2012, and it is now integrated into standard National Health Service (NHS) practice for pregnancies at risk of these disorders.

- In recessively inherited illnesses such as β-thalassaemia or cystic fibrosis, if the parents possess distinct mutations, the absence of the paternal allele in the maternal plasma suggests that the fetus will be unaffected.

- Should the paternal allele be present, an invasive procedure is necessary to ascertain whether the fetus has received the faulty maternal allele and is thus afflicted.

- The fetus's genotype can be ascertained non-invasively.

- An alternate method has been employed utilizing massively parallel sequencing (MPS), focusing on genomic areas associated with monogenic disorders.

- MPS using samples from pregnant women facilitates the detection of Down syndrome due to the presence of a markedly higher quantity of sequences from chromosome 21, notwithstanding the amalgamation of fetal and maternal DNA.

- Maternal plasma MPS enables the analysis of nearly all DNA molecules in a plasma sample, as opposed to being restricted to those with specific PCR primer binding sites, thereby providing a significantly more efficient approach than digital PCR for optimizing the diagnostic information derived from a plasma sample.

- At present, two primary types of MPS-based methodologies are employed to deliver plasma-DNA-based NIPT clinical services to patients:

  - Shotgun sequencing:

    - This method involves the random sequencing of DNA molecules present in a maternal plasma sample.

    - The percentage representation of DNA molecules sequenced from the chromosome of interest, such as chromosome 21, is compared with those sequenced from other regions of the genome.

    - This approach's advantage lies in the uniformity of the sequencing processes, regardless of the chromosomal targets' genomic positions.

    - Consequently, this method may be utilized for identifying chromosomal or genetic anomalies throughout the genome.

    - A drawback of this method is that genomic areas unrelated to NIPT are also analyzed due to the random nature of sequencing, resulting in unfocused sequencing expenses and information acquired.

  - Targeted sequencing:

    - This method preferentially targets genomic regions associated with chromosomes at risk of aneuploidy, along with a chosen set of reference regions, for sequencing.

    - The primary benefit of the targeted sequencing methodology is the ability to focus sequencing efforts on specific genomic regions of interest, hence minimizing the application of sequencing to areas not immediately pertinent to prenatal testing.

    - A drawback of the targeted sequencing methodology is that the targeting components, such as DNA hybridization probes or PCR primers, must be custom-designed for a specific test panel and require modification as the number of test targets expands.

- The expense of DNA sequencing remains substantial, regardless of whether targeted or shotgun methodologies are employed.

- Currently available data demonstrate highly favorable outcomes for the prediction of trisomy 21 and trisomy 18 when sequencing is effectively conducted.

- Initially, these tests shown lower reliability for detecting trisomy 13; however, advancements have led to improved outcomes following algorithm optimization.
- Detection rates for trisomy 21 and 18 in extensive studies utilizing various technologies have indicated sensitivity and specificity nearing 100% following successful sequencing.
- Potential sources of error
  - Early gestational age:
    - The concentration of cffDNA in maternal blood elevates with gestational age.
    - Early sampling in pregnancy increases the likelihood of false-negative results in Y chromosome 14 or RhD testing.
    - Aneuploidy testing procedures currently permit identification only when the fetal DNA percentage is a minimum of 4–5%, given the existing sequencing depth.
    - Aneuploidy tests utilizing MPS, accessible commercially, are often indicated for pregnant women from 10 weeks of gestation, necessitating a dating scan to confirm gestational age before to sample collection.
  - Obesity:
    - The percentage of maternal plasma DNA that is fetal is influenced by several maternal factors, including maternal weight.
    - Elevated maternal weight correlates with a reduced percentage of fetal DNA.
    - The cause remains ambiguous, however, it may involve elevated adipocyte turnover, resulting in increased maternal plasma DNA or augmented blood volume, leading to a dilutional impact.
    - Given that obesity correlates with a markedly reduced cffDNA proportion, potentially leading to less precise NIPT outcomes, this should be addressed in counseling or patient informational materials.
  - Multiple gestations:
    - In a monochorionic twin pregnancy, which is also monozygotic, both fetuses will either be afflicted or unaffected.
    - Given that the quantity of cffDNA is roughly twice that of a singleton pregnancy, cffDNA aneuploidy testing will not only be feasible but likely more efficacious than in singletons.
    - Nonetheless, in the case of dichorionic twins, which may exhibit discordance, maternal plasma DNA testing becomes more complex.
    - Targeted sequencing of maternal plasma can also ascertain the zygosity of twin pregnancies.
    - If the fetuses are identified as dizygotic, this method would enable the quantification of the fetal DNA contribution from each fetus.
    - This information will guarantee that the maternal plasma sample possesses adequate DNA from each fetus to produce a meaningful test outcome.
  - Placental mosaicism:
    - Substantial evidence indicates that the origin of cffDNA is the placenta.
    - Chorionic villus sampling (CVS) reveals that aberrant cell lines may exist in the placenta but not in the fetus, occurring in around 1% of CVS samples; this occurrence is referred to as 'restricted placental mosaicism.'
    - Instances of trisomic placental cells alongside a normal fetus may necessitate invasive testing confirmation prior to pregnancy termination.
    - Only over time can data from an adequate number of cases be gathered to evaluate the incidence of placental mosaicism potentially yielding erroneous results.

- – The predominant rationale for the purported 'false' (discordant) positives is confined placental mosaicism; that is, NIPT identifies mosaic aberrant cell colonies inside the placenta.
  - Maternal conditions:
    - – Maternal chromosomal anomalies, such as mosaicism or malignancy, may be infrequent sources of inconsistent outcomes.

■ Invasive testing and karyotyping yield information regarding all chromosomes; therefore, if the objective of the non-invasive test is to achieve this, sequencing material from all 46 chromosomes should be prioritized.

■ A primary benefit of extensive testing is the potential for serendipitously identifying a disease with catastrophic implications.

■ The primary drawback of non-specific screening for chromosomal aneuploidies, including but not limited to Down syndrome, is that pregnant women are often notified of results with ambiguous significance.

■ The identification of Down syndrome using maternal plasma DNA testing will transform the administration of prenatal diagnosis and screening in the UK, encompassing both the NHS and commercial sector.

■ This will significantly impact certain existing services, leading clinical biochemistry serum screening laboratories and cytogenetic and molecular genetics laboratories to anticipate a decline in sample volume.

■ Given that women are currently utilizing these tests, all obstetricians should be well-versed in the associated counseling problems.

QUESTIONS

1. Which of the following is the source of cell-free fetal DNA (cffDNA)?
   A. Fetal liver
   B. Fetal bone marrow
   C. Umbilical cord
   D. Placenta

2. What is the meaning of fetal fraction in NIPT?
   A. Proportion of fetal to total cell-free DNA
   B. Proportion of fetal to maternal cell-free DNA
   C. Proportion of fetal to (maternal + paternal) cell-free DNA
   D. Proportion of fetal cell-free DNA per 100 mL of maternal plasma

3. NIPT using cffDNA is used to detect all of the following conditions, except?
   A. X-linked genetic disorders
   B. Single-gene disorders such as Huntington's disease
   C. Achondroplasia and thanatophoric dysplasia
   D. Autism and attention deficit hyperactivity disorder (ADHD)

4. After what gestation is cffDNA detectable in maternal blood?
   A. 10 weeks
   B. 12 weeks
   C. 14 weeks
   D. 16 weeks

5. Which of the following is most commonly used to detect male fetal sex in the non-invasive cffDNA technique?

A. Real-time PCR

B. Digital PCR

C. MPS

D. Chromosomal microarray

6. Which of the following is most commonly used to detect aneuploidy (such as Down syndrome) in the non-invasive cffDNA technique?

A. Real-time PCR

B. Digital PCR

C. MPS

D. Gel electrophoresis

7. For aneuploidy detection, what is the minimum fetal DNA percentage required in the maternal sample above which processing and reporting of the sample is done?

A. 2%   C. 8%

B. 4–5%   D. 10%

8. What is the average fetal fraction detected in the maternal plasma between 10–20 weeks of gestation?

A. 4–5%   C. 10–15%

B. 8%   D. 15–18%

9. What percentage of CVS samples have confined placental mosaicism?

A. 1%   C. 5%

B. 3%   D. 10%

10. According to the latest reports, what is the detection rate and false-positive rate of NIPT for trisomy 21?

A. 99%/0.1%   C. 95%/3%

B. 90%/5%   D. 90%/10%

11. First-trimester combined test includes all of the following, except?

A. Maternal age

B. Nuchal translucency (NT)

C. Serum beta-hCG and PAPP-A levels

D. Serum beta-hCG and AFP levels

12. According to the latest reports, what is the detection rate and false-positive rate of first-trimester combined test for trisomy 21?

A. 99%/0.1%   C. 85%/3%

B. 90%/5%   D. 90%/10%

13. According to the latest evidence, what is the detection rate of NIPT for trisomy 21 in singleton pregnancies?

A. 87%   C. 93.7%

B. 90%   D. 99.2%

14. According to the latest evidence, what is the detection rate of NIPT for trisomy 21 in twin pregnancies?

A. 87%   C. 93.7%

B. 90%   D. 99.2%

15. According to the latest research, what is the overall incidence of chromosomal abnormalities in pregnancy?

A. 1 in 50 live births

B. 1 in 150 live births

C. 1 in 500 live births

D. 1 in 1000 live births

16. Chromosomal abnormalities contribute to what percentage of early pregnancy losses?

A. 10%   C. 50%

B. 20%   D. 80%

17. All of the following are examples of prenatal genetic screening tests, except?

A. Dual marker test

B. Nuchal translucency

C. cffDNA

D. Amniocentesis

18. Which of the following is an example of diagnostic genetic testing for chromosomal abnormalities?

A. CVS

B. cffDNA

C. Amniocentesis

D. A and C

E. All of the above

19. Which of the following factors falsely lower the cffDNA percentage in the maternal blood sample and hence increase the false-negative rates?

A. Multiple pregnancy

B. Maternal obesity (high BMI)

C. Early gestation <10 weeks

D. B and C

E. All of the above

20. Which of the following is the most common cause of false-positive rates of cffDNA in genetic screening?

A. Confined placental mosaicism

B. Vanishing twins

C. Maternal tumors

D. Maternal copy variants

21. A 38-year-old primigravida patient, with monochorionic twin pregnancy conceived by in vitro fertilization (IVF) presents to your antenatal outpatient (OPD) with her combined screening report. Her report is suggestive of normal nuchal translucency of both twins, but there is an increased risk of trisomy 21 on a dual marker test. The patient is very anxious and disturbed with her results. She has read about NIPT and is keen to proceed with the same. Which of the following statements regarding the role of NIPT in monochorionic twin pregnancies is incorrect?

A. In a monochorionic pregnancy (monozygotic/identical twins), both fetuses contribute an identical quantity of genetic DNA to the maternal circulation.

B. A monochorionic twin pregnancy does not influence the cell-free DNA analysis for aneuploidy risk.

C. Cell-free DNA testing should not be conducted in monochorionic twin pregnancies due to concerns over the accuracy of results.

D. In monochorionic twins, the accuracy of aneuploidy identification is comparable to that in singleton pregnancies.

22. A 30-year-old primigravida patient presents to your antenatal OPD with her combined screening test results. She is carrying a dichorionic diamniotic twin pregnancy which she conceived spontaneously. Her reports are suggestive of a high risk for trisomy 21 on a dual marker report. Her nuchal translucency is normal. She is very disturbed regarding her test results. She is very keen to opt for the cffDNA test as she wants a non-invasive test for confirmation. Which of the following statements regarding the role of cffDNA in dichorionic twin pregnancies is not described correctly?

A. In dizygotic twins, the individual cell-free DNA given by each fetus is often less than that of a singleton pregnancy.

B. Zygosity cannot be determined with NIPT.

C. Individual fetal fractions in dizygotic twin gestations can be quantified.

D. Single-nucleotide polymorphism (SNP) analyses enable the distinct assessment and analysis of the cell-free DNA pertaining to each twin.

23. Concerning the zygosity and chorionicity of twin pregnancies, which of the following statements is the least accurate?

A. Dizygotic ('non-identical') twins result from the fertilization of two separate eggs and typically possess dichorionic diamniotic extra-fetal membranes.

B. An early separation at the morula stage will yield dichorionic diamniotic tissues, analogous to those observed in a dizygotic twin pregnancy.

C. Approximately 60% to 70% of twin pregnancies are monozygotic and 20% to 30% are dizygotic twins, depending upon maternal age, utilization of reproductive treatments, and the race/ethnicity of the population.

D. Approximately 75% of monozygotic twins are monochorionic, while 25% are dichorionic.

24. In which of the following situations is testing for zygosity of twin pregnancies using cffDNA considered to be of clinical importance?

A. Instances in which chronicity assessment via ultrasound was not performed due to advanced gestational age at the commencement of care, unavailability of imaging, ambiguous results, or subsequent clinical observations indicating a potential misassignment of chorionicity.

B. Instances in which a fetal anatomical abnormality or growth restriction was present in just one of the two fetuses, raising concerns about the potential impact of a variably expressed or variably penetrant condition on both fetuses, as opposed to one being impacted and the other unaffected.

C. In instances where the concentration of cffDNA is inadequate for obtaining an aneuploidy result.

D. All of the above.

25. A 40-year-old primigravida patient presents to your antenatal OPD. She has conceived twins with IVF. Her early pregnancy viability scan shows an ongoing healthy singleton pregnancy with a vanishing twin. She presents with her combined screening test results which are suggestive of increased aneuploidy risk on a dual marker test. The nuchal translucency of the ongoing healthy pregnancy is normal. All of the following statements regarding the use of cffDNA testing in identifying a vanishing twin are true, except?

A. A vanishing twin can be detected via cffDNA screening.

B. Vanishing twins can be readily identified by counting-based NIPT when the analysis is limited to trisomies 21, 18, and 13.

C. The SNP-based NIPT will detect a vanishing dizygotic twin (with or without aneuploidy) if the maternal plasma contains adequate cffDNA.

D. Conflicting data exists about the significance of the vanishing twin phenomenon and its effects on pregnancy outcomes.

ANSWERS

1. D	10. A	19. D
2. A	11. D	20. A
3. D	12. B	21. C
4. A	13. D	22. B
5. A	14. C	23. C
6. C	15. B	24. D
7. B	16. C	25. B
8. C	17. D	
9. A	18. D	

27 SIP – Novel Therapies in Hemolytic Disease of the Fetus and Newborn (HDFN)

Source: The Use of Novel Therapies in the Management of Haemolytic Disease of the Fetus and Newborn (HDFN) Scientific Impact Paper No. 75 September 2025. https://www.rcog.org.uk/guidance/browse-all-guidance/scientific-impact-papers/the-use-of-novel-therapies-in-the-management-of-haemolytic-disease-of-the-fetus-and-newborn-hdfn-scientific-impact-paper-no-75/

IMPORTANT POINTS FROM THE GUIDELINE (SIP)

- Hemolytic disease of the fetus and newborn (HDFN) is an uncommon disorder that leads to the development of anemia in a fetus during gestation or in a newborn after delivery. If not addressed, this may result in stillbirth or neonatal mortality.

- HDFN occurs when a pregnant woman's antibodies traverse the placenta, enter the fetal circulation, and bind to antigens (acquired from the father) on the hemoglobin-containing red blood cells, resulting in their destruction and subsequent fetal anemia.

- This results in fetal hemolysis, anemia, and, if allowed to progress, may lead to hydrops due to high-output cardiac failure and fetal demise. Fetal hemolysis may potentially induce postnatal jaundice due to elevated unconjugated bilirubin levels resulting from hemoglobin degradation, leading to potential neurological impairment.

- This typically occurs after a sensitizing event, such as fetomaternal hemorrhage during gestation, during the time of parturition, or subsequent to an incompatible blood transfusion.

- Women regularly undergo blood testing at the onset of pregnancy to determine their ABO blood type and Rh antigens.

- Five primary Rhesus antigens exist: D, C, c, E, and e; with anti-D being the predominant cause of HDFN.

- If a woman is identified as RhD negative, a non-invasive blood test is conducted to determine whether the fetal blood group matches that of the woman.

- If a mother is RhD negative and the infant is RhD positive, the infant is at risk.

- The newborn has inherited the D antigen from the father, resulting in Rhesus incompatibility.

- Additional red blood cell antibodies, including anti-Kell and anti-Duffy, may also induce fetal anemia.

- Women most susceptible to HDFN are those that produce red cell alloantibodies against the Rhc, RhD, and Kell blood type antigens.

- IgG antibodies are the sole immunoglobulins capable of traversing the placenta through the transmembrane protein known as the fetal/neonatal Fc Receptor (FcRn), potentially resulting in the hemolysis of fetal red blood cells if the fetus expresses the matching red cell antigen.

- The initial maternal immune response to the RhD antigen is often subdued; however, the secondary immunological response in future pregnancies with a Rh-D positive fetus results in a more pronounced and earlier onset of anemia.

- Red cell antibodies are present in 2% of all pregnancies, while clinically relevant antibodies are identified in 0.4% of pregnancies.

- Fetal mortality has significantly decreased due to the implementation of standard antenatal blood type and routine antenatal anti-D prophylaxis (RAADP) during the third trimester.

- Nonetheless, despite anti-D prophylaxis, around 1 in 1000 women continue to experience D alloimmunization.

- Intrauterine blood transfusion (IUT) is presently the sole widely acknowledged therapeutic intervention to avert fetal demise and mitigate cognitive impairment in fetuses afflicted by HDFN.

DOI: 10.1201/9781003650355-27

- Maternal intravenous immunoglobulins (IVIGs) and, more recently, monoclonal antibodies have been proposed as non-invasive alternatives to mitigate or postpone the necessity for IUT.

- Fetal hemoglobin is expected to rise to around 150 g/L by the end of pregnancy.

- Fetal anemia results in an increase in peak systolic blood flow velocity in the fetal middle cerebral artery peak systolic velocity (MCA PSV), and as the anemia advances, it may lead to diminished tissue perfusion and hypoxia, ultimately causing end-organ dysfunction.

- Delayed manifestations of severe illness including fetal hydrops, fetal cardiomegaly, and ultimately fetal demise if not addressed.

- Hydrops may manifest with a fetal hemoglobin level of less than 40 g/L at 18 weeks and less than 80 g/L at term.

- Hemolysis results in elevated bilirubin levels, which during pregnancy is eliminated through the placenta; however, postnatally, it can inflict significant damage to the fetal neurological system, referred to as kernicterus.

- Bilirubin may accumulate in the basal ganglia and brainstem nuclei, resulting in athetoid cerebral palsy, auditory deficits, and psychomotor impairments.

- All pregnant women undergo screening for blood group, D status, and antibody presence during the first trimester and again at 28 weeks of gestation to identify pregnancies at risk for Rh incompatibility.

- Women with D-negative blood are assessed for fetal RhD status by non-invasive prenatal testing (NIPT), which involves analyzing cell-free fetal DNA in maternal blood to determine the fetal RhD genotype.

- Non-invasive fetal genotyping by cell-free fetal DNA (cffDNA) can be conducted on maternal blood to evaluate the risk of HDFN by detecting antigens for D, e, E, c, C, and K. This test exhibits high sensitivity and specificity. RhD, c, e, C, and E can be identified with high sensitivity following 11 weeks of gestation.

- Kell genotyping may be conducted after 20 weeks to mitigate the possibility of false negative results associated with earlier testing.

- If cffDNA NIPT is unavailable, paternal genotyping may be beneficial to ascertain if the father is homozygous or heterozygous; if the father is homozygous, the parents can be warned that all pregnancies will be at risk of HDFN.

- Pregnancies with alloantibody levels over a specific threshold are sent to a fetal medicine service for sequential ultrasound examinations to monitor the onset of fetal anemia by MCA Doppler velocities.

- An MCA-PSV ≥1.5 multiples of the median (MoM) predicts moderate to severe fetal anemia with a sensitivity of 100% and a false-positive rate of 12%.

- Fetal anemia can be detected on the CTG by the presence of diminished variability exhibiting a sinusoidal pattern.

- Women having a prior history of HDFN or increasing antibody levels/titres exceeding a designated threshold should be referred to fetal medicine during early pregnancy.

- Upon identifying elevated peak systolic velocities in the middle cerebral artery, referral to a tertiary fetal medicine facility for direct fetal blood sampling constitutes the most precise diagnostic approach for fetal anemia.

- This invasive technique entails a 1.3% risk of miscarriage or preterm birth and risk of further sensitization.

- IUT, the infusion of blood into the fetal umbilical vein at the placental insertion, during its intrahepatic pathway, or within a free loop of the cord under ultrasound guidance, is the primary treatment for HDFN.

- This invasive technique poses a risk of premature birth and miscarriage, contingent upon the gestational age at which it is conducted. The hazards are greatest before 22 weeks' gestation with the early onset of fetal anemia.

- Miscarriage rates are reported to be 8.5% before 20 weeks and 0.9% beyond 20 weeks. Complications encompass intrauterine infection (0.1%), rupture of membranes (1.4%), and iatrogenic preterm birth (when conducted after 24 weeks).

- The overall complication rate associated with the procedure is 3–5%.

- In the absence of hydrops, the survival rate after IUT exceeds 90%.

- The elevated fetal loss rates linked to early IUTs before to 22 weeks are due to the necessity for intraperitoneal transfusion instead of intravascular transfusion, since the fetal vasculature is insufficiently developed for cannulation during early gestations.

- Consequently, to enhance results, it is advisable to postpone the initiation of the first IUT to the latest feasible gestational age. IVIG possesses the capacity to facilitate this.

- Vaginal delivery is feasible after IUT provided the fetus is stable, with facilities providing labor induction at 36–37 weeks post-IUT.

- The reliability of MCA-PSV to diagnose anemia decreases following the initial transfusion, hence it is not that reliable in the later stages of the third trimester.

- The postnatal management of HDFN involves neonatal phototherapy or exchange transfusions to rectify fetal anemia and reduce fetal bilirubin levels. This is guided by a direct agglutinin assay from the umbilical cord.

- Maternal antibodies may persist for 6 months, necessitating continuous surveillance of the infant for kernicterus.

- Recombinant erythropoietin and IVIG are no longer utilized during the neonatal period due to their ineffectiveness and the associated heightened risk of necrotizing enterocolitis (NEC) in newborns with HDFN.

- Ninety-five percent of children receiving intrauterine therapy exhibit typical neurodevelopmental outcomes.

- The incidence of cerebral palsy among children born post-IUT is 2.4%.

- Severe early onset fetal anemia is not always amenable to transfusion due to the challenges in cannulating narrow early umbilical arteries, together with the diminished ability of a fetus under 24 weeks to endure anemia and hydrops. Anemia tends to manifest around 3 weeks earlier in any subsequent afflicted pregnancy. Therefore, IVIG serves as an alternate therapeutic option.

- IVIG is a concentrated solution of immunoglobulins obtained from the pooled plasma of 1000 to 10,000 healthy human blood donors. The IVIG product consists of immunoglobulins that closely resemble those seen in normal human plasma. Ninety percent comprises IgG, along with IgA, cytokines, and soluble receptors.

- The fundamental architecture of an immunoglobulin (IgG) is a Y shape, comprising two identical polypeptide heavy chains that constitute the trunk of the Y (the Fc portion, which interacts with Fc gamma receptors on immune cells and complement) and two identical polypeptide light chains that form the arms of the Y (the Fab fragment, which binds to the antigen).

- The Fc part of IVIG binds to FcRns found on nearly all immune cells, which may be either inhibitory or stimulatory. Immunoglobulins are essential in adaptive humoral immunity.

- Their mechanism of action includes:

  - The dilution of maternal circulating antibodies.

  - The competitive inhibition of the placental FcRn, so diminishing the maternal transplacental transfer of pathogenic IgG.

  - They additionally activate the inhibitory fc-gamma receptors on macrophages to attenuate action.

  - They obstruct the antibody receptors present on the surface of erythrocytes.

  - They can obstruct the FcRns of phagocytic cells to diminish the ingestion of autoantibody-coated cells.

- Recent studies indicate that commencing IVIG therapy at 13 weeks with a dosage of 1 g/kg/week may be advantageous and discontinuing therapy with the emergence of fetal anemia in favor of IUT.

- Evidence suggests that IVIG can be utilized alongside concurrent IUT to mitigate the disease process and extend the intervals between successive IUTs.

- IVIG may delay the gestational age at which clinically significant fetal anemia manifests and may postpone or obviate the necessity for an intrauterine transfusion until a gestational period with reduced transfusion risks.

- The NICE guideline on neonatal jaundice advises administering IVIG at a dosage of 500 mg/kg over 4 hours as a supplementary treatment to continuous intensified phototherapy in instances of Rhesus or ABO hemolytic disease when serum bilirubin levels increase by more than 8.5 µmol/L/hour.

- The neonatal administration of IVIG has demonstrated a reduction in the necessity for exchange transfusions, a decrease in length of hospitalization, and a diminished requirement for phototherapy.

- Nipocalimab, a specific immunomodulatory medication, is emerging as a potentially viable treatment for severe HDFN. Nipocalimab (M281) is a high-affinity, human, aglycosylated monoclonal antibody that specifically inhibits the neonatal FcRn to decrease circulating immunoglobulin G (IgG) levels, encompassing both auto- and alloantibodies.

- A multicenter randomized trial investigating nipocalimab for pregnancies at risk of severe HDFN is now in progress, and findings should be anticipated prior to its implementation in clinical practice.

QUESTIONS

1. What is the incidence of clinically significant red blood cell antibodies seen in pregnant women?

   A. 0.4%

   B. 1%

   C. 2%

   D. 4%

2. Despite anti-D prophylaxis, what is the incidence of anti-D alloimmunization in pregnant women?

   A. 1 in 1000

   B. 4 in 1000

   C. 1 in 100

   D. 2 in 100

3. What is the normal expected fetal hemoglobin at term?

   A. 80 g/L

   B. 100 g/L

   C. 150 g/L

   D. 180 g/L

4. At what level of fetal hemoglobin can hydrops occur at term?

   A. 40 g/L

   B. 80 g/L

   C. 100 g/L

   D. 150 g/L

5. What part of the fetal neurological system is commonly affected by kernicterus?

    A. Hippocampus

    B. Cerebellum

    C. Basal ganglia/brainstem nuclei

    D. Frontal lobe

6. Which of the following is the only widely recognized treatment option to prevent fetal death/neurological impairment in fetuses affected by HDN?

    A. Monoclonal antibodies

    B. IVIG

    C. IUT

    D. Anti-VEGF treatment

7. Doppler studies of which of the following vessels in the fetus is used to monitor the development of fetal anemia in patients with anti-D alloimmunization?

    A. Umbilical artery

    B. MCA

    C. Ductus venosus

    D. Uterine artery

8. What value of peak systolic velocity of MCA-PSV best predicts moderate-to-severe fetal anemia?

    A. >1 MoM

    B. >1.5 MoM

    C. >2 MoM

    D. >2.5 MoM

9. Which of the following is the most accurate method of diagnosis of fetal anemia?

    A. MCA-PSV >1.5 MoM

    B. Ductus venosus Doppler

    C. Fetal blood sampling

    D. Cardiotocogram (CTG)

10. What is the incidence of miscarriage/preterm birth with fetal blood sampling?

    A. 1 in 1000

    B. 4 in 1000

    C. 1.3%

    D. 4%

11. How is fetal anemia diagnosed on CTG?

    A. Persistent acute fetal bradycardia for 3 minutes

    B. Early variable decelerations for 90 minutes

    C. Presence of late decelerations

    D. Presence of reduced variability with a sinusoidal pattern

12. Which of the following women should be referred to specialized fetal medicine centers early in pregnancy?

    A. Women with a previous pregnancy history of HDFN

    B. Women with rising antibody levels/titres

    C. An antibody level/titre above a specific threshold

    D. All of the above

13. At what gestation is the risk of preterm birth and miscarriage seen to be maximum with IUT done for fetal anemia in patients with HDFN?

    A. Before 22 weeks

    B. Between 22 to 24 weeks

    C. Between 24 to 28 weeks

    D. After 28 weeks

14. What is the overall procedure complication rate with IUT?

    A. 1 in 1000   C. 3–5%

    B. 1%   D. 8–10%

15. In the absence of fetal hydrops, what is the fetal survival rate following IUT?

    A. 30%   C. 70%

    B. 50%   D. 90%

16. At what gestation should elective birth be offered to patients undergoing IUT for HDFN, in cases where the fetus is not compromised?

    A. 34–35 weeks   C. 36–37 weeks

    B. 35–36 weeks   D. 37–38 weeks

17. What is the incidence of cerebral palsy in babies of patients undergoing IUT during pregnancy?

    A. 1.6 per 1000   C. 1%

    B. 3.4 per 1000   D. 2.4%

18. Which of the following parameters is used to guide the postnatal treatment of HDFN?

    A. Neonatal ultrasound to confirm reversal of ascites/skin edema

    B. Direct agglutinin test (DAT) from the umbilical cord

    C. Neonatal MCA-PSV Doppler

    D. Neonatal hemoglobin levels

19. How long do the maternal antibodies causing HDFN persist in the neonate?

    A. 6 weeks   C. 6 months

    B. 3 months   D. 12 months

20. According to the NICE guideline on neonatal jaundice, what is the recommended dose of IVIG during the neonatal period?

    A. 250 mg/kg over 4 hours

    B. 500 mg/kg over 4 hours

    C. 1000 mg/kg over 4 hours

    D. 1500 mg/kg over 4 hours

21. What is the definition of severe HDFN?

    A. Fetal death or need for IUT before 20 weeks

    B. Fetal death or need for IUT before 22 weeks

    C. Fetal death or need for IUT before 24 weeks

    D. Fetal death or need for IUT before 28 weeks

22. All of the following are advantages of IVIG use in patients with HDFN, except?

    A. Delayed onset of fetal anemia (hence need for first IUT) to a later gestation

    B. Reduced occurrence of fetal hydrops

    C. Reduced need for neonatal exchange transfusion

    D. Reduced occurrence of neurodevelopmental problems in the neonates

23. What is the standard dose of IVIG used in HDFN?

    A. 0.4 g/kg maternal weight weekly

    B. 0.6 g/kg maternal weight weekly

    C. 0.8 g/kg maternal weight weekly

    D. 1 g/kg maternal weight weekly

24. Which monoclonal antibody is now emerging as a potential effective therapy for severe HDFN?

    A. Bevacizumab

    B. Rituximab

    C. Nipocalimab

    D. Trastuzumab

25. Which of the following non-Rh antigens are not associated with hemolytic disease in the newborn?

    A. Kell

    B. Duffy

    C. Lewis

    D. Kidd

26. When the fetus is in utero, how much fall in fetal hemoglobin can cause hydrops fetalis depicted by pleural and pericardial effusion, ascites, and diffuse edema on ultrasound?

    A. Hemoglobin deficit is more than 3 g/dL below the gestational age average

    B. Hemoglobin deficit is more than 7 g/dL below the gestational age average

    C. Hemoglobin deficit is more than 9 g/dL below the gestational age average

    D. Hemoglobin deficit is more than 11 g/dL below the gestational age average

27. Which of the following types of bilirubin is responsible for kernicterus in infants born with hemolytic disease in the newborn?

    A. Water soluble – conjugated bilirubin

    B. Water soluble – unconjugated bilirubin

    C. Water insoluble – conjugated bilirubin

    D. Water insoluble – unconjugated bilirubin

28. In terms of ABO incompatibility-induced hemolytic disease of the newborn, which of the following statements is incorrect?

   A. ABO incompatibility occurs in around 15–25% of pregnancies.

   B. ABO incompatibility-induced HDFN impacts merely 1% of these pregnancies.

   C. It cannot manifest during the first pregnancy.

   D. It is less severe than HDFN caused by Rh incompatibility.

29. Which of the following maternal blood group types has the highest risk of ABO incompatibility-induced hemolytic disease in the newborn?

   A. Blood group B

   B. Blood group A

   C. Blood group O

   D. Blood group AB

30. On antenatal ultrasound, which of the following is not correctly mentioned as a sign of hydrops fetalis in a fetus affected by hemolytic disease of the newborn?

   A. ≥ Two body cavities/compartments showing fluid collection

   B. Skin edema of scalp subcutaneous tissue showing thickness >10 mm

   C. Placentomegaly

   D. Polyhydramnios

31. Which of the following signs of hydrops fetalis is not seen easily in early pregnancy (as early as less than 14 weeks of pregnancy)?

   A. Ascites

   B. Skin edema

   C. Placentomegaly

   D. Pleural/pericardial effusion

32. In couples with ABO incompatibility-induced hemolytic disease of newborn, where the direct antiglobulin test is negative, which of the following tests in the neonate is recommended for diagnosis of HDFN?

   A. Neonatal bilirubin

   B. Neonatal hemoglobin

   C. Indirect antiglobulin test

   D. Neonatal MCA-PSV Doppler

33. Which of the following correctly describes the significant increase in bilirubin levels to diagnose hemolysis in the neonate after birth?

   A. Increase in total serum bilirubin >0.2 mg/dL per hour in the first 24 hours after birth

   B. Increase in total serum bilirubin >0.3 mg/dL per hour in the first 24 hours after birth

   C. Increase in total serum bilirubin >0.7 mg/dL per hour in the first 24 hours after birth

   D. Increase in total serum bilirubin >1.0 mg/dL per hour in the first 24 hours after birth

ANSWERS

1. A	12. D	23. D
2. A	13. A	24. C
3. C	14. C	25. C
4. B	15. D	26. B
5. C	16. C	27. D
6. C	17. D	28. C
7. B	18. B	29. C
8. B	19. C	30. B
9. C	20. B	31. D
10. C	21. C	32. C
11. D	22. D	33. B

28 SIP – Perinatal Risks of In Vitro Fertilization (IVF)

Source: In Vitro Fertilisation: Perinatal Risks and Early Childhood Outcomes Scientific Impact Paper No. 8 May 2012. https://www.rcog.org.uk/guidance/browse-all-guidance/scientific-impact-papers/perinatal-risks-associated-with-ivf-scientific-impact-paper-no-8/

IMPORTANT POINTS FROM THE GUIDELINE (SIP)

- Infertility is predicted to impact one in seven couples in the UK at some point during their reproductive lives.

- With more than 30 years of experience, in vitro fertilization (IVF) has become a standard medical procedure for addressing infertility, with births resulting from IVF estimated to represent over 1% of all births in the UK.

- The primary determinant of pregnancy and long-term outcomes is whether the pregnancy is a singleton or a multiple gestation, regardless of the conception method, whether natural or aided.

- Moreover, the risks escalate proportionally with the number of fetuses, and monozygosity is likewise linked to elevated odds of unfavorable outcomes.

- IVF seemingly doubles the risk of monozygotic twins compared to natural conception; however, the occurrence of monozygotic twins post-IVF remains quite low.

- Currently, around one in four IVF pregnancies in the UK culminate in multiple births due to the prevalent practice of transferring two or three embryos, with the bulk of multiple pregnancies arising from such transfers.

- Many parents view multiple pregnancies as an optimal outcome, and for most multiples, especially twins, there are typically no long-term negative effects.

- Currently, it is unfeasible to anticipate who would experience difficulties perinatally or subsequently in life.

- Thus, elective single embryo transfer and the restriction in the UK to the transfer of two embryos for women under 40 serve as a population-level strategy to mitigate the risks of prematurity and its related problems and socioeconomic expenses.

- Upon diagnosing a multiple pregnancy in a fertility facility, a referral to a specialized multiple birth clinic should be initiated.

- This would enable the couple to have counseling for selective fetal reduction for triplets and higher-order pregnancies, in addition to specialized prenatal screening and diagnosis.

- Multiple pregnancies inherently pose a distinct risk for preterm birth; nevertheless, there exists a modest yet statistically significant 23% elevation in the relative risk of preterm birth among IVF twins in comparison to naturally conceived twins, although the specific contributions of spontaneous or elective preterm births remain unidentified.

- Treatment necessitating donor oocytes or intracytoplasmic sperm injection (ICSI) can affect the risk.

- Moreover, early fetal death in a multiple gestation may elevate the chance of premature birth for the surviving singleton.

- Prematurity resulting from multiple pregnancies is a well-established risk factor for low birth weight (LBW) <2500 g, very low birth weight (VLBW) <1500 g, and extremely low birth weight (ELBW) <1000 g; however, singleton IVF pregnancies also exhibit a heightened risk of LBW in comparison to naturally conceived singletons.

- While prematurity somewhat affects the risk of LBW in singletons, the relative risk of infants being small for gestational age is elevated by around 40–60%, indicating that variables beyond premature birth contribute to this condition.

DOI: 10.1201/9781003650355-28

- Approximately 3% to 5% of all infants receive a diagnosis of a congenital abnormality shortly after delivery. IVF is linked to a 30–40% elevated risk of significant congenital abnormalities in comparison to natural conceptions.

- The elevated risk seems to be partially linked to underlying infertility or its causes, since couples who require over 12 months to conceive also demonstrate a heightened risk of malformations.

- The primary malformations observed in IVF pregnancies encompass various gastrointestinal, cardiovascular, and musculoskeletal disorders, notably septal heart defects, cleft lip, esophageal atresia, and anorectal atresia.

- In certain instances, infertility may have a hereditary basis, and effective IVF therapy may consequently enable intergenerational transmission.

- This has raised concerns that children conceived through these techniques may exhibit a higher incidence of genetic defects.

- Infertile men and women have a heightened incidence of structural chromosomal abnormalities: a 4.6% prevalence of autosomal translocations and inversions in oligospermic males, and a 1.14% prevalence of autosomal reciprocal balanced translocations in infertile women, compared to a general population prevalence of 0.16%.

- Nonetheless, these structural anomalies would often be identified and subsequent transmission prevented through preimplantation genetic diagnosis (PGD) after karyotyping men with azoospermia or severe oligospermia, as well as couples experiencing repeated implantation failure or miscarriage.

- Microdeletions on the long arm of the Y chromosome (Yq), specifically in the AZF region, may lead to spermatogenic failure and result in either oligospermia or azoospermia, the latter obstructing continued vertical transmission.

- Sons conceived from oligospermic males with Yq microdeletions will inherit this subfertile phenotype, and further expansions or de novo deletions may occur, leading to a more severe phenotype in the children.

- While other monogenic illnesses such as cystic fibrosis are linked to infertility due to the congenital lack of the vas deferens, vertical transmission of prevalent mutations can be circumvented by testing the female partner and conducting PGD if she is a carrier.

- There is growing evidence that epigenetics may play a role in aberrant embryo and trophoblast development, with IVF superovulation and culture conditions potentially generating epigenetic alterations and long-term genomic imprinting.

- Nine human imprinting disorders have been found to date; however, current evidence associates IVF with only three: Beckwith–Wiedemann syndrome (BWS), Angelman syndrome (AS), and, more recently, maternal hypomethylation syndrome.

- The total prevalence of these illnesses is minimal, at less than 1 in 12,000 births (BWS 1 in 13,700, and AS 1 in 16,000); hence, routine screening for imprinting problems in infants conceived by IVF is not advised.

- The aggregated findings indicate an approximate 70% elevation in the probability of perinatal mortality for IVF singletons relative to natural conceptions.

- Women who conceived by IVF had a statistically significant 4-fold elevated risk of stillbirth in comparison to fertile women.

- PGD/screening (PGS) necessitates the extraction of one or more blastomeres from the embryo for genetic analysis, facilitating the transfer of unaffected embryos.

- Despite the extraction of a varied quantity of material from the growing embryo, the general outlook for children aligns with that of conventional ICSI.

- The prolonged incubation of embryos in vitro from the conventional day 2 (cleavage stage) transfer to day 5 (blastocyst stage) has been promoted as a method to enhance embryo selection and, consequently, pregnancy rates. The embryo is grown sequentially in various mediums to promote in vitro growth.

■ A systematic review and meta-analysis have shown that the likelihood of live birth following fresh IVF is 40% greater with blastocyst-stage embryo transfer compared to cleavage-stage embryo transfer when an equivalent number of embryos are transferred.

■ Upon controlling for confounding variables, the incidence of preterm birth in singleton pregnancies was markedly elevated following blastocyst-stage transfer compared to cleavage-stage transfer; the likelihood of congenital abnormalities was also increased.

■ Elective single blastocyst transfer is an efficacious method to mitigate the risk of multiple births while preserving a high pregnancy rate.

■ Assisted hatching (AH), a procedure that involves the disruption of the zona pellucida to promote implantation, has recently demonstrated an increase in clinical pregnancy rates; however, it does not improve live birth rates or decrease the incidence of multiple pregnancies. The long-term effects on pregnancy and progeny remain uncertain.

■ The harvest of immature oocytes and their subsequent in vitro maturation (IVM) without ovarian stimulation is a novel advancement in assisted reproductive technology (ART). IVM provides the advantages of ovarian stimulation – specifically, an increased number of oocytes – while mitigating the associated hazards. Individuals with polycystic ovarian syndrome (PCOS) or polycystic ovaries are suitable candidates for iIVM.

■ The neuromotor, cognitive, language and behavioral outcomes in children conceived with IVF or ICSI appear comparable to those of children conceived spontaneously.

■ The sole persistent unfavorable result has been an elevated incidence of cerebral palsy, which is somewhat, though not entirely, attributed to the heightened chance of premature delivery.

■ The Barker hypothesis posits that detrimental prenatal settings may result in enduring effects in adulthood. For instance, maternal under-nutrition during gestation correlates with a heightened risk of coronary heart disease, type 2 diabetes, cerebrovascular accidents, and hypertension.

■ Peripheral adipose tissue mass was shown to be elevated in offspring conceived by IVF.

■ Cardiometabolic disparities also occur among children conceived via IVF, with an approximate increase of 4 mmHg in systolic blood pressure and 2 mmHg in diastolic blood pressure, along with an elevation in fasting glucose levels.

■ Early childhood development (weight gain) may serve as a predictor of cardiovascular risk factors (blood pressure and body fat composition) in children conceived by IVF.

■ These significant observations underscore the necessity for metabolic epidemiology investigations in adolescents and adults undergoing IVF.

■ Advanced maternal age is a risk factor for nearly all pregnancy and postnatal problems.

■ The mean age at which women pursue conception is steadily increasing, leading to a higher utilization of IVF among older women who are already at risk for pregnancy difficulties.

■ In older women undergoing IVF, there is an increased incidence of cesarean section delivery, obstetric hemorrhage, pre-eclampsia, pregnancy-induced hypertension, and gestational diabetes.

■ Due to their age, older women are more prone to pre-existing comorbidities that complicate their pregnancy trajectory and outcomes.

■ Women with substantial comorbidities, irrespective of age, must undergo pre-IVF evaluation and counseling.

■ As the age at which women pursue conception is postponed, a growing number of women are utilizing oocyte donation, a method formerly restricted to those with early ovarian insufficiency.

- A rise in early pregnancy and perinatal problems is seen, with the incidence of pregnancy-induced hypertension varying between 16% and 40%, particularly elevated among primiparous women.

- Notwithstanding these dangers, there is scant knowledge regarding the long-term consequences of egg donor pregnancies for both the woman and her child.

- Individuals with PCOS face heightened risks of gestational diabetes, pregnancy-induced hypertension, pre-eclampsia, and premature birth during pregnancy.

- Furthermore, a heightened risk of neonatal critical care hospitalization and elevated perinatal death, unrelated to multiple births, has been noted.

- These statistics underscore the significance of pre-ART counseling for women with PCOS and stress the necessity of weight management prior to ART.

- The utilization of first-trimester combined ultrasonography and biochemical screening for Down syndrome is currently advised.

- Pregnancy-associated plasma protein-A (PAPP-A) levels are markedly diminished in fresh transfer IVF pregnancies, resulting in a heightened risk of false-positive results and an increased likelihood of undergoing chorionic villous sampling or amniocentesis.

- This may indicate the comparative inaccuracy of ultrasound dating.

- Additional extensive research will be necessary before guidelines for modifying risk assessments for IVF pregnancies can be established.

- Currently, long-term follow-up studies on children conceived via IVF are predominantly reassuring after controlling for the confounding variables of preterm and multiple gestation.

- Nevertheless, ongoing enhancement of the technological procedure and clinical implementation of innovative advancements necessitates continuous monitoring.

QUESTIONS

1. What is the prevalence of infertility in couples in the UK at some stage during their reproductive life?

    A. One in two

    B. One in three

    C. One in five

    D. One in seven

2. IVF accounts for what percentage of births in the UK?

    A. 1%

    B. 3%

    C. 5%

    D. 10%

3. To what extent does IVF increase the risk of monozygous twins in comparison to natural conception?

    A. 2-fold

    B. 4-fold

    C. 6-fold

    D. 10-fold

4. To what extent is premature birth increased in IVF twins in comparison to naturally conceived twins?

   A. 10%

   B. 23%

   C. 35%

   D. 50%

5. By what extent does the relative risk of babies being born small for gestation age (SGA) increase in patients with multiple pregnancies?

   A. 20–30%

   B. 30–40%

   C. 40–60%

   D. >60%

6. What is the incidence of congenital anomalies in babies born to the general population?

   A. 1–2%

   B. 3–5%

   C. 7–8%

   D. 10%

7. To what extent does IVF increase the risk of congenital anomalies in babies in comparison to natural conceptions?

   A. By 10–20%

   B. By 30–40%

   C. By 50–60%

   D. By 80%

8. All of the following major congenital malformations increase in IVF babies, except?

   A. Gastrointestinal anomalies such as esophageal atresia, anorectal atresia

   B. Cardiovascular anomalies such as septal heart defects

   C. Musculoskeletal defects

   D. Neural tube defects

9. Congenital absence of vas deferens is commonly associated with which of the following single-gene disorders?

   A. Duchenne muscular dystrophy

   B. Cystic fibrosis

   C. Fragile X syndrome

   D. Huntington's disease

10. What is the incidence of genomic imprinting disorders in association with IVF?

    A. 1 in 1000

    B. 1 in 4000

    C. 1 in 8000

    D. 1 in 12,000

11. IVF is linked to all of the following genomic imprinting disorders, except?

    A. BWS

    B. AS

    C. Silver–Russell syndrome

    D. Maternal hypomethylation syndrome

12. To what extent is the perinatal mortality increased in IVF conceptions in comparison to natural conceptions?

    A. 15%

    B. 30%

    C. 50%

    D. 70%

13. To what extent is the risk of stillbirth increased in women with IVF?

    A. 2-fold

    B. 3-fold

    C. 4-fold

    D. 10-fold

14. Comparing day 5 blastocyst stage embryo transfer to day 2 cleavage stage transfer, by what percentage is the live birth rate increased?

    A. 10%

    B. 20%

    C. 40%

    D. 60%

15. Risk of which of the following conditions is increased in children born to women with IVF or ICSI in comparison to women who have conceived naturally?

    A. Neuromotor problems

    B. Cognitive problems

    C. Language and behavioral outcomes

    D. Cerebral palsy

16. What is the absolute increase in the risk of pre-eclampsia/gestational hypertension in patients conceived by IVF?

    A. 1%

    B. 2%

    C. 5%

    D. 10%

17. What is the absolute increase in the risk of gestational diabetes mellitus in patients conceived by IVF?

    A. 1%

    B. 2%

    C. 5%

    D. 10%

18. According to the latest research, what is the incidence of preterm labor in patients conceived with IVF?

   A. 3%

   B. 7%

   C. 11%

   D. 15%

19. All of the following odds–ratios for increase in risk of important obstetric complications in patients conceived by IVF are correct, except?

   A. Placenta previa OR 3.76

   B. Placenta accreta OR 2.27

   C. Placental abruption OR 1.87

   D. Fetal growth restriction OR 4.5

20. In patients conceived with ARTs, which of the following characteristics increases the risk of maternal complications especially pre-eclampsia, gestational diabetes, and thromboembolism?

   A. Age >35 years

   B. BMI >30 kg/m²

   C. Multiple pregnancies

   D. All of the above

   E. B and C

21. According to latest research, what is the overall incidence of miscarriage in patients conceived with artificial reproductive techniques?

   A. 15–20%

   B. 30%

   C. 40%

   D. 50–60%

ANSWERS

1. D	8. D	15. D
2. A	9. B	16. B
3. A	10. D	17. A
4. B	11. C	18. C
5. C	12. D	19. D
6. B	13. C	20. D
7. B	14. C	21. A

29 SIP – Prenatal Exome Sequencing

Source: Evidence to Support the Clinical Utility of Prenatal Exome Sequencing in Evaluation of the Fetus with Congenital Anomalies Scientific Impact Paper No. 64 February 2021. https://www.rcog.org .uk/guidance/browse-all-guidance/scientific-impact-papers/evidence-to-support-the-clinical-utility -of-prenatal-exome-sequencing-in-the-evaluation-of-the-fetus-with-congenital-anomalies-scientific -impact-paper-no-64/

IMPORTANT POINTS FROM THE GUIDELINE (SIP)

- Up to 3% of fetuses exhibit a congenital abnormality, many of which have an underlying genetic etiology.

- Aneuploidy and copy number variation occur in around 40% of these pregnancies, detectable using standard G-banding karyotyping and chromosomal microarray analysis (CMA).

- These techniques are currently the routine procedures conducted on fetal tissue (amniocytes or chorionic villi) in these cases.

- A significant number of instances may result from an underlying monogenic condition, identifiable through DNA sequencing.

- Next generation sequencing (NGS) is a potent genomic instrument capable of analyzing the 3 billion bases of the human genome at the resolution of a single base pair.

- NGS methodologies encompass targeted sequencing utilizing phenotype-specific gene panels, which may be restricted to particular criteria, such as skeletal deformities, or a more extensive 'clinical' panel that may comprise up to 6000 known genes.

- Sequencing may be conducted on the complete genome (whole genome sequencing) or the exome (exome sequencing [ES]), which can subsequently be analyzed using particular panels for a more focused methodology.

- The exome constitutes 1–2% of the genetic coding yet encompasses over 85% of identified disease-associated variations.

- Next-generation sequencing (NGS) has transformed the detection of uncommon genetic illnesses, achieving diagnostic rates of 40% in previously undetected pediatric developmental anomalies.

- There is a lack of clinical guidance about the application of prenatal ES to examine fetuses with congenital abnormalities.

- Alongside pathogenic variants implicated in the pertinent fetal structural abnormality (FSA), variants of unknown significance (VUS) with potential clinical implications were identified in 4% of instances.

- Extensive prospective investigations have demonstrated that prenatal ES offers supplementary clinical benefits beyond conventional genetic testing.

- Establishing a conclusive prenatal molecular diagnosis is crucial as it facilitates counseling, empowering parents to make educated autonomous decisions regarding their pregnancy and enabling physicians to manage antenatal and early postnatal care more efficiently.

- Moreover, approach circumvents an extended 'diagnostic journey' that numerous infants with monogenic diseases experience.

- This additional information enables clinicians to advise parents on the likelihood of recurrence in future pregnancies, so facilitating options for prenatal testing by invasive or non-invasive methods, as well as preimplantation genetic diagnosis.

- It is expected that the growing implementation of prenatal ES in clinical practice would enhance the interpretation of genetic variations.

- In the PAGE investigation, several novel prenatal manifestations of previously documented diseases, which were only characterized postnatally, were reported.

DOI: 10.1201/9781003650355-29

- This signifies the necessity to curate the fetal genome and guarantee that clinical and genetic data are incorporated into worldwide genomic databases for enhanced counseling and informed decision-making in prenatal sequencing.

- DECIPHER serves as the optimal database for documenting phenotype–genotype associations (https://decipher.sanger.ac.uk).

- Guidelines for prenatal ES are limited, and the sole published statement from the International Society of Prenatal Diagnosis, the Society of Maternal-Fetal Medicine, and the Perinatal Quality Foundation does not endorse the routine application of prenatal ES.

- Nonetheless, it concedes that there are situations in which it may be deemed appropriate after consulting experts.

- When implementing ES in clinical practice, several concerns must be addressed.

- Detailed pre- and post-test counseling must be conducted by experienced staff in ES technologies, alongside a multidisciplinary team (MDT) comprising a trained obstetrician, senior laboratory scientist, consultant geneticist, and genetic counselor, who should participate in both case selection and sequencing interpretation.

- Before initiating testing, it is imperative to secure informed written consent from the parents after they have reviewed a pertinent information leaflet and received details about relevant support organizations, such as antenatal results and choices.

- Accurate prenatal phenotyping by imaging should ideally be conducted by a specialist proficient in fetal dysmorphology to facilitate later variant interpretation.

- The extensive implementation of variant classification guidelines from the American College of Medical Genetics and the Association for Clinical Genetic Science has significantly enhanced the uniformity of variant interpretation, while trio testing and precise expert phenotyping have also augmented diagnostic yield.

- Trio testing, involving the fetus and both parents, is a suggested method for prenatal ES to facilitate expedited analysis by excluding family, predominantly benign, genetic variations.

- The prevailing agreement is that Class IV (over a 90% likelihood of becoming pathogenic) and Class V (pathogenic) variations should be disclosed if they correspond with the fetal phenotype.

- Variants of uncertain significance (VUS) will be presented solely if they are classified as 'hot' and align with the phenotype following MDT discussion.

- This is difficult in several situations due to the inconsistent expression of diseases and the occasional lack of knowledge regarding the long-term outcomes for fetuses with pathogenic mutations in certain genes.

- The reporting of non-actionable incidental discoveries resulting from prenatal ES, such as single gene neurodegenerative diseases, remains contentious and should not be included into UK clinical practice at this time.

- In summary, it is advisable to disclose any variance that may influence care during pregnancy or for the family, within the clinical context of the test performed or in the future.

- Conversely, it stipulates that the following should remain unreported: any finding not associated with potential phenotypes relevant to the pregnancy (future child) in question, or lacking clinically actionable implications for that child or family in the future, such as VUS that cannot be correlated with a potential phenotype based on the involved genes, and incidental pathogenic variants for which no intervention is available.

- Technical considerations encompass: (i) the necessity of acquiring adequate fetal DNA devoid of maternal cell contamination for expedited NGS analysis; and (ii) the creation of sophisticated bioinformatics programs to filter and annotate the variations.

- This will guarantee that variants deemed pertinent are prioritized for analysis.

- The trio technique is optimum for minimizing the number of variants requiring review and enables the timely return of data within a clinically relevant timeframe.

- Comparing the fetal exome with the parental exomes, inheritance filtering facilitates the identification of variants that may be responsible for the clinical presentation, as opposed to those that are merely a result of standard genetic variation.

- It is important to note the possibility of overlooking parentally inherited variations when the affected parent has a mild, inconspicuous phenotype.

- In cases where the trio approach is impractical, such as after assisted reproduction utilizing donor sperm or ova, a duo sample from the fetus and biological father should be collected as a minimum requirement.

- In the postnatal context, standard turnaround times for intricate genetic tests ranged from 3 to 6 months.

- Nonetheless, prenatal investigations indicated that delivering the results of ES within 2–3 weeks was achievable.

- Simultaneously doing CMA and ES can significantly decrease turnaround times.

- Prenatal ES was implemented in clinical practice in England on 1 October 2020.

- The evaluation for this service is conducted by the West Midlands, Oxford, Wessex, and North Thames Genomic Laboratory Hubs. Referrals from fetal medicine units are evaluated by local clinical genetics services, and possible cases are deliberated with the genomic laboratory hub before being approved for study.

- Rigorous qualifying requirements have been instituted to guarantee equitable access to this service, necessitating periodic assessment and updates.

- The PAGE and Columbia investigations significantly contribute to the bioinformatics pipeline and filtering methodologies.

- Cases necessitate evaluation by a MDT and referral via local clinical genetics services.

- Technical considerations regarding the provision of ES may impose an additional burden on the NHS.

- The NHS is a well-structured healthcare system with established MDTs and accredited laboratory systems, potentially facilitating the transition of fetal ES from research to clinical practice.

- Prenatal ES offers extensive information regarding the fetal genome.

- This technology affects the child, the future fetus, the parents, the extended family, and raises data privacy issues.

- In addition to the ambiguity posed by potential variations associated with fetal structural anomalies (FSA), there exists the possibility of secondary discoveries that may provide information regarding late-onset illnesses unrelated to the FSA.

- During trio testing, parental sequencing may uncover secondary or accidental findings, necessitating careful management of these results.

- The American College of Medical Genetics guidelines may be applicable for managing secondary results.

- In the United States, reporting of discovered variations in 56 genes is obligatory.

- This strict approach contradicts the UK system that allows individuals to 'opt out' of receiving such information.

- A further domain of ethical discourse pertains to the advisement on variant grading and the counseling of parental choices.

- It is essential for women and their partners to be informed of the options available to them about the continuation or termination of their pregnancy.

- Individuals seeking more assistance in the decision-making process should be directed to organizations such as Antenatal Results and Choices.

- A societal debate exists around the ownership of genetic information and the disclosure of variants that may impact the broader family; is such information permissible to reveal?

- Genetic counselors are advocating for the perception of genomic information as a shared asset when sharing it to other family members, which is essential in specific circumstances.

- ES has the capacity to reveal non-paternity and consanguinity, potentially leading to more complex discussions for physicians and parents.

- With advancements in genomics, the pathogenicity of genetic variations may occasionally be redefined retroactively.

- This may have enduring health implications, as well as repercussions for actions made, potentially resulting in irrevocable outcomes, such as abortion predicated on the genetic diagnosis of a pathogenic variation that is subsequently reclassified as non-pathogenic.

- All of these complex issues must be evaluated before initiating testing and addressed during pre-test counseling.

- Utilizing a targeted methodology (employing clinical exome instead of whole ES, or interpreting whole ES through a panel of genes identified prenatally) results in a diminished number of genes under examination.

- Consequently, the identification of secondary discoveries and VUS can be significantly restricted, so circumventing the majority of these concerns.

- This strategy may be contemplated in the future; however, diminishing the number of genes analyzed constrains the capacity to identify target genes that may remain undiscovered.

- While the ES methodologies are established in the specified molecular research laboratories, the clinical infrastructure for variant assessment via MDT clinical review panels is currently under development following national discussions and consultations within NHS England regions.

- As prenatal ES becomes increasingly established, the appropriate applications and limitations of the technique will become more evident (e.g. optimal diagnostic yield necessitates sequencing DNA from the fetus and both parents, and not all pathogenic mutations will be identified by ES).

- This, along with other evidence on the health, economic, and ethical dimensions of ES, will establish a foundation for nationally endorsed standards.

QUESTIONS

1. What is the incidence of congenital anomalies in the developing fetus on antenatal ultrasound examinations?

    A. 1 in 1000

    B. 1%

    C. 3%

    D. 10%

2. In fetuses with structural differences on antenatal ultrasound, what percentage of the chromosomal changes are detected by the standard genetic tests (chorionic villous sampling and amniocentesis)?

    A. 10%

    B. 25%

    C. 40%

    D. 60%

3. In fetuses with structural differences on antenatal ultrasound where the standard genetic test is negative, what percentage of pregnancies can have a genetic diagnosis with prenatal ES?

A. 10%

C. 40%

B. 25%

D. 60%

4. What percentage of the human genetic code is represented by the exome?

A. 1–2%

C. 20%

B. 10%

D. 85%

5. What percentage of clinically significant genetic disease-related variants are represented in the exome of the human genome?

A. 1–2%

B. 10%

C. 20%

D. 85%

6. Which of the following is the preferred database used for recording the phenotypic–genotypic correlations for genetic diseases in the UK?

A. PROSPERO

B. GENCODE

C. DECIPHER

D. CINAHL Ultimate

7. 'Trio testing' involves genetic testing of all of the following, except?

A. To examine the genetic material (DNA) of the patient (for example, the fetus)

B. To examine the genetic material (DNA) of the father

C. To examine the genetic material (DNA) of the mother

D. To examine the genetic material (DNA) of both paternal and maternal grandparents

8. According to available evidence in the literature about prenatal ES, in which of the following situations should the genetic defect be reported?

A. Any finding that is not linked to prospective phenotypes for the pertinent pregnancy (future offspring)

B. Any finding that does not possess clinically actionable consequences for the pregnancy (child) or family in the future, such as VUS that cannot be associated with a prospective phenotype based on the implicated genes

C. Any variation that may affect pregnancy care or familial health, within the clinical setting of the administered test or for prospective concerns

D. Any accidental pathogenic variations for which no therapeutic intervention exists

9. What is the estimated reporting time (turnaround time) for prenatal ES?

A. 24 hours

B. 2–3 days

C. 2–3 weeks

D. 2–3 months

10. Which of the following statements regarding CMA is incorrect?

   A. It encompasses whole-genome sequencing.

   B. It aids in the identification of copy number variations.

   C. It aids in identifying duplications and deletions of DNA segments.

   D. It precisely detects single-gene diseases and balanced chromosomal translocations.

11. According to recommendations pertaining to the current clinical practice in the UK, prenatal ES can be used in all of the following situations, except?

   A. Unexplained fetal phenotype

   B. When standard karyotyping or CMA fails to yield a conclusive genetic diagnosis

   C. To ascertain a genetic etiology of a clinically pertinent fetal structural abnormality identified via prenatal ultrasonography

   D. In instances of monogenic neurodegenerative diseases

12. Which of the following statements about ES is inaccurate when compared to targeted sequencing?

   A. ES identifies single-nucleotide variants in coding regions.

   B. The sequencing depth of ES ranges from 50 to 100 times.

   C. ES can identify all types of mutations, including single-nucleotide polymorphism (SNPs) and insertion or deletion mutations of DNA (INDELs), in specific locations.

   D. ES is not as cost-effective as targeted sequencing.

13. Which of the following statements about ES is inaccurate in comparison to genome sequencing?

   A. ES detects single-nucleotide variants in coding areas.

   B. The sequencing depth of ES ranges from 50 to 100 times.

   C. ES is more cost-effective when compared to genome sequencing.

   D. ES reveals single-nucleotide variations (SNVs) in both coding and non-coding areas and can also detect structural variants.

14. Which of the following cannot be detected by ES?

   A. Single-gene disorders

   B. Triple repeat disorders

   C. INDELs

   D. B and C

   E. All of the above

15. According to available evidence, which of the following is an important indication for the application of ES in clinical practice?

   A. Present pregnancy with a fetus displaying a single significant abnormality or many organ system abnormalities suggestive of a possible genetic etiology, despite non-diagnostic outcomes from CMA.

   B. Current pregnancy with no CMA results following a multidisciplinary review, which indicates that the fetal phenotype distinctly suggests a single-gene disorder.

   C. A previously misdiagnosed fetus displaying deformities suggestive of a genetic etiology, accompanied by the recurrence of unexplained similar anomalies in the current pregnancy.

   D. All of the above.

16. According to the American College of Medical Genetics and Genomics (ACMG) what is the recommended depth at which diagnostic ES should be performed?

   A. ≥90–95% of the sequence must be covered at least 10-fold, with an average depth of coverage of at least 100-fold

   B. ≥90–95% of the sequence must be covered at least 50-fold, with an average depth of coverage of at least 500-fold

   C. ≥90–95% of the sequence must be covered at least 100-fold, with an average depth of coverage of at least 1000-fold.

   D. ≥90–95% of the sequence must be covered at least 100-fold, with an average depth of coverage of at least 500-fold

ANSWERS

1. C	7. D	13. D
2. C	8. C	14. D
3. A	9. C	15. D
4. A	10. D	16. A
5. D	11. D	
6. C	12. C	

30 SIP – Preterm Birth

Source: Preterm Labour, Antibiotics, and Cerebral Palsy Scientific Impact Paper No. 33 February 2013. https://www.rcog.org.uk/guidance/browse-all-guidance/scientific-impact-papers/preterm-labour -antibiotics-and-cerebral-palsy-scientific-impact-paper-no-33/

IMPORTANT POINTS FROM THE GUIDELINE (SIP)

- Parturition occurring prior to 37 weeks of gestation is referred to as preterm birth.

- Preterm infants face a heightened chance of significant impairments, including cerebral palsy.

- A considerable number of infants born preterm without disabilities experience notable behavioral and educational challenges.

- Cerebral palsy encompasses a collection of illnesses affecting brain and nervous system functions, including movement, cognition, auditory perception, visual perception, and thought processes.

- It is the predominant cause of motor impairment in children, with an incidence of 1.5–3 occurrences per 1000 births.

- The likelihood of cerebral palsy is inversely related to gestational age at birth.

- Its frequency is 80 times greater in infants born before 28 weeks of gestation than in those delivered at term.

- Preterm birth is the most significant identified risk factor for cerebral palsy.

- Infection or inflammation is frequently linked to premature birth, particularly when membranes have ruptured, especially before 30 weeks of gestation, and should be regarded as a contributing factor, either directly or indirectly, to the elevated mortality and neurological morbidity in this population.

- The elevated risk of brain injury in preterm newborns may be directly associated with the adverse intrauterine inflammatory milieu, as well as the challenges posed by the subsequent neonatal critical care phase after preterm delivery.

- Research indicates that intrauterine infection or inflammation directly correlates with an increased risk of brain injury in preterm infants delivered spontaneously, characterized by a greater incidence of infection, compared to those delivered via physician-initiated methods, who exhibit a lower incidence of infection.

- Moreover, funisitis (inflammation of the umbilical cord's connective tissue) correlates with elevated cytokines (IL-6, IL-8, TNF-α, IL-1β) in amniotic fluid and fetal blood, which are linked to white matter injury and cerebral palsy.

- A recent systematic analysis indicated that clinical chorioamnionitis correlates with white matter injury and cerebral palsy, while histological chorioamnionitis is linked to periventricular leukomalacia.

- Recent research indicates a potential correlation between prenatal infections and various neurological and mental disorders throughout infancy and adulthood.

- A putative causal link exists between antibiotics and cerebral palsy; however, no direct association has been shown.

- Subclinical infection is associated with a significant percentage of preterm births; thus, the acute use of antibiotics could potentially eliminate the infection, extend the duration of pregnancy, and enhance neonatal outcomes.

- Alternatively, antibiotics may inhibit the infection, so extending the pregnancy, yet subjecting the fetus to a detrimental inflammatory milieu.

- A recent meta-analysis of antibiotic therapy throughout the prenatal period for asymptomatic women at risk of preterm birth demonstrated no decrease in preterm delivery rates.

- It has been suggested that antibiotics may elevate the risk of preterm birth in these situations, hence routine therapy is not advised.

DOI: 10.1201/9781003650355-30

- Bacterial vaginosis is established as a risk factor for preterm birth, maternal infectious morbidity, and miscarriage. However, clinical trials assessing antibiotic therapy during the antenatal period to mitigate these complications have produced inconsistent outcomes; thus, antibiotic therapy is not standard practice.

- The existing evidence, excluding long-term follow-up of the children, does not endorse the regular administration of antibiotics during the prenatal period for asymptomatic mothers.

- The use of antibiotics after preterm premature rupture of membranes (PPROM) is linked to statistically significant decreases in chorioamnionitis and a reduction in the frequency of infants born within 48 hours and 7 days post-randomization.

- The subsequent indicators of newborn morbidity were diminished: Neonatal infection, surfactant administration, oxygen therapy, and abnormal cerebral ultrasonography findings prior to hospital discharge; however, no decrease in perinatal mortality was noted.

- Co-amoxiclav was linked to a heightened risk of infant necrotizing enterocolitis.

- A meta-analysis of 11 trials indicated a decrease in maternal infection with preventive antibiotics, although it did not reveal any advantage or detriment for the predetermined newborn outcomes.

- There was an indication of potential harm with a nearly significant rise in infant death within the antibiotic group.

- The most compelling evidence about the impact of antibiotics provided during pregnancy on long-term childhood outcomes originates from the ORACLE Children Study (OCS), which tracked surviving children at the age of 7 in the UK through a parent-reported postal questionnaire.

- In children whose mothers experienced PPROM, the administration of antibiotics appeared to have minimal impact on their health and educational achievement at the age of 7. This finding was unexpected, given that antibiotics were anticipated to enhance clinical outcomes in this population, as positive amniotic fluid cultures are identified in 32% of women at presentation and up to 75% during subsequent labor.

- The reasons for this remain ambiguous but may be associated with the duration of antibiotic exposure, which was rather brief in this cohort of women, as almost 60% delivered within a week.

- Evidence suggests that antibiotics do not eliminate or prevent intra-amniotic infection.

- In children whose mothers experienced spontaneous preterm labor, the administration of erythromycin (with or without co-amoxiclav) correlated with an increase in the prevalence of functional impairment from 38% to 42%.

- The prevalence of children with cerebral palsy rose from 1.7% to 3.3% linked to erythromycin and from 1.9% to 3.2% related with co-amoxiclav.

- A proposal was made that a higher incidence of cerebral palsy in children was associated with women who had received both antibiotics.

- The reason for the higher risk of functional impairment and cerebral palsy associated with antibiotic receipt remains unclear.

- The prevalence of subclinical infection in this cohort is quite low, ranging from 13% to 22%.

- Consequently, the lack of benefit is not surprising; however, the evidence of harm is unexpected.

- Several explainations have been proposed, although none are confirmed.

- The most apparent explanation is a direct consequence of the antibiotics; however, this appears improbable as it was not observed in the PPROM cohort.

- The duration of antibiotic exposure for this cohort was relatively prolonged, with only 15–20% delivering within 7 days.

- An episode of preterm labor that resolves may indicate an infectious event, wherein maternal defenses, aided by antibiotics, counteract the insult, so extending the pregnancy, although it may not alleviate the concurrent intrauterine and fetal inflammation.

- An ongoing inflammatory environment may result in prenatal brain injury, thereby causing cerebral palsy.

- Ultimately, it is plausible that the occurrence of spontaneous preterm labor was not linked to infection, but rather to other diseases related to the so-called 'preterm parturition syndrome.'

- The reviewed evidence indicates that women experiencing spontaneous preterm labor with intact membranes and no signs of overt infection should not routinely receive antibiotics, as such treatment has been associated with an increased risk of functional impairment and cerebral palsy in their offspring.

- The decision to consistently give antibiotics for women with PPROM in the absence of overt infection is ambiguous, despite current guidelines advocating for their routine administration in acute scenarios.

- The advantages in certain short-term outcomes (such as extended pregnancy duration, decreased incidence of infection, reduced necessity for surfactant and oxygen therapy, and fewer infants exhibiting abnormal cerebral ultrasounds prior to hospital discharge) must be weighed against the absence of evidence supporting benefits in other areas, including perinatal mortality and long-term outcomes.

- Considering the absence of any long-term proven advantage, it would be reasonable to refrain from prescribing antibiotics to women with PPROM in the absence of infection, particularly in a high-income environment where assistance is accessible.

- A more compelling case exists for routine antibiotic treatment in low-income environments, when availability to alternative therapies (antenatal steroids, surfactant therapy, breathing, and antibiotic therapy) may be limited.

- Erythromycin has been designated as the preferred antibiotic following evaluation by the ORACLE.

- Co-amoxiclav should be contraindicated in women predisposed to premature delivery because of the heightened risk of neonatal necrotizing enterocolitis.

- It is prudent to refrain from using co-amoxiclav during pregnancy in cases where organisms exhibit sensitivity to alternative antibiotics.

- Antibiotics ought not to be used unless a definitive diagnosis of PPROM has been established.

- Women experiencing spontaneous preterm labor with intact membranes may be deemed at heightened risk for Group B *Streptococcus* infection (GBS).

- The RCOG does not endorse routine prophylaxis in this context.

QUESTIONS

1. What is the incidence of preterm premature rupture of membranes in the UK?

    A. <1% of all pregnancies

    B. 3% of all pregnancies

    C. 10% of all pregnancies

    D. 20–30% of all pregnancies

2. Which of the following is considered to be the strongest risk factor for cerebral palsy?

    A. Preterm birth

    B. Maternal hypothyroidism

    C. Maternal infections during pregnancy

    D. Hemolytic disease of newborn

3. What is the incidence of preterm birth in the UK?

    A. About 3% of live births

    B. About 8% of live births

    C. About 15% of live births

    D. About 20% of live births

4. What is the prevalence of cerebral palsy worldwide?

    A. 1.5–3 cases per 1000 live births

    B. 5–7 cases per 1000 live births

    C. 7–10 cases per 1000 live births

    D. 10–15 cases per 1000 live births

5. Which of the following is the most common cause of motor disability in childhood?

    A. Inherited conditions such as muscular dystrophy

    B. Movement disorders such as Huntington's disease

    C. Cerebral palsy

    D. Dyspraxia

6. Which of the following is the antibiotic of choice in women diagnosed with preterm premature rupture of membranes?

    A. Co-amoxiclav

    B. Vancomycin

    C. Erythromycin

    D. Benzyl-penicillin

7. Co-amoxiclav should be avoided in women at risk of preterm delivery due to an increased risk of which of the following adverse effects?

    A. Intraventricular hemorrhage

    B. Necrotizing enterocolitis

    C. Cerebral palsy

    D. Hypoxic-ischemic encephalopathy

8. Giving routine antibiotics has been proven beneficial for babies born to mothers belonging to which of the following groups?

    A. Women in spontaneous labor at term

    B. Women diagnosed with proven PPROM

    C. Asymptomatic women who are at risk of preterm birth

    D. Symptomatic women in preterm labor with intact membranes

9. According to RCOG guidelines, what is the recommended antibiotic dosage of choice in women diagnosed with preterm premature rupture of membranes?

    A. Erythromycin 333 mg 8 hourly for 7 days or until established labor, whichever is sooner

    B. Amoxicillin 250 mg 8 hourly for 10 days or until established labor, whichever is sooner

    C. Azithromycin 1 gm stat dose

    D. Erythromycin 250 mg 6 hourly for 10 days or until established labor, whichever is sooner

10. Which of the following statements regarding bacterial vaginosis in pregnancy is incorrect?

    A. It increases the risk of miscarriage.

    B. It increases the risk of preterm premature rupture of membranes and preterm birth.

    C. It increases the risk of maternal infectious morbidity.

    D. It is recommended to offer routine antibiotics to all women during pregnancy to prevent complications.

11. Which of the following outcomes is not improved in babies born to women with PPROM who are offered routine antibiotics?

    A. Prolongation of pregnancy

    B. Decreased requirement for surfactant and oxygen in babies after birth

    C. Decreased risk of perinatal mortality

    D. Decreased incidence of abnormal cerebral ultrasound of babies before discharge

12. According to World Health Organization (WHO) categorization of preterm births, which of the following is correct?

    A. Extremely preterm (<28 weeks)

    B. Very preterm (28 to <32 weeks)

    C. Moderate preterm (32 to <34 completed weeks of gestation)

    D. A and B

    E. All of the above

13. Which of the following vaccines are contraindicated during pregnancy?

    A. Intranasal live-attenuated influenza vaccine

    B. Yellow fever

    C. TDaP

    D. A and B

14. Which of the following factors is considered the strongest predictor of spontaneous preterm birth?

    A. Previous preterm birth

    B. Short cervical length

    C. Raised cervical-vaginal fetal fibronectin levels

    D. B and C

    E. All of the above

15. What is the clinically accepted definition of PPROM?

    A. PPROM is characterized by the spontaneous rupture of membranes prior to 37 weeks' gestation, occurring at least 1 hour before the initiation of contractions.

    B. PPROM is characterized by the spontaneous rupture of membranes prior to 37 weeks' gestation, occurring at least 2 hours before the initiation of contractions.

    C. PPROM is characterized by the spontaneous rupture of membranes prior to 37 weeks' gestation, occurring at least 6 hours before the initiation of contractions.

    D. PPROM is characterized by the spontaneous rupture of membranes prior to 37 weeks' gestation, occurring at least 12 hours before the initiation of contractions.

16. Which of the following ethnic groups are considered to be at highest risk of preterm birth?

    A. Black women

    B. Caucasians

    C. East-Asian

    D. Hispanics

17. Regarding recurrence of preterm birth in successive pregnancies, which of the following statements is not described correctly?

    A. The recurrence risk for women with a history of preterm delivery varies between 15% and over 50%.

    B. It is contingent upon the number and gestational age of prior deliveries.

    C. The likelihood of subsequent preterm births is directly proportional to the gestational age of the preceding preterm delivery.

    D. The fundamental mechanism of recurrence remains ambiguous.

18. According to available evidence, which of the following intrauterine infections is least likely to cause preterm birth?

    A. Maternal infection with bacterial vaginosis

    B. Maternal infection with *Ureaplasma urealyticum*

    C. Maternal infection with *Mycoplasma hominis*

    D. Maternal viral infection

ANSWERS

1. B	7. B	13. D
2. A	8. B	14. D
3. B	9. D	15. A
4. A	10. D	16. A
5. C	11. C	17. C
6. C	12. D	18. D

31 SIP – Reproductive Aging

Source: Reproductive Ageing Scientific Impact Paper No. 24 January 2011. https://www.rcog.org.uk/guidance/browse-all-guidance/scientific-impact-papers/reproductive-ageing-scientific-impact-paper-no-24/

IMPORTANT POINTS FROM THE GUIDELINE (SIP)

- The depletion rate of a woman's lifetime reserve of oocytes is inevitable.

- 'Unexplained infertility' is an uncommon diagnosis for couples with women in their 20s; however, it is the predominant cause of infertility in women over 35 years old.

- This rise results from the deterioration of oocyte 'quality' attributed to aging in women.

- Quality in this context denotes a multifaceted array of age-associated alterations in nuclear and cytoplasmic competence, influencing essential processes such as as spindle formation, chromosomal segregation, mitochondrial functionality, and cytoskeletal integrity.

- A poor-quality egg is less probable to undergo fertilization and, if fertilized, will provide an embryo that typically exhibits delayed division and a low likelihood of implantation.

- Women aged over 35 are at heightened risk for early pregnancy and associated obstetric and neonatal problems.

- The older women are at an increased risk of stillbirths, miscarriages, or ectopic pregnancies.

- Obstetric complications linked to advanced maternal age encompass gestational diabetes, placenta previa, placental abruption, hypertension, and cesarean delivery.

- Older women are more likely to be nulliparous, necessitate assisted reproductive technology for conception, and experience many pregnancies both naturally and through assisted reproductive methods, all of which are risk factors for heightened obstetric and neonatal morbidity.

- The ideal age for childbearing is between 20 and 35 years, considering both obstetric and reproductive health factors.

- Societal transformations over the last 40 years have led to a significant increase in the number of women postponing childbirth until their mid-30s or later.

- The majority can conceive naturally and deliver a healthy child at term if conception occurs at 35 years of age; however, the incidence of infertility, miscarriage, or fetal abnormalities escalates significantly thereafter, resulting in only two out of five individuals desiring a child at 40 years of age being able to achieve this goal.

- The average age of women undergoing in vitro fertilization (IVF) therapy in the UK is increasing, indicative of the rise in infertility associated with growing maternal age; nonetheless, success rates for women over 40 remain low.

- Women who consider family an essential aspect of their life fulfillment are advised to conclude childbearing by the age of 35.

- Numerous commercially available assays exist to assess ovarian reserve.

- Women undergoing assessments of their ovarian reserve must understand that these tests evaluate oocyte number rather than oocyte quality.

- Ovarian reserve refers to the number of oocytes present in a woman's ovaries at a specific moment in time.

- The ovarian reserve diminishes with age until menopause, at which point ovulation halts, leaving only a few hundred primordial follicles.

- The response to gonadotrophin stimulation fluctuates monthly within the same individual; therefore, maximally stimulating doses of gonadotrophins are frequently avoided clinically as a preventive measure against ovarian hyperstimulation syndrome, and transvaginal egg collection does not consistently retrieve all available oocytes in a cohort.

                                            DOI: 10.1201/9781003650355-31

- The quantification of serum follicle-stimulating hormone (FSH) concentration during the early follicular phase of the menstrual cycle has been fundamental in evaluating ovarian reserve in IVF practice for 30 years.

- As the oocyte pool decreases, increased pituitary stimulation is required to facilitate the establishment of a dominant follicle.

- Consequently, elevated levels of FSH indicate less ovarian reserve.

- The application of FSH measures in this context is flawed, as concentrations fluctuate due to pulsatile secretion from the pituitary, and no consensus on a cut-off level indicative of bad outcomes has been established.

- Nearly all IVF centers routinely assess early follicular phase FSH and depend on the data to inform clinical decision-making.

- Recent advancements in reliable antibody-based assays for inhibin B and anti-Müllerian hormone (AMH) have enabled the assessment of these granulosa cell products as indicators of ovarian reserve.

- Inhibin B is synthesized by tiny antral follicles in response to FSH stimulation, whereas AMH is predominantly produced by pre-antral follicles and is independent of FSH.

- AMH provides the most accurate prognostic value for evaluating ovarian reserve in women.

- AMH concentrations are relatively steady during the cycle, exhibiting minimal change from cycle to cycle; thus, blood sampling is simplified.

- Ovarian reserve can be evaluated by high-resolution transvaginal ultrasound to enumerate tiny antral follicles of 2–10 mm in diameter.

- Antral follicle count (AFC) is associated with oocyte yield in IVF and with several biochemical indicators.

- The disadvantages encompass the test's reliance on the operator and the necessity of visiting the ultrasonography facility, while newer studies have failed to demonstrate any advantage over AMH testing.

- All the aforementioned tests indicate the quantity of primordial follicles left in the ovaries rather than assessing their quality.

- The quantity of oocytes is directly associated with their quality, as evidenced by the recognized decrease in fertility and rise in chromosomal abnormalities in embryos from older women with diminished oocyte counts; however, this correlation does not necessarily extend to younger IVF patients, who may possess high-quality oocytes despite a low yield.

- Pre-IVF evaluations of ovarian reserve are inadequate indicators of pregnancy success.

- This is not unexpected, as numerous additional variables collectively influence the probability of live birth.

- The success of IVF will be affected by the embryology laboratory conditions, sperm quality, uterine and tubal variables such as hydrosalpinx or anatomical anomalies, endometrial receptivity, and the maternal response to pregnancy.

- None of these is significantly modified, if at all, by ovarian reserve.

- The primary factors influencing the likelihood of live birth are woman's age and oocyte yield.

- A diminished ovarian reserve in a young woman may necessitate additional specialist evaluation, including high-resolution transvaginal ultrasound for AFC and assessments to exclude recognized etiologies of premature ovarian failure.

- Advancements in oocyte vitrification enable young, healthy women to preserve oocytes until their less reproductive years.

- The probability of achieving a healthy pregnancy from a vitrified oocyte is minimal (4%), necessitating the collection and freezing of numerous eggs to provide a viable opportunity for future success.

- The optimal age for oocyte vitrification is likely below 30 years, leading to the medicalization of relatively young women.

- An unrealistic dependence on their reserve of vitrified oocytes may cause women to postpone childbearing for extended periods, ultimately resulting in disappointment when the preserved oocytes subsequently fail to fertilize or implant.

- An alternative method for addressing infertility due to ovarian aging is the utilization of oocytes from a younger, viable donor.

- Oocyte donors must undergo superovulation through the administration of reproductive medications, succeeded by transvaginal oocyte retrieval.

- This imposes a significant cost, deterring many potential volunteers due to the extent of intervention necessary.

- Another strategy to address the unavoidable decline in oocyte quality in older patients is to conduct embryo biopsy and testing; specifically, to evaluate IVF embryos for aneuploidy by preimplantation genetic screening (PGS), thereafter replacing only euploid embryos.

- Research has also been conducted on cytoplasmic transfer strategies to enhance the quality of mitochondria obtained from oocytes of young donors.

- Cytoplasmic transfer may enhance the likelihood of fertilization and implantation while circumventing the disadvantages of oocyte donation, enabling the woman to conceive a genetically related child.

- Reproductive aging affects male fertility and the health of their progeny.

- Although numerous men retain fertility into their fifth decade and beyond, the prevalence of spermatogenesis problems escalates with increasing age.

- Men over 40 years of age adversely affect a couple's fertility and fecundity, particularly when the female partner is similarly of advanced age.

- Advancing paternal age may correlate with reduced serum androgen levels, less sexual activity, changes in testicular morphology, and a decline in semen quality (volume, motility, and morphology).

- Advanced paternal age affects sperm DNA integrity and is believed to exert epigenetic influences.

QUESTIONS

1. What percentage of couples seeking fertility treatment in the UK are diagnosed with unexplained infertility?

    A. 10%

    B. 25%

    C. 40%

    D. 50%

2. What percentage of women after the age of 40 years will be able to have a healthy pregnancy and delivery at term?

    A. 10%

    B. 25%

    C. 40%

    D. 50%

3. In women strongly keen to plan a family, by what age should they be best advised to complete childbearing?

   A. 30 years

   B. 35 years

   C. 40 years

   D. 42 years

4. Which of the following commercially available tests for testing ovarian reserve can assess oocyte quality?

   A. AFC

   B. AMH

   C. FSH

   D. None of the above

   E. A and B

5. Which of the following tests has the best predictive value in assessing the ovarian reserve in women?

   A. AFC

   B. AMH

   C. FSH

   D. Serum inhibin B levels

6. Which factor is regarded as the most reliable indicator of ovarian response to stimulation in IVF?

   A. AFC

   B. AMH

   C. FSH

   D. Serum estradiol levels

7. AMH is produced from which of the following?

   A. Pre-antral follicle

   B. Antral follicle

   C. Zona pellucida

   D. Corona radiata

8. What is the normal AMH level in a young woman of reproductive age?

   A. 1–4 ng/mL

   B. 4–7 ng/mL

   C. 7–9 ng/mL

   D. >10 ng/mL

9. For young women of reproductive age, what is the best age for oocyte vitrification?

   A. <25 years

   B. <30 years

   C. Between 30–35 years

   D. Between 35–37 years

10. Regarding measurement of AFC for women of reproductive age group, which of the following statements is incorrect?

    A. It is measured by transvaginal scan.

    B. It is measured during the late-follicular phase of the menstrual cycle.

    C. It is the quantity of small follicles (2–10 mm) seen on ultrasonography, which are prospective egg-containing follicles.

    D. It is the sum of antral follicles in both ovaries.

11. According to latest reports in women who have undergone oocyte freezing, what is the clinical pregnancy rate per oocyte?

    A. 4–12%

    B. 15–20%

    C. 20–30%

    D. 70–80%

12. According to the latest research, what is the reported live birth rate in women who have undergone oocyte freezing?

    A. 4–12%

    B. 15–20%

    C. 25–30%

    D. 35–40%

13. Which of the following mechanisms is considered to be the most important cause of reproductive aging in women?

    A. Oxidative stress

    B. Mitochondrial defects

    C. Telomere shortening

    D. Meiotic chromosome segregation errors

14. Early menarche increases the risk of all of the following, except?

    A. Developing breast cancer

    B. Developing osteoporosis

    C. Developing cardiovascular diseases

    D. Developing metabolic disorders

15. Which factor in females is deemed the most significant determinant of heterogeneity in the onset of menopause?

    A. Birth weight

    B. Initial supply of follicles at the time of birth

    C. Body mass index (BMI)

    D. Chronological age of the woman

16. Which of the following factors increase the risk of premature and early menopause?

    A. Nulliparity

    B. Early menarche

    C. Breastfeeding for more than 6 months

    D. A and B

    E. All of the above

17. Which of the following correctly defines premature ovarian insufficiency (POI)?

    A. POI can be diagnosed in women under 40 who exhibit oligomenorrhea or amenorrhea for a minimum of 6 months, accompanied by FSH levels over 10 IU/L.

    B. POI can be diagnosed in women under 40 who exhibit oligomenorrhea or amenorrhea for a minimum of 4 months, accompanied by FSH levels exceeding 25 IU/L.

    C. POI can be diagnosed in women under 35 who exhibit oligomenorrhea or amenorrhea for a minimum of 6 months, accompanied by FSH levels over 10 IU/L.

    D. POI can be diagnosed in women under 35 who experience oligomenorrhea or amenorrhea for a minimum of 4 months, accompanied by FSH levels exceeding 25 IU/L.

18. What is the sole genetic marker currently utilized for the evaluation of individuals with suspected premature ovarian failure?

    A. The 5'-UTR contains a triplet-base repeat (CGG) in the FMR1 gene (fragile X mental retardation 1), situated on the long arm of the X chromosome at locus Xg27.3

    B. Non-reciprocal translocation between chromosomes 14 and 15

    C. Expansion of the CTG repeat in the DMPK gene

    D. Expansion of the GAA repeat within the FXN gene

19. Which of the following statements is incorrect about telomeres?

    A. They are repeating DNA sequences, generally 'TTACCG'.

    B. They shorten in length with age.

    C. They serve a protective function to avert the destruction of chromosomal ends.

    D. An enzyme known as 'telomerase' can preserve or lengthen telomeres.

ANSWERS

1. B	8. A	15. B
2. C	9. B	16. D
3. B	10. B	17. B
4. D	11. A	18. A
5. B	12. C	19. A
6. A	13. A	
7. A	14. B	

32 SIP – Reproductive Outcomes after Cervical Disease Treatments

Source: Reproductive Outcomes after Local Treatment for Preinvasive Cervical Disease Scientific Impact Paper No. 21 July 2016. https://www.rcog.org.uk/guidance/browse-all-guidance/scientific-impact-papers/reproductive-outcomes-after-local-treatment-for-preinvasive-cervical-disease-scientific-impact-paper-no21/

IMPORTANT POINTS FROM THE GUIDELINE (SIP)

- The implementation of systematic call and recall screening programs in the UK has led to a significant reduction in the incidence and death of invasive cervical cancer.

- The objective of the screening program is to detect preinvasive cervical disease (cervical intraepithelial neoplasia [CIN]).

- The therapy for CIN often involves excision, yielding excellent success rates.

- The average age of women receiving treatment for preinvasive cervical disease aligns with the age of women experiencing their first childbirth; therefore, evidence regarding the effects of cervical treatment on future fertility and pregnancy should be accessible for effective patient counseling at colposcopy and antenatal clinics.

- In the UK, outpatient long loop excision of the transformation zone (LLETZ) is the primary treatment, however certain units provide ablative therapy.

- A 2014 meta-analysis determined that local therapy for CIN does not negatively impact fertility.

- The pregnancy rate was greater for treated women compared to untreated ones.

- This may be attributed to the treatment's effect on fertility or to specialists advising postponement of pregnancy until after the initial postoperative phase.

- The scant available evidence precluded the categorization of risk based on cone length and treatment frequency.

- The effect of recurrent and proportionately extensive excisions on fertility is still ambiguous.

- A systematic review and meta-analysis indicated comparable rates of overall and first-trimester miscarriages between treated and untreated women; however, cervical therapy notably elevated the risk of second-trimester miscarriage relative to untreated controls.

- The meta-analysis indicated that women who received treatment exhibited elevated incidence of ectopic pregnancy and pregnancy termination in comparison to untreated persons.

- Excisional treatment elevates the risk of preterm birth (under 37 weeks of gestation), low birthweight (below 2500 g), and preterm prelabor rupture of membranes (PPROM).

- Their frequency and severity escalated with treatment modalities that excise substantial quantities of cervical tissue.

- There is growing evidence that the extent of cervical excision or destruction, as well as the cone length and volume, may serve as predictors for subsequent preterm birth.

- A meta-analysis indicated that excisional treatments over 10 mm in length heightened the risk of preterm, whereas smaller excisions did not.

- The risk escalated incrementally with the depth of the cones: the absolute risk was 9.6% for medium-sized cones (10–14 mm), 15.3% for big cones (15–19 mm), and 18% for very large cones (20 mm or larger).

- A further study indicated that the risk of preterm birth escalated thrice when the excision volume above 6 cm³ and/or the length exceeded 12 mm.

- It is predicted that each millimeter increase in cone length elevates the probability of preterm birth by 6%.

- The ratio of cervical volume to length excised may more accurately correlate with results than the actual excision length, given the significant variability in pretreatment cervical measurements.

DOI: 10.1201/9781003650355-32

- Women who underwent cold knife conization (CKC) were 3-fold more likely to deliver prior to 32–34 weeks of gestation (severe preterm) and almost 5-fold more likely to deliver before 28–30 weeks of gestation (extreme prematurity).

- Perinatal mortality was elevated following CKC.

- The incidence of these serious adverse events did not rise following LLETZ or laser ablation.

- The mechanism underlying the heightened risk of second-trimester loss and preterm delivery linked to CIN and its treatment remains unclear.

- It has been hypothesized that localized cervical intervention could eliminate a significant number of mucus-secreting endocervical glands, hence negatively impacting sperm motility, while pronounced cervical os stenosis may also impede conception.

- Although the acquired mechanical weakening of the cervix resulting from surgery may appear to be a reasonable inference, more nuanced mechanisms could be at play.

- Ascending vaginal infection into the fetoplacental unit and the resultant inflammation are believed to contribute to preterm labor.

- During pregnancy, the uterus is safeguarded by the cervix through its mucus plug, the localized production of antimicrobial peptides and proteins, and a predominately benign *Lactobacillus* vaginal microbiota.

- Lactobacilli suppress pathogen proliferation by sustaining an unfavorable pH and secreting species-specific metabolites and bacteriocins that restrict the growth of competing organisms.

- Resecting a portion of the cervix or being infected with human papillomavirus (HPV) may compromise the host's defense mechanisms, alter the chemical microenvironment, and hinder the maintenance of a pregnancy to full term.

- The risk of premature delivery following cervical therapy is 15%.

- Vaginal progesterone, as opposed to systemic progesterone, lowers the risk of premature birth in women with a shortened cervix overall.

- Numerous obstetricians feel that preterm labor subsequent to cervical therapy is attributable to 'cervical incompetence,' which may be rectified with cerclage.

- Nonetheless, cerclage is unsuitable for all women with a history of cervical therapy, as roughly 85% of them will achieve term delivery.

- Cervical cerclage does not diminish the risk of preterm labor in the general obstetric population when the sole risk factor is an incidentally identified short cervix in the second trimester; however, it does lower the risk in women with a short cervix who have a history of mid-trimester losses or preterm deliveries.

- Excisional methods, especially LLETZ, have predominantly supplanted destructive treatments in industrialized nations.

- The resulting specimen yields critical prognostic data regarding the grade, completeness of excision (excision margins), lack of (micro)invasion, and the stratified risk of future preterm based on the specimen's length.

- Repeated excisions increase both the frequency and severity of unfavorable reproductive outcomes.

- The colposcopist must therefore optimize treatment following a thorough colposcopy on the initial try, as margins significantly elevate the chance of high-grade recurrence.

- Prudence is advised when contemplating CIN treatment in nulliparous women.

- Treatment must be customized to properly address the condition while also minimizing reproductive complications.

- The HPV vaccine is expected to diminish the occurrence of preinvasive lesions necessitating therapy and further mitigate negative reproductive outcomes.

QUESTIONS

1. Which of the following is the preferred method of treatment for CIN in the UK?

    A. Laser ablation

    B. Laser conization

    C. CKC

    D. Outpatient LLETZ

2. According to the available research, women treated for CIN are at an increased risk of all of the following, except?

    A. Ectopic pregnancy

    B. Mid-trimester miscarriage

    C. First-trimester miscarriage

    D. Termination of pregnancy

3. To what extent is the risk of mid-trimester miscarriage increased after conization is performed for CIN in women of reproductive age group?

    A. 2-fold

    B. 4-fold

    C. 8-fold

    D. 10-fold

4. Which of the following statements regarding the effects of CKC on pregnancy outcomes is incorrect?

    A. Effects are dependent upon the amount of cervical tissue excised.

    B. Women undergoing CKC are three times more likely to deliver before (32–34 weeks).

    C. Women undergoing CKC are five times more likely to deliver before (28–30 weeks).

    D. It does not increase the perinatal mortality in newborns.

5. Above what length of cervical tissue excised during the excisional treatments for CIN, is the risk of prematurity increased?

    A. 5 mm

    B. 10 mm

    C. 15 mm

    D. 20 mm

6. Above what volume of cervical tissue excised during the excisional treatments for CIN, is the risk of prematurity increased 3-fold?

    A. $3\,cm^3$

    B. $6\,cm^3$

    C. $8\,cm^3$

    D. $10\,cm^3$

7. By what percentage does the risk of preterm birth increase with every 1 mm increase in cone length excised during excisional treatments for CIN?

    A. 2%   C. 10%

    B. 6%   D. 15%

8. What is the overall risk of preterm birth after a cervical treatment performed for CIN?

    A. 5%

    B. 10%

    C. 15%

    D. 25%

9. Which of the following are the possible reasons for preterm birth after an excision treatment for CIN?

    A. Mechanical weakness of the cervix

    B. Histological alterations in the repaired cervix, influencing tensile strength

    C. Diminished cervical antimicrobial functions, including mucus plug generation, permitting microbial entry into the uterine canal

    D. All of the above

    E. A and C

10. Which of the following interventions have evidence in preventing preterm birth in women who are incidentally detected with a short cervix on a routine mid-trimester scan?

    A. Cervical cerclage

    B. Vaginal progesterone

    C. Oral progesterone

    D. Cervical pessary

ANSWERS

1. D	5. B	9. D
2. C	6. B	10. B
3. B	7. B	
4. D	8. C	

33 SIP – Risk-Reducing Salpingo-Oophorectomy (RRSO)

Source: Risk-Reducing Salpingo-Oophorectomy and the Use of Hormone Replacement Therapy below the Age of Natural Menopause Scientific Impact Paper No. 66 October 2021. https://www.rcog.org.uk/guidance/browse-all-guidance/scientific-impact-papers/risk-reducing-salpingo-oophorectomy-and-the-use-of-hormone-replacement-therapy-below-the-age-of-natural-menopause-scientific-impact-paper-no-66/

IMPORTANT POINTS FROM THE GUIDELINE (SIP)

- In the UK, due to historically limited access to genetic testing, risk-reducing salpingo-oophorectomy (RRSO) has been provided to women from high-risk families with an estimated lifetime ovarian cancer risk of 10% or greater who could not obtain gene testing.

- RRSO is the most efficacious approach for preventing ovarian cancer and is economically viable for women with a lifetime ovarian cancer risk of 4–5% or higher.

- RRSO may also be provided to women with moderate risk gene mutations such as RAD51C, RAD51D, and BRIP1 (5–13% lifetime ovarian cancer risk), as well as to selected women with a notable family history of ovarian cancer (e.g. one or two first-degree relatives with ovarian cancer) who are categorized as intermediate risk (5–10% lifetime risk).

- PALB2 has been established as a gene associated with intermediate risk for ovarian cancer, leading some to advocate for RRSO in affected women, while others have insufficient evidence for this intervention.

- RRSO may be contemplated for women with PALB2 mutations after a non-directive counseling approach that considers supplementary risk and protective factors, ideally conducted around or post-menopause.

- Family history must be integrated into the personalized risk assessment procedure for all women.

- As the adoption of RRSO for ovarian cancer prevention rises, a greater number of women will encounter the enduring effects of premature surgical menopause.

- If not contraindicated, it is essential that hormone replacement therapy (HRT) is provided following premenopausal oophorectomy until the age of natural menopause.

- Women must obtain evidence-based information and multidisciplinary guidance, including advice on HRT, symptom management, specialized counseling, and ongoing support to address diverse physical, mental, and long-term health ramifications.

- RRSO has historically been provided and demonstrated to be both clinically efficacious and cost-efficient in BRCA1/BRCA2 mutation carriers and in women with Lynch syndrome (carriers of mismatch repair gene mutations [MLH1, MSH2, or MSH6]).

- A simultaneous hysterectomy is performed in individuals with Lynch syndrome due to their 40–60% lifetime risk of endometrial cancer.

- It is generally recommended at ages 35–40 for BRCA1 carriers, 40–45 for BRCA2 carriers, 40–50 for RAD51C/RAD51D carriers, and around or beyond menopause (ages above 45–50) for PALB2 carriers.

- In BRIP1 carriers and mutation-negative women at intermediate risk (5–10% lifetime ovarian cancer risk) with a significant family history, it may be postponed until ages 45 to 50.

- Women receive optimal care in specialized high-risk clinics or through multidisciplinary teams that include gynecologists or gynecological oncologists with a focus on high-risk women's health, alongside psychologists, clinical nurses, and menopause specialists.

- Links to clinical genetics, as well as breast and colorectal teams, should also be included.

- Individuals who are carriers of BRCA1 and BRCA2 mutations do not exhibit an elevated risk for endometrial cancer.

DOI: 10.1201/9781003650355-33

- Iatrogenic menopause resulting from RRSO may be linked to vasomotor symptoms, mood alterations, sleep disturbances, diminished libido, vaginal dryness, dyspareunia, and inferior sexual functioning relative to women who preserve their ovaries. The utilization of HRT alleviates all these problems.

- Sexual dysfunction after RRSO has been recorded in up to 74% of women, in contrast to the general population's incidence of 40–45%.

- Research within the general population indicates that premenopausal oophorectomy correlates with a heightened risk of cardiovascular disease, resulting in an absolute mortality increase of up to 3% from heart disease in low-risk women who have undergone early surgical menopause without HRT.

- Women at low risk who have undergone early surgical menopause without HRT are at an elevated risk of stroke, neurocognitive impairment, dementia, and parkinsonism.

- Estrogen-only hormone replacement therapy (E-HRT) is recommended for women who have undergone hysterectomy alongside RRSO.

- In individuals with an intact uterus, estrogen is administered alongside a progestogen (E+P-HRT) to safeguard against endometrial hyperplasia and cancer.

- Progestogens may be administered cyclically to provoke regular withdrawal bleeds or continuously in a formulation that eliminates bleeding.

- Estrogens may be administered orally or transdermally (subcutaneous implants are no longer available in the UK).

- Transdermal estrogens exhibit a reduced risk of venous thromboembolism (VTE), stroke, and myocardial infarction compared to oral formulations.

- Vaginal estrogen does not cause an elevated risk of endometrial hyperplasia.

- Progestogens may be administered orally, transdermally, or via a progestogen-releasing intra-uterine device directly within the uterus. The latter is linked to a reduced incidence of side effects compared to systemic progestogen.

- Oral micronized progesterone may possess a superior risk profile compared to synthetic progestogens.

- Tibolone is a synthetic steroid exhibiting estrogenic, progestogenic, and androgenic properties. This can be utilized as continuous combined HRT to address vasomotor, psychosocial, and libido issues post-surgical menopause, while preserving bone mass and mitigating the risk of vertebral fractures.

- Premenopausal oophorectomy decreases free androgen index values by 50%.

- Testosterone treatment may be advantageous for women suffering from diminished energy and libido, even with sufficient estrogen replacement.

- Transdermal testosterone enhances sexual activity, orgasms, and libido.

- In the UK, there are no licensed treatments for women; therefore, care should be administered in specialized facilities, ensuring access to hormone assays and monitoring for unwanted effects.

- Off-license formulations of testosterone comprise gels and subcutaneous implants; their usage should be assessed after 3 to 6 months and is typically restricted to a duration of 24 months.

- In a low-risk general population of women, E+P-HRT is linked to an elevated risk of breast cancer, with a meta-analysis indicating that E-HRT may also heighten risk, but to a significantly lesser extent than E+P-HRT.

- Insufficient data on BRCA carriers have not demonstrated a notable difference in breast cancer risk between E-alone or E+P preparations (relative to non-users); nevertheless, further long-term data and bigger, well-structured trials are necessary to validate this finding.

- Among women with low-risk E-HRT exhibits a superior risk profile compared to E+P-HRT. Additional data on high-risk BRCA women is required.

- For breast cancer patients with just vaginal or urogenital symptoms, non-hormonal interventions, including lubricants and moisturizers, are the primary alternatives.

- Ospemifene, a novel selective estrogen receptor modulator exhibiting estrogenic effects in the vagina, may be advantageous for symptomatic vulvovaginal atrophy (VVA). Nevertheless, sufficient data concerning women with breast cancer is deficient. Therefore, its use is currently not advised for this demography of women.

- Intravaginal administration of dehydroepiandrosterone (DHEA) has demonstrated clinical efficacy for the symptoms of VVA; however, its usage is not currently advised for women with a history of breast cancer due to inadequate safety data.

- In cases where non-hormonal alternatives are ineffective and symptoms are severe, short-term topical estrogen at the minimal effective vaginal dosage may be contemplated, contingent upon expert consultation, including for patients with estrogen receptor-positive breast cancer with a favorable prognosis.

- It is recommended to administer vaginal estrogen in conjunction with tamoxifen rather than with aromatase inhibitors. The impact of systemic estrogen absorption may be mitigated by tamoxifen's mechanism of action at the receptor level in breast tissue.

- While the overall risk of endometrial cancer does not rise following RRSO, there is a deficiency of specific data about the risk of endometrial cancer associated with HRT use in BRCA carriers or women at elevated risk for ovarian cancer.

- In accordance with recommendations for individuals at low risk, only combined regimens should be administered to women possessing a uterus.

- In healthy postmenopausal women, continuous combined HRT is linked to a marginally reduced incidence of endometrial hyperplasia or cancer compared to cyclical regimens.

- Oral HRT is linked to an elevated risk of VTE, particularly within the initial year of treatment, and seems to be greater with estrogen plus progestogen HRT compared to estrogen-only HRT.

- The risk of VTE with conventional therapeutic doses of transdermal HRT is comparable to the baseline population risk.

- Transdermal HRT should be preferred over oral formulations for women at heightened risk of VTE, particularly those with a body mass index exceeding 30 kg/m^2.

- There are few contraindications, mostly a history of breast cancer and a personal history of VTE or thrombophilia. Nonetheless, the latter may be deemed appropriate for transdermal HRT following a discussion of the benefits and hazards, along with consultation from hematology specialists on an individual basis.

- HRT should not be administered in cases of undiagnosed abnormal vaginal bleeding, or in the presence of suspected or active endometrial cancer.

- Following the initiation of HRT, it is recommended to reassess therapy after three months and subsequently on an annual basis.

- Although routine testing may be unnecessary, investigations should be initiated by particular symptoms or concerns, such as unexpected bleeding.

- Serum hormone levels are typically uninformative for guiding treatment decisions.

- Assessing and providing guidance on cardiovascular risk factors is essential.

- Evaluation of osteoporosis risk should be conducted.

- Dual energy X-ray absorptiometry (DEXA) scanning for bone mineral density (BMD) should be contemplated 1–2 years post-RRSO, particularly if there are supplementary risk factors for compromised bone health.

- If BMD is normal and HRT has been administered, the utility of a second DEXA scan is minimal.

- Women with diagnosed osteoporosis, a significant familial predisposition, or those at heightened risk from aromatase inhibitor therapy for breast cancer should get initial and periodic DEXA scans every 2 to 5 years.

- Routine monitoring of endometrial thickness is unnecessary during the administration of topical or systemic HRT.
- Alternatives to HRT include:
  - Pharmacological treatments such as selective serotonin reuptake inhibitors (SSRIs), selective noradrenaline reuptake inhibitors (SNRIs), clonidine, gabapentin, and beta-blockers.
  - Venlafaxine 37.5 mg, escalated to 150 mg/day, paroxetine 10 mg/day, or citalopram 10–30 mg/day are the most efficacious medications.
  - Clonidine 100 µg per day significantly reduced the frequency of hot flushes and enhanced quality of life in women with breast cancer compared to placebo, albeit it may entail intolerable adverse effects.
  - Cognitive behavioral therapy.
  - Psychoeducation and mindfulness.
  - Physical exercise.
  - Phytoestrogens are contraindicated for breast cancer survivors.
  - Vaginal lubricants and moisturizers help alleviate vaginal dryness during coitus.
- To mitigate the risk of bone demineralization and enhance cardiovascular health post-RRSO, women are recommended to adopt a healthy lifestyle, engage in weight-bearing exercises, refrain from smoking and excessive alcohol consumption, and sustain a normal body weight (corresponding to a body mass index of 18.5–24.9 kg/m²).
- It is recommended to supplement a total daily intake of 1200 mg of calcium and 600–1000 IU of vitamin D3.

QUESTIONS

1. What is the overall lifetime risk of ovarian cancer in the general population?
   A. 0.1%
   B. 1.4%
   C. 2–3%
   D. 5%

2. Which of the following is considered the strongest risk factor of ovarian cancer?
   A. Nulliparity
   B. Family history of ovarian cancer
   C. Intake of oral contraceptive pills
   D. Avoidance of breastfeeding post-delivery

3. What is the lifetime risk of developing epithelial cancer in individuals with hereditary ovarian cancer syndromes who have a minimum of two first-degree relatives diagnosed with epithelial ovarian cancer?
   A. 1–4%
   B. 4–5%
   C. 10%
   D. 13–50%

4. Which of the following gynecological cancers is the most common cause of death?

    A. Endometrial cancer

    B. Cervical cancer

    C. Breast cancer

    D. Ovarian cancer

5. Which of the following is the most effective method of prevention of ovarian cancer in BRCA1 and BRCA2 carriers?

    A. Taking oral contraceptive pills

    B. Lifestyle modification

    C. RRSO

    D. Annual transvaginal scan and serum CA-125 levels

6. In BRCA1 and BRCA2 carriers, what is the residual risk of primary peritoneal cancer after RRSO?

    A. <1%

    B. 2–4%

    C. 5–10%

    D. 15%

7. In high-risk families in the UK, what is the estimated lifetime risk of ovarian cancer?

    A. 2–4%

    B. 10%

    C. 15%

    D. 20%

8. What is the lifetime risk of endometrial cancer in patients with Lynch syndrome?

    A. 10–20%

    B. 20–40%

    C. 40–60%

    D. 80%

9. In women who are carriers of BRCA1, what is the suggested age for performing RRSO?

    A. From 35–40 years

    B. From 40–45 years

    C. From 40–50 years

    D. >45–50 years

10. In women who are carriers of BRCA2, what is the suggested age for performing RRSO?

    A. From 35–40 years

    B. From 40–45 years

    C. From 40–50 years

    D. >45–50 years

11. In women who are carriers of RAD51C and RAD51D with increased risk of ovarian cancer, what is the suggested age for performing RRSO?

A. From 35–40 years

B. From 40–45 years

C. From 40–50 years

D. >45–50 years

12. In women who are carriers of BRIP1 and PALB2 with increased risk of ovarian cancer, what is the suggested age for performing RRSO?

A. From 35–40 years

B. From 40–45 years

C. From 40–50 years

D. >45–50 years

13. In women with Lynch syndrome, who are carriers of MLH1, MSH2, MSH6, what is the suggested age of performing RRSO with concomitant hysterectomy?

A. From 35–40 years

B. From 40–45 years

C. From 40–50 years

D. >45–50 years

14. Patients with Lynch syndrome are at an increased risk of all of the following cancers, except?

A. Colorectal cancer

B. Endometrial cancer

C. Ovarian cancer

D. Breast cancer

15. What is the reported incidence of sexual dysfunction after RRSO?

A. Up to 40%

B. Up to 60%

C. Up to 75%

D. Up to 90%

16. What is the reported absolute increase in mortality due to heart disease in low-risk women who have undergone premenopausal oophorectomy?

A. <1%

B. Up to 3%

C. Up to 10%

D. Up to 15%

17. What is the recommended timing of initiation and duration of HRT after RRSO?

A. After ruling out contraindications, it should be initiated 4–6 weeks postoperatively and continued until natural age of menopause (about 51 years).

B. After ruling out contraindications, it should be initiated immediately postoperatively and continued until natural age of menopause (about 51 years).

C. After ruling out contraindications, it should be initiated 4–6 weeks postoperatively and continued for 5 years.

D. After ruling out contraindications, it should be initiated immediately postoperatively and continued for 5 years.

18. A 38-year-old patient presents to your outpatient department (OPD) with history of breast lump that she felt on routine self-breast examination. On examination, it looked suspicious and hence biopsy is advised. A diagnosis of ductal carcinoma of breast is made. The patient is referred to the family genetics department, where she and her sister are tested to be positive for BRCA1 gene. The patient is planned for a bilateral mastectomy and RRSO. She is keen to know about HRT after her surgery. Which of the following statements regarding HRT is not true?

   A. E-HRT is recommended for women who have undergone hysterectomy and RRSO.

   B. For individuals with an intact uterus, estrogen is administered in conjunction with a pro-gestogen (E+P-HRT) to safeguard against endometrial hyperplasia and cancer.

   C. Transdermal estrogens present a comparable risk of VTE, stroke, and myocardial infarction as oral formulations.

   D. Vaginal estrogen does not correlate with an elevated risk of endometrial hyperplasia.

19. All of the following statements regarding tibolone as HRT are true, except?

   A. It is a synthetic steroid.

   B. It possesses anti-androgenic properties.

   C. It may be utilized as continuous combined HRT to address vasomotor, psychosocial, and libido issues subsequent to surgical menopause.

   D. It can preserve bone density and diminish the likelihood of vertebral fractures.

20. By what percentage does premenopausal oophorectomy reduce the free androgen index?

   A. 20%   C. 40%

   B. 30%   D. 50%

21. What is the mechanism of action of ospemifene?

   A. Selective glucocorticoid receptor agonist

   B. Selective serotonin receptor agonist

   C. Selective estrogen receptor modulator

   D. Selective progesterone receptor modulator

22. After starting HRT, how frequently should the therapy be reviewed?

   A. Review therapy after 1 month and semi-annually thereafter

   B. Review therapy after 3 months and semi-annually thereafter

   C. Review therapy after 6 months and annually thereafter

   D. Review therapy after 3 months and annually thereafter

23. Regarding alternative therapies for HRT, which of the following statements is not true?

   A. Pharmacological treatments, such as venlafaxine at 37.5 mg titrated to 150 mg/day, parox-etine at 10 mg/day, or citalopram at 10–30 mg/day, are the most efficacious agents.

   B. Phytoestrogens are recommended for those who have survived breast cancer.

   C. Cognitive behavioral therapy and exercise are efficacious in ameliorating endocrine and urinary problems.

   D. Vaginal lubricants may help alleviate vaginal dryness.

24. What is the recommended daily dose of calcium and vitamin D3 to maintain bone health in women who have undergone RRSO?

   A. 500 mg/day of calcium and 500 IU/day of vitamin D3

   B. 1000 mg/day of calcium and 1000 IU/day of vitamin D3

   C. 1200 mg/day of calcium and 600–1000 IU/day of vitamin D3

   D. 1000 mg/day of calcium and 2000 IU/day of vitamin D3

25. Which of the following is an absolute contraindication to HRT?

    A. Personal history of VTE

    B. Personal history of thrombophilias

    C. BMI >30 kg/m²

    D. Undiagnosed abnormal vaginal bleeding

26. A 39-year-old patient presents to your gynecology OPD with a breast lump. She is examined by the breast cancer specialist team and offered a biopsy as the lump felt suspicious on examination. The biopsy report is suggestive of ductal carcinoma of the breast. The patient and her family is referred for genetic counseling and testing for BRCA genes. Upon testing, the patient is found to be positive for BRCA1 gene. The patient is keen to know, to what extent does RRSO reduce the risk of ovarian/fallopian/peritoneal cancer?

    A. By about 40%

    B. By about 50%

    C. By about 60%

    D. By about 80%

27. What percentage of patients who are BRCA1 and BRCA2 positive undergoing RRSO are diagnosed with serous tubal intraepithelial carcinoma (STIC) of the fallopian tube?

    A. <1%

    B. 4–10%

    C. 15%

    D. 20–30%

28. Regarding the role of HRT in patients who are BRCA gene positive, which of the following statements is false?

    A. HRT is recommended until the age of natural menopause (51 years) after RRSO.

    B. The particular variant of the BRCA mutation may affect the risk of breast cancer linked to HRT.

    C. Breast tumors in BRCA2 carriers are often negative for estrogen and progestin receptors and exhibit reduced susceptibility to hormonal influence compared to those originating in BRCA1 carriers.

    D. HRT does not influence breast cancer mortality.

ANSWERS

1. B	11. C	21. C
2. B	12. D	22. D
3. D	13. A	23. B
4. D	14. D	24. C
5. C	15. C	25. D
6. B	16. B	26. D
7. B	17. B	27. B
8. C	18. C	28. C
9. A	19. B	
10. B	20. D	

34 SIP – Sentinel Lymph Node Biopsy (SLNB) in Endometrial Cancer

Source: Sentinel Lymph Node Biopsy in Endometrial Cancer Scientific Impact Paper No. 51 July 2016. https://www.rcog.org.uk/guidance/browse-all-guidance/scientific-impact-papers/sentinel-lymph-node-biopsy-in-endometrial-cancer-scientific-impact-paper-no51/

IMPORTANT POINTS FROM THE GUIDELINE (SIP)

- Sentinel lymph node biopsy (SLNB) entails the excision of a SLN, which is the initial node implicated in the dissemination of a tumor from the primary cancer to the lymphatic system.

- If this result is negative, it is inferred that the other nodes are not implicated.

- Sentinel nodal status may impact the delivery of adjuvant therapy, including radiation, chemotherapy, or a combination of both.

- Among gynecological malignancies, SLNB may significantly influence outcomes in women with endometrial cancer.

- Additionally, sentinel node biopsy is conducted in several women with breast cancer and is being recognized as the standard practice for women with vulvar cancer in the UK.

- The fundamental treatment for the majority of women with endometrial cancer is surgical intervention, specifically a total hysterectomy and bilateral salpingo-oophorectomy, with or without lymph node dissection.

- Minimally invasive surgery, now the favored technique, has been linked to diminished pain levels, shorter hospital stays, and expedited return to everyday activities in comparison to open surgery.

- Randomized controlled trials of complete pelvic lymph node dissection have not demonstrated a significant overall survival benefit; nevertheless, lymph node metastases remains a critical prognostic marker in endometrial cancer.

- It is crucial to distinguish lymph node sampling from systematic dissection.

- Lymph node sample entails the excision of a select number of nodes, typically when they are suspected to be positive for metastatic dissemination, usually determined through palpation and visual evaluation of nodal dimensions.

- A systematic lymph node dissection entails the excision of all nodes within a nodal drainage basin, regardless of their size.

- A lymph node dissection that removes micro-metastases is improbable to provide therapeutic advantage; nonetheless, it may reveal more aggressive malignancies necessitating additional interventions, such as chemotherapy.

- A SLNB should ideally offer a more sensitive approach for evaluating the dissemination of early-stage endometrial cancer compared to lymph node dissection, facilitating targeted adjuvant treatments such as radiotherapy or chemotherapy.

- Evidence indicates a greater detection rate of lymph node metastases with SLNB compared to conventional lymphadenectomy.

- The incidence of leg lymphoedema subsequent to node dissection is frequently underestimated, with rates ranging from 5% to 38%.

- The substitution of lymph node dissection with SLNB diminishes both acute and chronic morbidity in various malignancies.

- It can be inferred that SLNB in endometrial cancer correlates with decreased morbidity relative to complete lymphadenectomy.

- EBRT diminishes the likelihood of locoregional recurrence but does not significantly affect cancer-related mortality or overall survival rates.

- It is linked to considerable morbidity and a decline in quality of life.

DOI: 10.1201/9781003650355-34

- In comparison to postoperative radiation, the administration of combination chemotherapy yielded a substantial enhancement in overall and progression-free survival rates.

- The majority of women diagnosed with endometrial cancer will present with grade 1 or 2 endometrioid tumors.

- The likelihood of nodal involvement in this cohort of women is minimal.

- The prevalence of pelvic node positive is documented as 0%, 3%, and 11% in women with no, inner third, and outer third myometrial invasion, respectively.

- The likelihood of extrauterine dissemination significantly escalated with tumor grade.

- The preoperative grade determined by endometrial biopsy may not consistently correspond to the final grade of the hysterectomy material, with 15% to 27% of women seeing an upgrade.

- Women diagnosed with grade 3 endometrioid cancer, as well as those with more aggressive tumor types such as serous and clear cell tumors, face a significantly elevated risk of extrauterine dissemination.

- As many as 70% of women with serous carcinoma and 50% with clear cell carcinoma present with stage III or IV illness.

- The lymphatic drainage of the uterus typically occurs via the parametrium to the pelvic sidewall, encompassing dissemination to the iliac and obturator nodes.

- Metastatic illness may subsequently disseminate from the pelvic sidewall to the common iliac and ultimately para-aortic lymph nodes.

- Alternative drainage, encompassing the uterine fundus, may also occur via the ovarian arteries directly to the superior para-aortic nodes.

- It seems rational that fundal tumors may disseminate via the ovarian vessels directly to the aortic nodes situated above the inferior mesenteric artery at the renal vein level, particularly on the left side.

- This indicates that if the sentinel node is located in the para-aortic region, it may be overlooked by methods that entail injecting a substance into a location that drains to the pelvic nodes.

- The incidence of isolated metastases to the high para-aortic area ranged from 1% to 6%.

- Various techniques exist for administering radioactive tracers or colored dyes.

- These encompass cervical injection, hysteroscopic injection, and sub-serosal myometrial injection.

- Cervical injection is the most accessible due to the ease of reaching the cervix.

- This approach resembles that employed for SLNB in cervical cancer.

- The primary issue with cervical injection alone is the risk of overlooking metastatic dissemination via the ovarian drainage pathway to the para-aortic area, resulting in false-negative outcomes.

- The use of a fundal injection alongside the cervical injection did not seem to yield an increased detection rate.

- No definitive evidence exists regarding the preferred injection sites and depths.

- Injection into the cervical stroma, just beneath the epithelium, appears to be the most often employed method.

- Cervical injection appears to have detection rates ranging from 80% to 100%.

- Several studies have employed the hysteroscopic injection approach into the endometrium to locate the SLN.

- This technique is proposed to correctly represent the true drainage patterns of individual endometrial cancer by seeing the tumor.

- The approach is logistically the most intricate, and concerns have been expressed that hysteroscopic injection may pose the risk of propagating malignant cells via the fallopian tubes.

- The detection rate does not seem to exceed that of the other two methods and has been documented to range from 50% to 82%.

- Some researchers choose subserosal myometrial injection.

- This approach is believed to enhance detection of both pelvic drainage and para-aortic routes; nevertheless, it necessitates surgical injection of the tracer into the uterine body, rendering the use of technetium-99m (99mTc) technically challenging.

- The preoperative injection of 99mTc under ultrasound guidance may render this procedure painful for the patient and complicate the injection into the posterior portion of the uterine corpus.

- The detection rate appears to rise with the number of injections administered at various locations within the uterine corpus.

- Detection rates fluctuate significantly, ranging from 0% to 92%.

- Sentinel node mapping entails the injection of a tracer substance near the original tumor, subsequent detection of the tracer, and excision of the lymph node for histological examination.

- 99mTc may be provided either the day prior to or on the same day as surgery, facilitating the preoperative identification of sentinel node/s on both sides using single-photon emission computed tomography (SPECT) scan.

- This facilitates precise preoperative identification of the node/s.

- The 99mTc is identified intraoperatively via a gamma probe.

- Numerous centers utilize 99mTc in conjunction with a blue dye to visually identify the lymphatic pathways leading to the sentinel nodes.

- At times, a sentinel node may not be detected on one side of the pelvis; in such cases, a formal lymph node dissection is typically performed on that side.

- Factors contributing to the inability to identify a node encompass issues with the injection at the primary tumor site and obstruction of lymphatic pathways caused by the tumor.

- This phenomenon particularly arises with substantial primary tumors.

- A range of blue dye compounds is available, including isosulfan blue 1%, methylene blue 1%, and patent blue 2.5%.

- The blue dye is administered 10–20 minutes before the commencement of surgery, permitting the dye to permeate the lymphatic systems and reach the lymph nodes.

- This approach offers the benefits of user-friendliness and the absence of requirement for specialized equipment.

- Disadvantages encompass the necessity to access the entire retroperitoneal area to visualize the nodes and the reliance on a certain degree of subjectivity in visual evaluation.

- A minority (less than 1%) of women receiving injections may experience an adverse reaction, including anaphylaxis.

- The utilization of near-infrared (NIR) imaging for the detection of fluorescent dyes, such as ICG, represents an innovative technology with preliminary evidence indicating it may surpass the efficacy of blue dye alone.

- This approach integrates the advantages of the blue dye technique (visibility) with nuclear medicine methods (signal penetration into intact tissue) into a singular modality, relying on the capacity of certain dyes or fluorophores, such as ICG, to glow in the near-infrared light spectrum.

- Fluorescence occurs when a laser emitted from a near-infrared imager stimulates the dye, resulting in a wavelength that is transformed into a fluorescent image.

- The imager can be incorporated into the laparoscope or robotic system.
- The dependability of SLNB depends on the sentinel node detection rate, procedural sensitivity, and false-negative rate.
- In the setting of SLNB, false positives are virtually non-existent, resulting in a specificity of 100%.
- Current standards for SLNB stipulate that if a sentinel node is not detected on one side of the pelvis, a complete pelvic lymphadenectomy should be performed on that side.
- This would represent a substantial alteration in practice for certain individuals in the UK, particularly among low-risk women.
- Given the little morbidity associated with the SLNB technique, it may be advantageous for all women to undergo SLNB to assist in identifying those necessitating chemotherapy or radiotherapy.

QUESTIONS

1. According to latest guidelines, SLNB should be offered to which of the following women diagnosed with endometrial cancer?

    A. Women with low or intermediate risk of metastasis

    B. Women who are unfit for systematic lymphadenopathy

    C. Grade 1 and 2 endometroid cancer apparently confined to the uterus

    D. All of the above

    E. B and C

2. What is the estimated incidence of isolated metastases to the para-aortic lymph nodes in patients diagnosed with endometrial cancer?

    A. <1%

    B. 1–6%

    C. 10%

    D. 15%

3. According to latest guidelines, which of the following is the preferred site for injection of the tracer for SLNB in patients with endometrial cancer?

    A. Cervix

    B. Hysteroscopic-guided injection into the tumor site

    C. Sub-serosal myometrial injection

    D. Fundal myometrial injection

4. For detection of the sentinel node through a cervical injection, which of the following is the preferred site where the tracer is injected into the cervix?

    A. Ectocervix

    B. Endocervical canal

    C. Cervical stroma

    D. Transformation zone

5. According to the National Comprehensive Cancer Network (NCCN) guidelines, which of the following is most commonly used as a tracer during SLNB in patients with endometrial cancer?

   A. 99mTc colloid

   B. Methylene blue 1%

   C. Isosulfan blue 2.5%

   D. Fluorescent dye indocyanine green

6. According to latest guidelines, which of the following has the highest detection rate for SLN, during SLNB in patients with endometrial cancer?

   A. 99mTc colloid

   B. Methylene blue 1%

   C. Isosulfan blue 2.5%

   D. Fluorescent dye indocyanine green

7. The reliability of SLNB in context of endometrial cancer, depends upon all of the following factors, except?

   A. Detection rate of the sentinel node

   B. The sensitivity of the procedure

   C. The false-negative rate

   D. The false-positive rate

8. What is the specificity of SLNB?

   A. 70%   C. 90%

   B. 80%   D. 100%

9. According to the SENTI-ENDO study, what is the overall detection rate of SLNB in the right and left hemipelvis?

   A. 55–60%   C. 85–90%

   B. 75–80%   D. >90%

10. In what percentage of cases is there failed SLN mapping?

    A. 1%   C. 6%

    B. 3%   D. 10%

11. A 60-year-old postmenopausal woman, diagnosed with a grade 1 endometroid type of endometrial cancer, undergoing total laparoscopic hysterectomy, is planned for SLNB. Upon injecting the dye, there is no SLN detected on the right hemipelvis (failed SLN mapping). According to the NCCN guidelines, what is the recommended option in her surgery?

    A. No need of full pelvic lymph node dissection in the right hemipelvis

    B. No need of full pelvic lymph node dissection in the right and left hemipelvis

    C. Perform para-aortic lymphadenectomy (at the discretion of the surgeon)

    D. It is recommended to perform full pelvic lymph node dissection in the right hemipelvis (side-specific lymphadenectomy)

12. A 62-year-old postmenopausal woman, diagnosed with a grade 2 endometroid type of endometrial cancer, undergoing total laparoscopic hysterectomy, is planned for SLNB. Upon injecting the dye, a positive SLN is detected on the right hemipelvis. According to the NCCN guidelines, what is the recommended option in her surgery?

    A. No need of full pelvic lymph node dissection in the right hemipelvis

    B. No need of full pelvic lymph node dissection in the right and left hemipelvis

    C. Perform para-aortic lymphadenectomy (at discretion of the surgeon)

    D. Side-specific lymphadenectomy to be performed

13. What percentage of women injected with isosulfan blue dye as a tracer for SLNB, are at risk of anaphylaxis?

    A. 1 in 1000

    B. 1%

    C. 3%

    D. 10%

14. Which of the following side effects are seen with injection of 1% methylene blue solution as tracer for SLNB?

    A. Serotonin syndrome

    B. Paradoxical methemoglobinemia

    C. Risk of metastasis of tumor cells

    D. All of the above

    E. A and B

15. According to the NCCN guidelines, which of the following statements regarding the role of frozen section of SLN in patients with endometrial cancer is incorrect?

    A. Only nodes deemed suspicious should be submitted for frozen section analysis.

    B. It is recommended routinely for all SLNs on a regular basis.

    C. The outcomes of the frozen section dictate the necessity for para-aortic lymph node dissection.

    D. The frozen section exhibits low sensitivity for detecting metastases.

ANSWERS

1. D	6. D	11. D
2. B	7. D	12. C
3. A	8. D	13. B
4. C	9. B	14. E
5. A	10. C	15. B

35 SIP – Sex Steroid Treatment in Young Girls

Source: Sex Steroid Treatment for Pubertal Induction and Replacement in the Adolescent Girl Scientific Impact Paper No. 40 June 2013. https://www.rcog.org.uk/guidance/browse-all-guidance/scientific -impact-papers/sex-steroid-treatment-for-pubertal-induction-and-replacement-in-the-adolescent-girl -scientific-impact-paper-no-40/

IMPORTANT POINTS FROM THE GUIDELINE (SIP)

- Females with hypogonadism necessitate sex steroid replacement to facilitate pubertal development comparable to that of females with normal gonadal function.

- Many girls exhibiting pubertal delay may inevitably necessitate a condensed regimen of sex steroid replacement to align their development with that of their peers.

- The primary considerations encompass the timing for initiating estrogen therapy in girls with confirmed estrogen deficiency, the duration of unopposed estrogen required to replicate normal puberty, potential interactions with other pubertal treatments such as growth hormone, and the strategy for maintenance therapy after reaching the adult dosage.

- The primary objective of inducing puberty in girls with hypogonadism is to facilitate the timely development of secondary sexual characteristics, particularly breast and uterine maturation.

- This results in menstruation, the onset of the pubertal growth spurt, and ultimately, the attainment of maximal bone mass, which persists until about the age of 30.

- The initial effects of estrogen will manifest as breast budding, observed in 50% of females by the age of 11.3 years.

- By the age of 13.3, 50% of girls reach breast stage four, characterized by near complete growth and high areola.

- The mean age of menarche in the UK is 13 years.

- Concerning bone development, low-dose estrogen promotes height velocity, whereas high-dose estrogen leads to the closing of the epiphyseal growth plates.

- Most breast development happens over the 2 years preceding menarche.

- This would equate to 2 years of unopposed estrogen in therapeutic terms.

- Girls with a total lack of breast growth should be referred for comprehensive evaluation starting at age 13, whereas those with primary amenorrhea but normal breast development should be referred by age 15.

- The latter presentation suggests an absence of estrogen shortage and encompasses structural factors like Rokitansky syndrome, as well as euestrogenic causes of amenorrhoea, such as polycystic ovary syndrome (PCOS).

- The administration of exogenous estrogen for the induction of puberty should strive to accomplish the developmental milestones of puberty promptly.

- In young females with established estrogen deficiency, low-dose estrogen therapy may commence at the age of 10.

- In this scenario, a complete duration of 2–3 years of unopposed estrogen might be attained prior to the introduction of progesterone to induce the initial withdrawal bleed at age 13.

- Progesterone treatment should consistently occur several months after estrogen, so the combined oral contraceptive pill is never employed for initiating puberty.

- A prevalent scenario involves a female exhibiting delayed puberty during her adolescence, with estrogen exposure occurring at least 4 years later than expected. The initial dosage and rate of escalation for estrogen will be customized according on the age at presentation and the individual's specific concerns.

- Regardless of the tardiness of a girl's presentation, it is generally feasible to let a duration of 6–12 months of unopposed estrogen prior to the introduction of progestogens.

DOI: 10.1201/9781003650355-35

- The delayed delivery of estrogen frequently results in compromised breast growth, suggesting the existence of an ideal period for optimal breast and uterine development.

- The early administration of progestogen may negatively impact breast growth.

- Nonetheless, the combined oral contraceptive should be strictly avoided for the commencement of puberty at any age.

- Administering estrogen must be conducted in collaboration with a pediatric endocrinologist.

- In the UK, ethinyl-estradiol is frequently utilized, likely due to perceived peer group approval; nevertheless, current studies advocate for the usage of transdermal matrix patches.

- Conjugated equine estrogen is frequently utilized in the United States.

- Oral estradiol is an inconvenient choice due to challenges in attaining low initial doses.

- There is growing evidence that ethinylestradiol is less effective than transdermal oestradiol regarding blood pressure and bone density; hence, transdermal oestradiol is presently the preferred formulation.

- Progestogen is used only following an appropriate period of unopposed estrogen or in the event of breakthrough unplanned hemorrhage.

- Northisterone, the most potent progestogen, may be deemed excessive in this context.

- Medroxyprogesterone acetate or micronized progesterone, when administered for 12–14 days per cycle, may result in less negative effects.

- The progestogen may be administered every 2–3 months to decrease the incidence of withdrawal hemorrhage.

- Progestogen coverage can also be attained using the oral contraceptive pill.

- Combined oral contraceptive pills containing ethinylestradiol, due to their unphysiological formulation, fail to deliver optimal estrogen replacement in young women and should be utilized solely for contraceptive purposes, such as in females with ovarian failure, hypothalamic amenorrhea, or hypogonadotropic hypogonadism where the restoration of normal ovarian function is feasible.

- In individuals who additionally require growth hormone therapy, there is a propensity to postpone the administration of estrogen until the age of 12; however, earlier intervention with adequately modest levels of estrogen is currently believed to have no detrimental impact on final height and should be contemplated.

- In summary, the prevailing consensus supports the initiation of puberty with transdermal oestradiol patches, commencing at a dosage of 6.25 µg for younger cohorts and 12.5 µg for older cohorts.

- The time of dose escalation should be individualized, considering the potential for further growth.

- This treatment must only commence with the consultation of a pediatric endocrinologist.

QUESTIONS

1. During normal pubertal development, which of the following is the first sign of estrogen effect in females?

   A. Menstruation

   B. Pubic and axillary hair

   C. Growth spurt

   D. Breast budding

2. How much time before menarche does the majority of breast development occur during normal pubertal development in females?

   A. 6–9 months

   B. 1 year

   C. 2 years

   D. 3 years

3. Which of the following statements regarding the definition of delayed puberty in females is true?

   A. Females exhibiting a total lack of breast development at the age of 13 years.

   B. Females exhibiting normal breast development who have primary amenorrhea by the age of 15 years.

   C. Females exhibiting primary amenorrhea at the age of 14 years.

   D. A and B.

   E. All of the above.

4. For induction of puberty by using exogenous estrogen, by what age should low-dose estrogen administration start?

   A. 8 years

   B. 9 years

   C. 10 years

   D. 13 years

5. Which of the following should NOT be used for inducing puberty in young girls with delayed puberty?

   A. Low-dose oral estrogen

   B. Transdermal estradiol patches

   C. Combined oral contraceptive pills

   D. Gonadotropins

6. Which of the following is the preparation of choice for administration of low-dose estrogen for induction of puberty in young girls with delayed puberty in the UK?

   A. Oral estradiol

   B. Transdermal estradiol patches

   C. Conjugated equine estrogen

   D. Combined oral contraceptives

7. Which of the following progesterone options are recommended for use in young girls with delayed puberty for the purpose of induction of puberty?

   A. Norethisterone

   B. Micronized progesterone

   C. Medroxyprogesterone

   D. All of the above

   E. B and C

8. Combined hormonal oral contraceptive pills can be used for estrogen replacement in all of the following conditions, except?

   A. Premature ovarian failure

   B. Hypogonadotropic hypogonadism

   C. Hypothalamic amenorrhea

   D. Young girls with delayed pubertal development

9. Adipose tissue is a source of which of the following forms of estrogen which supports bone development?

   A. Estriol

   B. Estradiol

   C. Estrone

   D. Estetrol

10. What is the starting dose of low-dose estrogen (through transdermal patches) for use in younger girls with delayed puberty for the purpose of induction of puberty?

   A. 5 µg

   B. 6.25 µg

   C. 10 µg

   D. 12.5 µg

11. Regarding induction of puberty in young girls with delayed pubertal development, which of the following statements is NOT true?

   A. Low-dose estrogen, administered via transdermal patches, is recommended and should be initiated by the age of 10 years.

   B. Progesterone should be initiated 2–3 years subsequent to estrogen to induce the initial withdrawal bleed at the age of 13 years.

   C. Combined oral contraceptives are the primary approach for administering estrogen and progesterone to induce puberty in young females.

   D. A pediatric endocrinologist should be consulted to commence therapy.

ANSWERS

1. D	5. C	9. C
2. C	6. B	10. B
3. D	7. E	11. C
4. C	8. D	

36 SIP – Stem Cell Therapies in OBGYN

Source: Stem Cell Therapies in Obstetrics and Gynaecology: The Female Urogenital Tract and the Fetus as Sources and Targets for Molecular and Regenerative Medicine Scientific Impact Paper No. 38 May 2013. https://www.rcog.org.uk/guidance/browse-all-guidance/scientific-impact-papers/stem-cell-therapies-in-obstetrics-and-gynaecology-scientific-impact-paper-no-38/

IMPORTANT POINTS FROM THE GUIDELINE (SIP)

- Reproductive tissues are widely acknowledged as sources of stem/progenitor cells and as targets for regenerative therapy.

- Stem cells derived from reproductive tissues have been utilized or explored for their potential applications in other domains, such as hematological disorders, which have conventionally been addressed with hematopoietic stem cells (HSC) from adult sources, often necessitating toxic adjuvant therapies, or in bone tissue engineering.

- Stem cells possess two characteristics:
  - The primary characteristic is the capacity for self-renewal or the ability to undergo several cell divisions while preserving an undifferentiated state.
  - The second pertains to multipotency, the ability to develop into a mature cell type.

- Totipotent stem cells, derived from the morula, possess the capability to develop into both embryonic and extraembryonic cell types, thereby generating a full and viable organism.

- Pluripotent stem cells originate from totipotent cells and can differentiate into tissues from any of the three germ layers, encompassing fetal tissues such as amniotic fluid cells, the amnion, umbilical cord, and placenta.

- Embryonic stem cells are pluripotent and originate from the inner cell mass of a blastocyst.

- Multipotent stem cells differentiate into diverse tissues derived from a single germ layer, such as mesenchymal or HSC.

- Unipotent cells, such as muscle satellite cells, exclusively generate their own cell type but exhibit superior self-renewal compared to fully differentiated cells.

- Theoretically, the more primitive or 'potent' a stem cell is, the more susceptible it is to unregulated cell proliferation, hence increasing its potential for oncogenesis.

- While apprehensions exist about the oncogenic potential of pluripotent stem cells, including embryonic and induced pluripotent stem cells, non-pluripotent cell sources are not intrinsically carcinogenic.

- Research is now underway in gynecology on regenerative medicine techniques aimed at repairing or replacing damaged or diseased urogenital tract organs, including the urinary sphincter, pelvic floor, uterus, ovaries, and vagina.

- In obstetrics, stem cell transplantation has primarily concentrated on fetal therapy.

- In the last 10 years, stem cells have been extracted from embryonic, fetal, extra-fetal organs, and adult gonads.

- Extra-fetal tissues, including the amniotic membranes and placenta, originate from the inner cell mass of the blastocyst, which develops into the embryo, yolk sac, mesenchymal core of the chorionic villi, chorion, and amnion.

- Due to their common origin, amniotic fluid and the placenta possess a diverse array of progenitor cells.

- This encompasses mesenchymal, hematopoietic, trophoblastic, and potentially more primordial stem cells.

- Despite variations in the chemical and cellular content of amniotic fluid based on gestational age and fetal health, mesenchymal stem cells (MSC) can be reliably extracted at every stage of gestation.

DOI: 10.1201/9781003650355-36

- MSC from placental and amniotic fluid have demonstrated the ability to differentiate into various cell types of mesodermal lineage, along with a limited number of cells from ectodermal and endodermal lineages.

- Amniotic fluid has yielded additional cell types, including a population of CD117 positive cells that exhibit pluripotential markers, demonstrate self-renewal exceeding 50 population doublings while preserving telomere length, are non-tumorigenic, and possess the capacity to differentiate into tissues of all three germ layers.

- Their potential for autologous and allogeneic cell sources in regenerative medicine applications is under investigation; nevertheless, this necessitates a facility dedicated to their characterization, immunological characteristics, and storage.

- Fetal stem cells have been extracted from multiple regions of the fetus.

- HSC from the bone marrow and liver during early gestation are well characterized, but placental HSC have been described more recently.

- Primitive human fetal mesenchymal stem cells (hfMSC) have been extracted from nearly all regions of the developing fetus, have enhanced proliferative potential, express markedly elevated levels of telomerase, and possess longer telomeres in comparison to adult stem cells.

- Moreover, they efficiently differentiate into neural and muscular lineages and exhibit superior osteogenic differentiation compared to later perinatal and adult sources of MSC, indicating their potential for postnatal applications in bone tissue engineering.

- Primitive hfMSC are efficiently transduced by integrating vectors and lack expression of HLA-II and costimulatory molecules CD80 and CD86, signifying their applicability for ex vivo gene therapy and allogeneic applications.

- The utilization of fetal and perinatal stem cells in regenerative medicine necessitates regulation by suitable institutional and regulatory bodies.

- Protocols for the best collection of these tissues should maximize both the quantity and quality of stem cells obtained before their storage in Good Manufacturing Practice (GMP) facilities.

- Umbilical cord blood (UCB) banking is a recognized procedure in numerous centers globally, serving as a source of HSC and MSC, with proven efficacy for allogeneic postnatal treatment of hematological disorders, including leukemia and bone marrow failure.

- The extraction of stem cells from fetal tissue after a medically authorized pregnancy termination should be directed by the precise cell type sought, particularly if the retrieved cells are designated for a specific application.

- hfMSC have been harvested from the liver for intrauterine transplantation aimed at osteogenesis imperfecta and for the treatment of haemoglobinopathies, both of which must be processed under GMP conditions.

- The majority of fetal components can be utilized as a source for donor cells, including the central nervous system for neural stem cells and the skin for epidermal progenitors.

- Biomaterials seek to address stress urinary incontinence (SUI) by offering structural and mechanical support to the bladder neck.

- This is performed through the injection of autologous stem or urethral tract progenitor cells, which have been culture-expanded prior to re-transplantation, into the urethral sphincter.

- This seeks to restore and renew the content and function of the rhabdomyosphincter muscle.

- A tissue-engineered, urothelial-lined bladder offers a functional barrier against urine exposure and may mitigate several severe problems linked to traditional entero-cystoplasty.

- The prerequisites for such 'engineered' tissue are more intricate than mere structural support; they must replicate the functions of a normal, healthy bladder wall by integrating compliance, typically provided by the detrusor smooth muscle, with a urinary barrier, usually conferred by the specialized urothelial lining.

- Three distinct procedures have been explored to enhance or repair the urinary bladder:
  - Utilization of acellular natural or synthetic biomaterials.
  - Implantation of scaffolds pre-incubated with autologous cells in vitro.
  - Integrating tissue-engineered urothelium with a host vascularized smooth muscle segment ('composite cystoplasty').

- Two specific prerequisites exist for the application of biomaterials in pelvic organ prolapse (POP) and urinary incontinence (UI).
  - The primary requirement is to offer mechanical support to the pelvic organs.
  - The second objective is to produce new muscle that can function cohesively with the existing organs, such as new sphincters.
  - The primary drawbacks of synthetic meshes for POP and pelvic floor-related UI are the risks of erosion and extrusion problems.
  - Biomaterials designed to substitute meshes must possess the tensile strength of meshes while also being bioabsorbable.
  - To achieve the objective of developing an optimized biomaterial for restoring pelvic floor function and addressing stress UI (SUI) in all patients, additional in vivo testing is required.

- Factors influencing uterine integrity, including congenital or acquired abnormalities and diseases, can undermine a woman's reproductive capacity.
  - The uterus serves as a source of progenitor cells that augment self-repair capabilities.
  - Cell treatment is proposed as a method to restore uterine tissues in women experiencing uterine factor infertility.

- The primary treatment for vaginal agenesis is vaginal dilation therapy.

- Vaginal reconstruction is frequently conducted as a remedy for vaginal agenesis utilizing non-vaginal tissue substitutes, such parts of the large intestine or skin.

- These materials are neither functionally nor anatomically optimal.

- The aim of IUSCT (in utero stem cell transplantation) is to rectify a genetic abnormality at an early stage of disease progression by transplanting normal functioning stem cells.

- The objectives of IUSCT include:
  - Substituting absent or abnormal proteins prior to irreversible organ damage.
  - Salvaging a fetus from a perinatally deadly disease.
  - Enhancing postnatal survival.
  - Maintaining essential capabilities.

- The prenatal environment provides the optimal opportunity for curing diseases that induce end-organ damage in utero, as it allows for the rectification of pathology during the initial phases of cellular impairment.

- Tolerance for transplanted cells may be established in the pre-immune fetus prior to the onset of antigen recognition at the conclusion of the first trimester, hence promoting engraftment in an immature bone marrow environment with minimal competition from host cells.

- The physical limitation on the quantity of donor stem cells that can be extracted and transplanted gives fetal size a marked advantage over the significantly bigger neonate.

- This advantage permits a higher concentration of stem cells to be attained within the target organ in comparison to a bigger postnatal recipient.

- Restrictive barriers, such as the blood–brain barrier, exhibit increased permeability throughout early development, potentially facilitating more effective stem cell engraftment in the fetus.

- The most compelling rationale for IUSCT is to address disorders that may lead to prenatal mortality, such as α-thalassaemia, and those that result in irreversible end-organ damage, such as certain mucopolysaccharidoses (MPS).

- In obstetrics, specifically fetal medicine, the advancements in prenatal molecular diagnostics and the emergence of stem cell transplantation and ex vivo gene transfer may significantly influence the treatment of various hereditary genetic problems.

- Clinical success has been documented for immunodeficiency disorders and skeletal dysplasia, while new data from preclinical models in mice and nonhuman primates will guide future clinical applications of this technique for other hereditary conditions.

- Considering the impact of β-globinopathies and advancements in preclinical research, it is probable that haemoglobinopathies will be among the initial disorders to achieve extensive clinical translation.

- Women receiving a prenatal diagnosis of severe or terminal genetic disorders are presently confronted with the decision to either bear an afflicted infant, with only palliative postnatal care accessible, or to terminate the pregnancy, potentially allowing for future preimplantation genetic diagnosis and embryo selection.

- The previously unrecognized potential of IUSCT may represent the sole treatment alternative.

- Conversely, evidence supporting the attainment of a complete cure is scant, and therapeutic advantages may only manifest following multiple pre- and postnatal administrations.

- Consequently, incomplete IUSCT may transform the result from perinatal demise to the survival of a severely damaged child needing postnatal therapy.

- Bystander maternal impacts will also be a significant factor that may diminish the inclination to treat the fetus.

- Potential harmful consequences may be associated with the method of material injection, including transplacental cell trafficking.

- Clinicians should be cognizant of the diverse ethical considerations involved when IUSCT is discussed.

- A multidisciplinary approach is advised, incorporating candid discussions of known limitations, potential advantages, and unknown or unquantifiable hazards.

- Centers of excellence in fetal medicine and therapeutic research should spearhead the development of scientific knowledge in this domain and establish clinical guidelines for forthcoming studies, in consultation with regulatory and ethical authorities.

QUESTIONS

1. Embryonic stem cells belong to which of the following cell classes?

   A. Totipotent

   B. Pluripotent

   C. Multipotent

   D. Unipotent

2. Muscle satellite cells belong to which of the following cell classes?

   A. Totipotent

   B. Pluripotent

   C. Multipotent

   D. Unipotent

3. Amniotic fluid stem cells are positive for which of the following receptors?

 A. CD28

 B. CD56

 C. CD117

 D. CD8

4. Regarding CD117-positive cells (derived from amniotic fluid), which of the following statements is incorrect?

 A. They possess pluripotency.

 B. They exhibit self-renewal capabilities.

 C. They preserve telomere length during proliferation and differentiation.

 D. They possess carcinogenic potential.

5. In comparison with their adult counterparts, all of the following characteristics regarding primitive hfMSC are true, except?

 A. They possess significant proliferative capacity

 B. They possess elevated levels of telomerase

 C. They exhibit elongated telomeres

 D. They are significantly immunogenic due to a high expression of HLA-II antigens

6. According to available research, MSC used for treating osteogenesis imperfecta by intrauterine transplantation is obtained from which of the following sources with higher osteogenic ability?

 A. Adipose tissue

 B. Placenta

 C. Adult bone marrow

 D. Fetal liver

7. Which of the following is the first-line management for vaginal agenesis?

 A. Vaginal reconstruction

 B. Vaginal dilation therapy

 C. McIndoe procedure

 D. Vecchietti's technique

8. Intrauterine stem cell transplantation can have a role in the management of which of the following congenital conditions?

 A. Osteogenesis Imperfecta

 B. Severe combined immunodeficiency syndrome

 C. Lysosomal storage disorders (LSD)

 D. All of the above

 E. B and C

9. What is the preferred site for injecting stem cells in intrauterine stem cell transplantation?

 A. Umbilical arteries

 B. Intrahepatic portion of umbilical vein

 C. Fetal bone marrow

 D. Ductus arteriosus

10. According to the available research, what is the fetal loss rate associated with in utero stem cell transplantation?

   A. <1%

   B. 2–3%

   C. 5%

   D. 10%

11. Regarding utilizing the fetal stage for stem cell transplantation in comparison to postnatal treatments to manage certain congenital genetic conditions, all of the following are advantages of IUSCT, except?

   A. It facilitates the correction of pathology during the early stages of cellular dysfunction.

   B. The fetal stage exhibits reduced immunogenicity relative to the postnatal stage, hence enhancing tolerance to transplanted cells.

   C. The fetus is smaller in size when compared to the newborn, hence permitting the transplantation of a reduced dosage of MSC per unit weight.

   D. Restrictive barriers, such as the blood–brain barrier, are underdeveloped (more porous) during the embryonic stage, potentially enhancing the efficacy of stem cell engraftment in the fetus.

ANSWERS

1. B	5. D	9. B
2. D	6. D	10. A
3. C	7. B	11. C
4. D	8. D	

37 SIP – Subclinical Hypothyroidism

Source: Subclinical Hypothyroidism and Antithyroid Autoantibodies in Women with Subfertility or Recurrent Pregnancy Loss Scientific Impact Paper No. 70 June 2022. https://www.rcog.org.uk/guidance /browse-all-guidance/scientific-impact-papers/subclinical-hypothyroidism-and-antithyroid-autoanti-bodies-in-women-with-subfertility-or-recurrent-pregnancy-loss-scientific-impact-paper-no-70/

IMPORTANT POINTS FROM THE GUIDELINE (SIP)

- Thyroid dysfunction is prevalent among women of reproductive age.

- The proper functioning of the thyroid gland facilitates healthy conception and excellent pregnancy outcomes.

- In the Western world, thyroid hormone deficiency, or hypothyroidism, is typically attributed to autoimmune thyroid disease (ATD) or Hashimoto's thyroiditis.

- Iodine deficiency is the predominant cause of hypothyroidism globally, whereas iatrogenic hypothyroidism resulting from radioiodine therapy or surgical intervention for hyperthyroidism is another significant etiological factor.

- Autoimmune hypothyroidism results from thyroid-specific antibodies targeting thyroid peroxidase (anti-TPO), the enzyme essential for thyroid hormone synthesis, and thyroglobulin (anti-Tg), the precursor for the manufacture and storage of thyroid hormones.

- The engagement of these antibodies with TPO and Tg induces a lymphocytic response, leading to thyroid gland fibrosis and a decrease in thyroid hormone synthesis.

- Thyroid autoantibodies may exert a broader impact on fertility and pregnancy, potentially contributing to a more generalized autoimmune process.

- Hypothyroidism is diagnosed when serum thyroid-stimulating hormone (TSH) levels exceed the reference range, indicating pituitary stimulation of an impaired thyroid gland.

- Treatment for hypothyroidism involves synthetic hormone replacement using levothyroxine (L-T4), often administered as a once-daily pill, replicating the physiological effects of endogenous thyroxine (T4) generated by the thyroid gland.

- An adequate dietary intake of iodine is essential for the proper synthesis of thyroid hormones.

- Iodine is prevalent in milk, various dairy products, and fish; yet, in numerous areas, diets lack sufficient iodine unless salt is iodized.

- Pregnancy necessitates heightened iodine intake due to two primary physiological alterations: the active transport of iodine to the fetoplacental unit and augmented iodine excretion in urine resulting from higher glomerular filtration and diminished renal tubular absorption.

- The decline in plasma iodine concentrations leads to a 3-fold increase in the thyroid gland's iodine uptake from the bloodstream.

- In the presence of pre-existing iodine deficit, the thyroid gland undergoes hypertrophy to adequately sequester iodine.

- The advised iodine consumption during pregnancy and breastfeeding is 250 µg per day.

- During early pregnancy, thyroid hormone synthesis increases, partly due to the elevated release of placental human chorionic gonadotrophin (hCG), which bears structural similarity to TSH and can activate the thyroid gland.

- However, these compensatory mechanisms are insufficient in the context of existing iodine shortage or elevated levels of thyroid autoantibodies.

- Consequently, euthyroid women may experience subclinical hypothyroidism (SCH), and those with pre-existing SCH may advance to overt hypothyroidism (OH).

DOI: 10.1201/9781003650355-37

- Globally, there is significant disparity in clinical practices regarding thyroid function tests and the ensuing diagnosis and treatment of thyroid dysfunction, particularly with the management of SCH and ATD.

- The absence of consensus is particularly evident in populations deemed high-risk, such as women with subfertility or those who have undergone recurrent pregnancy loss (RPL).

- The diagnosis of SCH should ideally be established using two distinct thyroid function tests conducted 3 months apart, in accordance with the 2019 National Institute for Health and Care Excellence (NICE) guidelines.

- SCH is a biochemical diagnosis characterized by elevated blood TSH levels beyond the established laboratory reference range, alongside normal levels of circulating thyroid hormones (free T4 and free T3).

- SCH is typically asymptomatic and may indicate the initial phases of thyroid malfunction, potentially advancing to overt disease.

- Historically, TSH levels ranging from 4.0 to 5.0 mIU/L were deemed normal for preconception and pregnancy. Nonetheless, there is a growing trend in practice to use a lower criterion for defining SCH.

- This has led to TSH readings over 2.5 mIU/L (both preconception and during the first trimester of pregnancy) being deemed abnormal. This criterion specifically applies to women deemed at high risk, including those with a history of subfertility or RPL.

- Reference ranges for serum TSH and fT4, specific to population, trimester, and laboratory, should be utilized as applicable when diagnosing SCH both preconception and throughout pregnancy.

- Classification of SCH:
  - Normal TSH: 2.5–4.0 mIU/L.
  - Mild-to-moderate SCH: TSH values exceeding 4.0 mIU/L and up to 10.0 mIU/L.
  - A TSH level exceeding 10.0 mIU/L, even in conjunction with a normal free T4, is deemed indicative of OH.

- In the absence of internal or transferable pregnancy-specific TSH reference ranges, an upper reference limit of 4.0 mIU/L may be applied.

- Untreated mild to severe SCH (TSH >4.0–10.0 mIU/L) correlates with early pregnancy loss; however, data is inadequate to establish a similar link for upper normal TSH levels (2.5–4.0 mIU/L).

- Evidence of low quality suggests that LT4 medication in women with mild to moderate SCH may enhance pregnancy and live birth rates; however, there is inadequate evidence of benefit for women with higher normal TSH levels.

- No definitive cut-off value exists to determine TPOAb positive; reference ranges provided by manufacturers for various assays should be utilized.

- The relationship between SCH and subfertility remains ambiguous.

- Routine preconception thyroid function tests (TSH and free T4) should be administered to women with a history of RPL and those with subfertility receiving assisted reproductive technology. A standard TFT should be documented in the 12 months before conception to enhance pregnancy outcomes.

- Women identified as TPOAb-positive should have a normal thyroid function test documented within the 6 months before conception, due to the increased risk of development to SCH and OH.

- Currently, there is inadequate data to endorse universal screening for all women attempting to conceive.

- The initial dosage of LT4 for women with untreated mild to moderate SCH is 1.0 to 1.2 µg/kg of body weight per day.

- In cases of SCH diagnosed and treated prior to conception in women experiencing subfertility or RPL, an empirical increase in levothyroxine dosage should commence upon confirmation of pregnancy.

- The suggestion is to administer twice the dosage on 2 days of the week (often Saturdays and Sundays) to replicate the 20–30% heightened thyroid requirement during pregnancy.

- An alternative method involves an empirical daily dose escalation of 25 μg for women receiving 100 μg or less, and 50 μg daily for those on more than 100 μg of levothyroxine.

- TSH levels should be assessed at 7 to 9 weeks of gestation and followed consistently until 34 weeks of gestation.

- Women diagnosed with SCH, who have not commenced treatment, should get a TSH measurement at the earliest opportunity, ideally between 7 and 9 weeks of gestation, and consider LT4 therapy if results fall beyond the reference range.

- Women undergoing LT4 medication during pregnancy should have their care collaboratively supervised with an endocrinologist or a practitioner proficient in handling thyroid disorders in pregnancy.

- LT4 therapy does not confer any advantage in enhancing pregnancy outcomes for euthyroid women who test negative for TPOAb.

- ATD refers to the existence of circulating antithyroid autoantibodies that specifically target the thyroid gland, potentially affecting thyroid function or remaining asymptomatic.

- TPOAb, thyroglobulin antibodies (TgAb), and TSH receptor antibodies (TRAb) are the three most clinically significant antithyroid autoantibodies, with TPOAb being the most prevalent and often assessed.

- TPOAb are regarded as the most sensitive indicator for identifying thyroid autoimmunity.

- Understanding the TPOAb status facilitates the categorization of women for thyroid function surveillance throughout pregnancy.

- Conducting routine preconception TPOAb testing (in conjunction with TFT) for women with infertility or a history of RPL, as opposed to standard TFTs, commencing in early pregnancy, is an acceptable approach until clinical and cost-effectiveness evaluations are accessible.

- If a woman tests positive for TPOAb, serum TSH concentration should be measured promptly during pregnancy, ideally between 7 and 9 weeks of gestation, and subsequently in each trimester, due to the possibility of development of SCH and OH.

- Additional research is required to ascertain the function of LT4 therapy in women exhibiting upper normal TSH levels who are TPOAb positive. Current evidence does not endorse this as standard practice.

- Additional research is necessary to ascertain the influence of selenium or steroids on enhancing pregnancy outcomes in euthyroid women who test positive for TPOAb.

- Insufficient evidence exists to establish a correlation between ATD and diminished reproductive potential; nonetheless, the presence of TPOAb may influence thyroid function during the use of assisted reproductive technology (ART).

- Consistent data indicates that the presence of thyroid antibodies correlates with an elevated risk of miscarriage.

- Elevated TSH levels have been identified as a predictor of fertilization failure in women undergoing in vitro fertilization (IVF), underscoring the significant role of thyroid hormones in oocyte physiology.

- TSH levels are considerably elevated in women whose oocytes do not fertilize.

- Numerous studies have indicated elevated miscarriage rates correlated with increased TSH levels.

- Consistent data indicates that elevated TPO antibodies along with SCH correlates with heightened risks of miscarriage and pregnancy problems, particularly in women with mild-to-moderate SCH.

- Most evidence indicates that ART and pregnancy outcomes are comparable among women with serum TSH levels below 2.5 mIU/L and those with upper normal TSH concentrations.

- Moreover, LT4 therapy for women with upper normal TSH levels has not demonstrated efficacy. Evidence of low quality indicates that LT4 medication in women with mild to moderate SCH (classified as TSH >4.0 mIU/L) is linked to improved pregnancy and live birth rates.

- Treatment should only commence prior to conception or during pregnancy when SCH is diagnosed based on TSH levels exceeding pregnancy and population-specific laboratory reference limits, or above 4.0 mIU/L if such ranges are not available.

QUESTIONS

1. What is the most common cause of hypothyroidism in the Western world?

    A. Hashimoto's thyroiditis

    B. Radioiodine therapy-induced hypothyroidism

    C. Iodine deficiency

    D. Thyroid cancer

2. What is the most common cause of hypothyroidism worldwide?

    A. Hashimoto's thyroiditis

    B. Radioiodine therapy-induced hypothyroidism

    C. Iodine deficiency

    D. Thyroid cancer

3. A 36-year-old patient presents to you with history of recurrent miscarriages. Her GP had offered her tests for RPL and has referred her to you to discuss the further care plan. Her antiphospholipid antibodies are negative, her glucose tolerance test is normal, her routine blood tests along with her pelvic ultrasound are normal. Her thyroid-stimulating hormone is high and her blood test is positive for anti-TPO antibodies. What is your working diagnosis in her case?

    A. Autoimmune thyroiditis (Hashimoto's disease)

    B. Iodine deficiency

    C. Subclinical hypothyroidism

    D. Goitre

4. What is the recommended daily iodine intake during pregnancy and lactation?

    A. 150 µg

    B. 250 µg

    C. 350 µg

    D. 450 µg

5. Which of the following factors increase the iodine demand during pregnancy?

    A. Active transfer of iodine to the fetoplacental unit

    B. Elevated iodine excretion in urine due to increased glomerular filtration and reduced renal tubular absorption

    C. Elevated release of bHCG hormone during pregnancy

    D. All of the above

    E. A and B

6. According to the NICE guidelines, which of the following is the recommended method to diagnose SCH?

   A. Two separate tests for thyroid function taken 4 weeks apart

   B. Two separate tests for thyroid function taken 6 weeks apart

   C. Two separate tests for thyroid function taken 3 months apart

   D. Two separate tests for thyroid function taken 6 months apart

7. All of the following statements regarding SCH are true, except?

   A. It is a biochemical diagnosis.

   B. It exhibits normal serum TSH levels alongside diminished amounts of circulating thyroid hormones (free T4 and free T3).

   C. SCH is typically asymptomatic.

   D. It may indicate the first phases of thyroid dysfunction, which can advance to manifest disease.

8. In women with RPLs and history of subfertility, what is the recommended range of TSH to be maintained preconceptionally and during the first trimester of pregnancy?

   A. <1.5 mIU/L

   B. <2.5 mIU/L

   C. <3.5 mIU/L

   D. <4.0 mIU/L

9. At least how many months before conception must a normal thyroid function test be recorded in women with RPL and history of subfertility?

   A. Within 3 months preconceptionally

   B. Within 6 months preconceptionally

   C. Within 12 months preconceptionally

   D. Within 18 months preconceptionally

10. At least how many months before conception must a normal thyroid function test be recorded in women who are positive for anti-TPO antibodies?

    A. Within 3 months preconceptionally

    B. Within 6 months preconceptionally

    C. Within 12 months preconceptionally

    D. Within 18 months preconceptionally

11. What is the recommended starting dose of levothyroxine (LT4) in women with untreated mild-to-moderate SCH?

    A. 0.5–0.7 µg/kg body weight per day

    B. 1.0–1.2 µg/kg body weight per day

    C. 1.5–2.0 µg/kg body weight per day

    D. 2.0–2.2 µg/kg body weight per day

12. A 33-year-old multigravida patient, presents to you in your outpatient department (OPD) with her thyroid function tests. The test is suggestive of high TSH levels of 8 mIU/L, with normal FT3 and FT4 levels. Her anti-TPO antibodies are negative. She is otherwise asymptomatic. What is your working diagnosis in her case?

   A. Autoimmune thyroiditis (Hashimoto's disease)

   B. Iodine deficiency

   C. Subclinical hypothyroidism

   D. Goitre

13. A 35-year-old multigravida patient with history of RPL, presents to you in your OPD with her thyroid function test. The test is suggestive of high TSH levels of 9 mIU/L, with normal FT3 and FT4 levels. Her anti-TPO antibodies are negative. She is otherwise asymptomatic. She is diagnosed as subclinical hypothyroid by her endocrinologist and started on levothyroxine (75 μg, daily). She has just tested positive on her home pregnancy test. What is your recommended management regarding the dosage of levothyroxine?

   A. Doubling the dose 2 days per week once pregnancy is confirmed

   B. Doubling the dose on alternate days of the week once pregnancy is confirmed

   C. Increase her dose by 25 μg 2 days per week once pregnancy is confirmed

   D. Increase her dose by 50 μg 2 days per week once pregnancy is confirmed

14. A 35-year-old multigravida patient with history of RPL, presents to you in your OPD with her thyroid function test. The test is suggestive of high TSH levels of 9 mIU/L, with normal FT3 and FT4 levels. Her anti-TPO antibodies are negative. She is otherwise asymptomatic. She is diagnosed as subclinical hypothyroid by her endocrinologist and advised to take levothyroxine (75 μg, daily), which she refused to start. She has just tested positive on her home pregnancy test. What is your recommendation for follow-up of her thyroid profile?

   A. Offer TSH measurement at 7–9 weeks of gestation

   B. Offer TSH measurement at 12 weeks of gestation

   C. Offer TSH measurement at the end of each trimester

   D. Offer TSH measurement monthly during her pregnancy

15. A 37-year-old multigravida patient with history of RPL, presents to you in your OPD with her thyroid function test. The test is suggestive of high TSH levels of 9 mIU/L and she has tested positive for anti-TPO antibodies. She has just tested positive on her home pregnancy test. What is your recommendation for follow-up of her thyroid profile?

   A. Offer TSH measurement at 7–9 weeks of gestation and subsequently in each trimester

   B. Offer TSH measurement at 12 weeks of gestation

   C. Offer TSH measurement at 7–9 weeks of gestation and then repeat in third trimester

   D. Offer TSH measurement monthly during her entire pregnancy

16. Which of the following antithyroid antibodies is the most prevalent and commonly tested in ATD?

   A. TPOAb   C. TRAb

   B. TgAb   D. All of the above

17. Which of the following is the most sensitive marker for the detection of thyroid autoimmunity?

   A. TgAb   C. TPOAb

   B. TRAb   D. TSH levels >10 mIU/L

18. What is the prevalence of TPOAb positivity in the general population?

    A. <5%

    B. 6–20%

    C. 10–31%

    D. 17–33%

19. What is the prevalence of TPOAb positivity in women with subfertility?

    A. <5%

    B. 6–20%

    C. 10–31%

    D. 17–33%

20. What is the prevalence of TPOAb positivity in women with a history of RPL?

    A. <5%

    B. 6–20%

    C. 10–31%

    D. 17–33%

21. Which of the following drugs is not a cause of hypothyroidism?

    A. Lithium

    B. Amiodarone

    C. Beta-blockers

    D. Tyrosine kinase inhibitors

22. Which of the following is not a criterion for initiating levothyroxine medication, as per the American Thyroid Association (ATA) and the American Association of Clinical Endocrinology (AACE)?

    A. TSH exceeds 7 mIU/L

    B. Manifestation of hypothyroid symptoms

    C. Positive TPO antibody

    D. Females of childbearing age

23. In elderly individuals with SCH and TSH levels <10 mIU/L undergoing levothyroxine therapy, which characteristics correlate with an increased mortality risk?

    A. Advanced age

    B. Senile dementia

    C. History of cerebrovascular disease

    D. All of the above

24. Each of the following are non-thyroidal etiologies of a rise in TSH that may lead to the misdiagnosis of SCH, with the exception of?

    A. Chronic kidney failure

    B. Adrenal insufficiency

    C. Increasing age

    D. Specific drugs such as glucocorticoids

ANSWERS

1. A
2. C
3. A
4. B
5. E
6. C
7. B
8. B

9. C
10. B
11. B
12. C
13. A
14. A
15. A
16. A

17. C
18. B
19. C
20. D
21. C
22. A
23. D
24. D

38 SIP – Surgery for Endometriomas

Source: The Effect of Surgery for Endometriomas on Fertility Scientific Impact Paper No. 55 September 2017. https://www.rcog.org.uk/guidance/browse-all-guidance/scientific-impact-papers/the-effect-of-surgery-for-endometriomas-on-fertility-scientific-impact-paper-no-55/

IMPORTANT POINTS FROM THE GUIDELINE (SIP)

- Endometriomas are linked to diminished monthly fertility rates, although a direct causative relationship has not been clearly proven.

- Repeated or substantial ovarian surgery adversely affects ovarian reserve, which must be taken into account while determining treatment options, particularly about additional surgery.

- The theoretical advantage of conducting surgery to enhance pelvic anatomy and accessibility is conceivable but lacks robust scientific validation.

- Until substantial evidence from extensive randomized controlled trials utilizing contemporary therapeutic techniques is obtained, numerous concerns regarding the appropriate management of an endometrioma will persist.

- Endometriosis is an inflammatory disorder defined by the presence of endometrial-like tissue in locations outside the uterine cavity.

- An estimated 6–10% of women, primarily of reproductive age, are affected by the illness, with a notably higher prevalence in specific categories, including those experiencing infertility.

- Ovarian endometriomas may occur in 17–44% of women with endometriosis and are frequently linked to the severe manifestation of the condition.

- The specific processes of endometriosis are not fully understood; nevertheless, it is generally accepted that most endometriotic lesions arise from retrograde menstruation and may be linked to immunological dysfunction, which might hinder the clearance of endometrial implants.

- Endometriotic ovarian cysts, referred to as 'endometriomas,' are mostly believed to form via the invagination of endometriotic tissue or cells through the ovarian serosa, particularly during the remodeling of the ovarian cortex post-ovulation.

- The existence of ovarian endometriomas is typically linked to the revised American Society of Reproductive Medicine (rASRM) staging of moderate-to-severe illness.

- Several theories regarding infertility associated with endometriosis have been suggested, including chronic inflammation, tubo-peritoneal anatomical distortion, and diminished endometrial receptivity, which result in impaired oocyte and embryo quality, as well as reduced ovarian reserve; however, the exact mechanism remains undetermined.

- Endometriosis is linked to immune system dysfunction.

- Peritoneal fluid from women with endometriosis has enhanced quantities of immune cells, such as macrophages, mast cells, natural killer cells, and T cells, alongside heightened levels of growth factors, chemokines, and cytokines.

- The augmented inflammatory condition can compromise oocyte quality and disrupt ovarian function, leading to impaired folliculogenesis and fertilization.

- An altered follicular environment, characterized by increased levels of progesterone and interleukin-6 and decreased levels of vascular endothelial growth factor (VEGF), may contribute to changes in the oocyte, resulting in diminished fertilization capacity and reduced embryo quality with low implantation potential.

- The existence of ovarian endometriomas, particularly when bilateral, can influence ovarian reserve, hence affecting the ovarian response to gonadotrophins during assisted reproductive technology (ART).

- Follicle depletion may result from damage caused by the inflammatory response associated with endometriosis and heightened oxidative stress in tissues, resulting in fibrosis.

DOI: 10.1201/9781003650355-38

- Potentially hazardous substances, including free iron, may permeate the cyst wall of the endometrioma, and prolonged mechanical stretching of the ovarian cortex might adversely affect the ovarian reserve.

- The most significant concern is the detrimental impact of ovarian surgery on ovarian reserve, particularly when conducted multiple times.

- Treatment of incidental disease in otherwise asymptomatic women is presently not advised, as the development and natural progression of endometriomas remain poorly comprehended.

- Ovarian endometriomas are optimally managed with cystectomy during surgery, rather than drainage and coagulation, as this approach is linked to a reduced recurrence risk and an elevated rate of spontaneous postoperative pregnancies, especially for cysts measuring 3 cm or larger.

- The evidence on the influence of an endometrioma on ovarian response during IVF is inconclusive.

- The size of the endometrioma, particularly when it exceeds 3 cm in diameter, may adversely affect ovarian responsiveness.

- The ovarian response was diminished, evidenced by a reduced number of oocytes recovered and an elevated cancelation rate in women with an endometrioma, despite a comparable total dosage of gonadotrophins administered.

- In comparison to women with peritoneal endometriosis without an endometrioma, IVF outcomes (live birth, pregnancy, miscarriage and cycle cancelation rates, and average number of oocytes retrieved) were comparable in women with an endometrioma.

- Implantation rates diminished in healthy receivers when oocytes originated from donors with endometriosis, indicating that the condition adversely affected oocyte quality.

- However, as per the European Society of Human Reproduction and Embryology (ESHRE) guidelines for endometriosis management, no significant differences have been evidenced in extensive databases encompassing recent IVF cycles, including those from the Human Fertilisation and Embryology Authority and the Society for Assisted Reproductive Technology.

- The surgical intervention for endometriomas before IVF is commonly performed, while its efficacy and necessity remain contentious.

- The possible physiological compensation by the healthy ovary for the impaired ovary, along with the increased doses of follicle-stimulating hormone necessary for ovarian stimulation, may explain the comparable IVF outcomes observed in women who have received surgical interventions for their endometriomas.

- A Cochrane review encompassing two small randomized controlled trials has indicated comparable pregnancy rates for surgical interventions (cystectomy or aspiration) and expectant care.

- Although pregnancy rates do not differ between cystectomy and aspiration of an endometrioma, cystectomy correlates with diminished ovarian response during controlled stimulation, resulting in fewer mature oocytes retrieved, thereby raising concerns regarding its potential negative impact on ovarian reserve.

- The ESHRE guideline panel determined that doing a cystectomy for an endometrioma exceeding 3 cm before IVF therapy does not enhance pregnancy rates.

- Surgery preceding ART may be contemplated for the management of endometriosis-related pain, to enhance follicle accessibility during oocyte retrieval, or to address any malignancy concerns.

- An endometrioma may potentially disrupt ovarian responsiveness to controlled stimulation and oocyte viability, while also presenting risks and technical challenges during oocyte retrieval.

- These include the possibility of injury to surrounding organs due to modified pelvic anatomy from adhesions, infection and abscess formation, contamination of follicular fluid with endometrioma material, advancement of endometriosis, further endometrioma growth and rupture, undetected malignancy, and cancer development in later life.

- A systematic analysis assessing the possible dangers of conservative therapy in women with diagnosed endometriomas undergoing IVF determined that there is inadequate data on the risks of diminished ovarian responsiveness and decreased oocyte competence.

- The ESHRE guideline group emphasized the necessity of adequately counseling women with the risks of diminished ovarian function post-surgery, including the potential risk associated with oophorectomy.

- The treatment options encompass expectant and surgical management, with the recommended approach determined by the woman's symptoms, fertility prognostic factors such as age and ovarian reserve, prior treatment history particularly regarding past surgical interventions, the characteristics of the cyst, and the woman's preferences.

- The determination to undertake surgery for an endometrioma necessitates meticulous consideration of multiple prognostic factors that may affect the efficacy of an ART cycle, including the woman's age, ovarian reserve, unilateral or bilateral nature of the condition, quantity and dimensions of the cysts, symptomatic presentation, presence or absence of concerning radiological characteristics, degree of extraovarian involvement, and prior history of ovarian surgery.

- Asymptomatic women, those of advanced reproductive age, individuals with diminished ovarian reserve, bilateral endometriomas, or a history of previous ovarian surgery may find it advantageous to initiate IVF straightaway, as surgical intervention could further impair ovarian function and postpone treatment commencement.

- Surgery may be deemed the primary option for extremely symptomatic women, those with preserved ovarian reserve, unilateral and sizable cysts, and should be contemplated for cysts exhibiting suspicious radiological and clinical characteristics.

- Endometriomas may be linked to extraovarian conditions, such as intestinal disorders and deeply infiltrating endometriosis.

- The excision of deeply infiltrating endometriosis has not demonstrated an enhancement in reproductive outcomes.

- While surgical removal of endometriotic nodules may offer symptomatic relief, it also poses considerable surgical risks, which should be thoroughly communicated to the patient.

QUESTIONS

1. What is the prevalence of endometriosis in women of reproductive age?

   A. 6–10%

   B. 25%

   C. 40%

   D. >50%

2. What percentage of women with endometriosis have severe disease with ovarian endometriomas?

   A. 6–10%

   B. 10–15%

   C. 17–44%

   D. 40–60%

3. The pathognomonic mechanisms with regard to the development of endometriosis include all of the following, except?

   A. Retrograde menstruation

   B. Immune failure in eliminating endometrial implants

   C. Invagination of endometriotic tissue or cells through the ovarian serosa during the remodeling of the ovarian cortex post-ovulation results in the formation of endometriomas

   D. The invagination of endometrial cells into the myometrium, prompted by tissue damage or dysfunction at the interface between the endometrium and myometrium

4. According to the rASRM classification of endometriosis, presence of ovarian endometriomas represents which of the following?

   A. Mild disease

   B. Mild-to-moderate disease

   C. Moderate disease

   D. Moderate-to-severe disease

5. Which of the following is the proposed mechanism of endometriosis-related infertility?

   A. Chronic inflammation

   B. Tubo-peritoneal anatomic distortion and reduced endometrial receptivity

   C. Poor oocyte and embryo quality and ovarian reserve

   D. All of the above

   E. A and B

6. Regarding the effect of endometriosis on oocyte and embryo quality, all of the following are true, except?

   A. Altered follicular environment

   B. Increased levels of progesterone

   C. Increased levels of interleukin-6

   D. Increased levels of VEGF

7. A 26-year-old patient presents to your gynecology outpatient department (OPD) as she is keen to start a family. Her cycles are regular and she has no significant past medical or surgical history. On routine transvaginal scan, a small left-sided endometrioma (size <2 cm) is noted incidentally. Considering that she is asymptomatic, what is your recommended management in her case?

   A. Offer dienogest for 6 months

   B. Offer laparoscopic cystectomy

   C. Offer laparoscopic drainage of endometrioma

   D. Offer conservative management to try for natural conception

8. In terms of surgical management of endometriosis, which of the following is NOT true?

   A. Restores pelvic anatomy

   B. May enhance spontaneous pregnancy rates

   C. Can reverse inflammatory and biomolecular alterations to affect fertilization and implantation

   D. Can diminish ovarian reserve

9. A 32-year-old patient presents to your gynecology OPD with complaints of extremely painful periods, troubling her for the last 6–9 months. Her GP offered her a transvaginal scan which is suggestive of a 5 cm left-sided endometrioma. She also gives a history of deep dyspareunia. She has been married for the last 3 years and is keen to start a family. What is your recommended management in her case?

   A. Offer ovulation induction and follicle monitoring

   B. Offer laparoscopic cystectomy

   C. Offer laparoscopic drainage of endometrioma

   D. Offer conservative management to try for natural conception

10. Comparing cystectomy with drainage as a treatment option of ovarian endometriomas, which of the following is true?

    A. Cystectomy does not impact ovarian reserve

    B. Cystectomy exhibits a lower recurrence rate

    C. Cystectomy may have a comparable postoperative spontaneous pregnancy rate to that of drainage/coagulation

    D. Cystectomy does not influence anti-Müllerian hormone levels

11. During oocyte retrieval, what is the estimated incidence of risk of infection of endometrioma?

    A. <2%

    B. 2.8–6%

    C. 7–10%

    D. >10%

12. During oocyte retrieval, what is the estimated incidence of follicular fluid contamination?

    A. <2%

    B. 2.8–6%

    C. 7–10%

    D. >10%

13. What is the estimated risk of ovarian malignancy later in life in patients with endometriomas?

    A. 1 in 1000

    B. 1–2%

    C. 4%

    D. 7%

14. A 43-year-old woman married for last 15 years, presents to your OPD as she is keen to conceive. She has a known case of endometriosis for which she had undergone laparoscopic left-sided cyctectomy about 6 years ago. Her latest AMH is low (<0.3 ng/mL). Her latest transvaginal scan is suggestive of small bilateral endometriomas. She has no significant past medical history. What is the recommended management option in her case?

    A. Offer bilateral laparoscopic cystectomy

    B. Offer bilateral laparoscopic drainage of the endometriomas

    C. Offer referral for IVF directly

    D. Offer dienogest for 6 months followed by ovulation induction

15. A 32-year-old patient is keen to plan a pregnancy. She has been married for 4 years. She presents to your gynecology OPD with complaints of deep dyspareunia since marriage. On per vaginum examination, the uterus is retroverted and a thickening of the left uterosacral ligament is felt. There is also fullness noted in the left adnexa. She is diagnosed with left-sided endometrioma with a size of 4 cm. She is planned for laparoscopy. Intraoperatively, deep endometriotic implants are noted in uterosacral ligaments, with left-sided 4 cm chocolate cyst, with partial obliteration of the pouch of Douglas. According to the rASRM classification her score is 25. What is her stage of endometriosis?

A. Stage 1

B. Stage 2

C. Stage 3

D. Stage 4

16. Regarding the endometriosis fertility index (EFI), which of the following statements is incorrect?

A. It forecasts the probability of spontaneous conception rates following surgery conducted for endometriosis.

B. It considers patient attributes such as age, prior infertility history, and specifics of past pregnancies.

C. A functional evaluation of the fallopian tubes and ovaries post-surgery is included in the grading system.

D. The scoring system excludes intraoperative surgical findings and the location/severity of endometriotic lesions.

17. What is the risk of malignant transformation in endometriomas?

A. <1%

B. 2.5%

C. 4–5%

D. 7%

ANSWERS

1. A	7. D	13. B
2. C	8. C	14. C
3. D	9. B	15. C
4. D	10. B	16. D
5. D	11. A	17. B
6. D	12. B	

39 SIP – Targeted Therapies for Ovarian Cancer

Source: Targeted Therapies for the Management of Ovarian Cancer Scientific Impact Paper No. 12 September 2013. https://www.rcog.org.uk/guidance/browse-all-guidance/scientific-impact-papers/ targeted-therapies-for-the-management-of-ovarian-cancer-scientific-impact-paper-no-12/

IMPORTANT POINTS FROM THE GUIDELINE (SIP)

- Annually in the United Kingdom, around 6500 women are diagnosed with ovarian cancer, resulting in approximately 4400 fatalities.

- A significant number of women exhibit advanced illness with minimal likelihood of treatment.

- The 5-year survival rate for advanced ovarian cancer from 2005 to 2009 was 43%.

- The prevailing method of care involves a mix of major surgery and platinum-based chemotherapy.

- Despite notable progress in surgical and chemotherapeutic techniques resulting in marginal enhancements in outcomes, a considerable risk of recurrence and therapeutic resistance persists, highlighting the want for improved treatment modalities.

- Novel physiologically targeted medicines have demonstrated efficacy in several malignancies, including leukemia, colon, kidney, and breast cancers.

- These drugs specifically target tumor cells and/or the microenvironment by leveraging distinct genetic aberrations inside the tumor, a strategy that offers the potential for enhanced selectivity and reduced toxicity compared to conventional treatments such as chemotherapy.

- Progress in comprehending the biology of ovarian cancer has resulted in clinical trials for targeted therapies, with angiogenesis inhibitors and poly-adenosine diphosphate–ribose polymerase (PARP) inhibitors being the most advanced.

- Epithelial ovarian cancer has historically been regarded as a single illness.

- Nonetheless, it is a heterogeneous disease comprising various histological subtypes characterized by unique clinical behaviors and molecular pathway defects (high-grade serous – p53, BRCA, homologous recombination deficiency; low-grade serous – BRAF, KRAS, NRAS, HER2; clear cell – PIK3CA, PTEN; endometrioid – PIK3CA, PTEN; and mucinous – KRAS, HER2).

- Clinical trials targeting particular subtypes of ovarian cancer are in progress.

- Drug targets encompass chemicals linked to tumor cells (such as folate receptors, mTOR inhibitors, and MEK inhibitors) and endothelial cells (including bevacizumab and vascular disrupting agents [VDAs]).

- Antiangiogenic medicines, such as bevacizumab and vascular endothelial growth factor receptor (VEGFR) inhibitors, along with PARP inhibitors, represent the most advanced new therapies.

- Angiogenesis, the development of new blood vessels, is an essential factor in cancer proliferation and metastasis.

- Bevacizumab, a monoclonal antibody targeting vascular endothelial growth factor (VEGF), has demonstrated promising efficacy in ovarian cancer.

- Two phase II clinical studies of bevacizumab demonstrated that monotherapy with anti-VEGF agents is a potential approach for recurrent ovarian cancer.

- Two randomized phase III trials, the Gynaecologic Oncology Group (GOG) trial 02185 and the International Collaborative Ovarian Neoplasm (ICON) 7 trial, have examined the addition of bevacizumab to the regimen of carboplatin and paclitaxel, followed by maintenance therapy, as first-line treatment for advanced epithelial ovarian cancer.

- The bevacizumab dosage administered in ICON7 was 7.5 mg/kg, which is half of the 15 mg/kg dosage utilized in GOG-0218.

DOI: 10.1201/9781003650355-39

- Both studies exhibited markedly significant enhancements in progression-free survival (PFS).

- Bevacizumab is associated with adverse effects such as hypertension and thrombosis.

- Bevacizumab is acknowledged to elevate the risk of gastrointestinal perforation and fistula development.

- The European Medicines Agency (EMA) has sanctioned the administration of bevacizumab in conjunction with carboplatin and paclitaxel as first-line therapy, as well as for the treatment of initial platinum-sensitive recurrence in combination with carboplatin and gemcitabine.

- On 13 June 2018, the Food and Drug Administration (FDA) sanctioned bevacizumab (Avastin, Genentech Inc.) for individuals with epithelial ovarian, fallopian tube, or primary peritoneal cancer, in conjunction with carboplatin and paclitaxel, succeeded by monotherapy with bevacizumab, for stage III or IV malignancies post-initial surgical resection.

- Individuals with BRCA mutations possess abnormalities in the homologous recombination DNA repair pathway (HRD) and have a 10–40% lifetime risk of developing ovarian cancer.

- PARP inhibitors function by inducing particular DNA damages that necessitate operational BRCA1 and BRCA2 for DNA repair mechanisms.

- Patients with BRCA-associated malignancies exhibit the absence of wild-type BRCA1 or BRCA2 in tumor cells, while normal cells maintain one wild-type copy of the corresponding gene.

- The distinction between tumor and normal cells allows PARP inhibitors to selectively eliminate tumor cells while preserving normal cells. This notion is referred to as 'synthetic lethality.'

- The epidermal growth factor receptor (EGFR) and the human epidermal growth factor 2 receptor (HER2) are tyrosine kinase receptors that play a role in cell proliferation and survival.

- Preclinical research indicated that EGFR and HER2 are possible targets in ovarian cancer.

- Nonetheless, the outcomes of trials involving erlotinib, gefitinib (EGFR inhibitors), trastuzumab (targeting HER2), and pertuzumab (HER2 dimerization inhibitor) have been comparatively unsatisfactory.

QUESTIONS

1. What is the 5-year survival rate of ovarian cancer in the UK?

    A. 20–25%

    B. 40–45%

    C. 50–70%

    D. Up to 80%

2. A defect in which of the following gene molecular pathways is associated with high-grade serous epithelial ovarian cancer?

    A. p53

    B. PTEN

    C. BRAF

    D. HER-2

3. A defect in which of the following gene molecular pathways is associated with low-grade serous epithelial ovarian cancer?

    A. p53

    B. PTEN

    C. BRAF

    D. BRCA

4. A defect in which of the following gene molecular pathways is associated with clear cell epithelial ovarian cancer?

   A. p53

   B. PTEN

   C. BRAF

   D. BRCA

5. A defect in which of the following gene molecular pathways is associated with mucinous epithelial ovarian cancer?

   A. p53

   B. BRCA

   C. BRAF

   D. HER-2

6. Which of the following monoclonal antibodies targeting VEGF has proven to be very effective against ovarian cancer?

   A. Rituximab

   B. Bevacizumab

   C. Trastuzumab

   D. Adalimumab

7. All of the following are proven adverse effects of bevacizumab except?

   A. Hypertension

   B. Thromboembolism

   C. Gastrointestinal perforation and fistula formation

   D. Hyponatremia and hypocalcemia

8. Regarding the use of PARP inhibitors in patients with recurrent ovarian cancer, which of the following statements is incorrect?

   A. They inhibit poly (ADP-ribose) polymerase (PARP), an enzyme implicated in DNA repair, so preventing cancer cells from repairing the DNA damage.

   B. They selectively eliminate BRCA-mutated cells that rely on the PARP enzyme for DNA repair.

   C. Only olaparib has received FDA approval for use in recurrent ovarian cancer.

   D. Their uncommon yet severe adverse effect is the potential to cause acute myeloid leukemia.

9. Which of the following PARP inhibitors is not approved for recurrent BRCA mutated ovarian cancer and recurrent platinum-sensitive ovarian cancer?

   A. Olaparib

   B. Niraparib

   C. Rucaparib

   D. Talazoparib

10. Regarding the use of HER2 receptor inhibitors in ovarian cancer, which of the following statements is correct?

    A. HER2 expression in epithelial ovarian cancer is primarily noted in the serous subtype, particularly in older patients, those with advanced stages, and individuals demonstrating high-grade differentiation.

    B. They possess substantial evidence in the management of advanced-stage epithelial ovarian malignancies.

    C. They seemingly lack a role in the therapy of HER2- positive breast cancer.

    D. Pertuzumab is a monoclonal antibody approved by the Food and Drug Administration (FDA) for the treatment of HER2- positive ovarian cancer.

11. Which of the following drugs is not correctly matched with its relevant mechanism of action?

    A. Olaparib – PARP inhibitor

    B. Trastuzumab – HER2 receptor inhibitor

    C. Sirolumus – mTOR inhibitor

    D. Pertuzumab – VEGF inhibitor

12. What is the mechanism of action of trebananib as an alternate treatment strategy for ovarian cancer?

    A. It is an anti-VEGF/VEGFR angiogenic inhibitor

    B. It is a non-VEGF angiogenic inhibitor

    C. It is a PARP inhibitor

    D. It is a EGFR inhibitor

13. Which of the following is an example of monoclonal antibody to the folate receptor, that has a potential role in treatment of ovarian cancer?

    A. Cetuximab

    B. Farletuzumab

    C. Panitumumab

    D. Matuzumab

14. Which of the following monoclonal antibody to IGF-1 receptor is under trial to be potentially added to the chemotherapy regimen for management of optimally debulked patients with ovarian cancer?

    A. Panitumumab

    B. Matuzumab

    C. Ganitumab

    D. Bevacizumab

ANSWERS

1. B	6. B	11. D
2. A	7. D	12. B
3. C	8. C	13. B
4. B	9. D	14. C
5. D	10. A	

40 SIP – Therapies Targeting the Nervous System for Chronic Pelvic Pain (CPP) Treatment

Source: Therapies Targeting the Nervous System for Chronic Pelvic Pain Relief Scientific Impact Paper No. 46 January 2015. https://www.rcog.org.uk/guidance/browse-all-guidance/scientific-impact-papers /therapies-targeting-the-nervous-system-for-chronic-pelvic-pain-relief-scientific-impact-paper-no-46/

IMPORTANT POINTS FROM THE GUIDELINE (SIP)

- Chronic pelvic pain (CPP) is characterized by the Royal College of Obstetricians and Gynaecologists as 'intermittent or persistent discomfort in the lower abdomen or pelvis of a woman lasting at least 6 months, not solely occurring during menstruation or intercourse and not linked to pregnancy.'

- Women with CPP may endure persistent or intermittent pain, which can be spontaneous or linked to particular behaviors such as urination (dysuria), defecation (dyschezia), or sexual intercourse (dyspareunia).

- CPP is linked to a substantial decline in quality of life, and psychological distress is often observed in these women.

- Although CPP is often linked to many gynecological conditions such as endometriosis, adenomyosis, chronic pelvic inflammatory disease, and pelvic organ prolapse, an underlying pathology is frequently unidentifiable, resulting in chronic pelvic pain syndrome (CPPS).

- The experience of pain requires the engagement of the central nervous system (CNS), and there is growing evidence that pain, regardless of its apparent source, can be both produced and sustained by the CNS itself.

- Moreover, chronic pain is linked to enduring alterations in both the structure and function of the CNS, which are largely consistent regardless of the specific pain condition.

- Compelling data currently indicates that abnormalities in the CNS manifest in numerous gynecological disorders linked to CPP, such as endometriosis, vulvodynia, interstitial cystitis/ bladder pain syndrome (IC/BPS), and dysmenorrhea.

- Furthermore, CNS dysfunction may contribute to numerous symptoms linked to CPP, such as impaired organ function regulation resulting in urinary frequency or retention and diarrhea or constipation, as well as endocrine dysfunction, notably changes in the hypothalamic–pituitary– adrenal axis activity, which could lead to heightened susceptibility to infections and autoimmune disorders.

- Although certain therapeutic alternatives may be appropriately started by a gynecologist, it is important to recognize that persistent pain is likely to be complex.

- Optimal outcomes are likely achieved with management by a multidisciplinary team, which may encompass specialists in hormonal, medicinal, invasive/surgical, and psychological therapies.

- More invasive therapies should be reserved for patients who are resistant to standard treatment for any identified pathology or when no such pathology can be identified.

- Alternative options, such as antidepressants, anticonvulsants, and local stimulation (transcutaneous electrical nerve stimulation [TENS]), may be initiated upon a patient's presentation with CPP and continued during further investigation and/or treatment.

- Antidepressant and anticonvulsant medications have proven fundamental in the treatment of chronic pain, especially neuropathic pain.

- Antidepressants seem to function by modifying the activity of pain inhibitory systems through the modulation of serotonin, noradrenaline, dopamine, and acetylcholine, and possibly by direct anti-inflammatory, opioidergic, or N-methyl-D-aspartate (NMDA) antagonistic mechanisms.

- Their analgesic efficacy is distinct from their antidepressant efficacy and frequently manifests at lower dosages than those necessary to elicit an antidepressant effect.

DOI: 10.1201/9781003650355-40

- Anticonvulsant medications seem to function via a mix of mechanisms, including the blockage of voltage-gated sodium and calcium channels, as well as interactions with the γ-aminobutyric acid (GABA) system.

- Generally, both categories of medications are generally tolerated, exhibiting relatively minimal side effects, predominantly drowsiness and nausea, but specific adverse effects differ among the treatments.

- The diverse modes of action imply that if one treatment fails, another may succeed, and combination therapy may be effective even with partial efficacy.

- Likewise, if the bad effect profile of a certain medication is deemed unacceptable, an option that may be more suitable for the patient is likely available.

- It is important to note that a dose–response curve presumably exists for both medication groups; hence, dosages should be incrementally elevated if an initial response is not noticed.

- The application of antidepressants in the treatment of chronic urological pelvic pain lacks sufficient backing from a substantial number of rigorously conducted randomized controlled studies; yet, it was recognized that there is some evidence of efficacy for amitriptyline and sertraline.

- There is even less evidence to substantiate the use of anticonvulsant medicine in CPP.

- The administration of botulinum toxin (onabotulinumtoxin A or Botox®, Allergan, Marlow, UK) injections for the alleviation of CPP is on the rise, while the studies providing supporting data are currently inadequate.

- In addition to its direct impact on muscles, botulinum toxin is believed to influence the CNS, a phenomenon that is significant yet not entirely comprehended.

- Studies on botulinum toxin in women with overactive bladder indicate that it is a well-tolerated intervention with the capacity to markedly enhance quality of life, hence warranting further exploration of its application in vulvodynia and CPP.

- Three more pharmaceutical interventions aimed at the neurological system have been explored for the alleviation of CPP.

- Notably, melatonin dramatically alleviated daily pain, menstrual discomfort, dyschezia, and dysuria in a sample of 40 women with CPP and laparoscopically diagnosed endometriosis. This finding may not be universally applicable to women with CPP in the absence of endometriosis.

- Lofexidine hydrochloride, an α2-adrenoceptor agonist, was examined in a group of women with CPP and no discernible disease on laparoscopy, due to its immediate antinociceptive effects and its ability to inhibit vasospasm in the utero-ovarian region. This trial found no meaningful difference relative to the placebo.

- Dexamfetamine sulfate, a sympathomimetic amine, has been documented as an effective treatment for CPP, but solely in conjunction with the unusual condition of idiopathic orthostatic edema.

- Consequently, additional randomized controlled trials are necessary before this treatment may be endorsed for CPP broadly.

- The external use of electrical and magnetic stimulation can modify neurophysiology either locally (at the pain location) or centrally (in the brain or spinal cord), potentially resulting in analgesia.

- Moreover, electrical stimulation may be applied directly to the peripheral nerves, spinal cord, or brain.

- TENS is a recognized method of analgesia employed during labor.

- The precise mechanism by which it produces an analgesic effect remains unidentified.

- It was long presumed to function through the 'gate-control' theory, in which stimulation of large diameter Aβ fibers suppresses the activity of smaller fibers (Aδ and C, which transmit pain) from the same segments.

- Electrical stimulation of tiny fibers alone can induce both segmental and extra-segmental inhibition, resulting in analgesia.

- Moreover, the application of low-frequency electrical stimulation enhances the production of endogenous opioids, therefore, diminishing pain in both acute and chronic contexts.

- It has demonstrated efficacy in alleviating pain in males with CPPS/prostatitis.

- Considering the pain localization in women with CPP, intravaginal electrical stimulation (IVES) has been suggested as an alternative approach.

- Initial findings indicated that IVES is linked to a substantial decrease in pain and dyspareunia, with the alleviation of pain sustained at a 7-month follow-up.

- Recently, IVES for CPP was evaluated in a randomized experiment controlled by a placebo (sham stimulation).

- This established that active stimulation was more effective than sham, resulting in a considerable decrease in pain intensity by the conclusion of the 5-week treatment regimen.

- This study lacked long-term follow-up.

- Several mechanisms have been suggested through which magnetism may affect pain, including: i) selective reduction of neuronal depolarization by modifying membrane resting potential, ii) enhancement of blood flow (potentially expediting tissue repair and eliminating harmful mediators), iii) alteration of ion binding kinetics, thereby modulating the release of cytokines and other inflammatory mediators.

- In patients with CPP, pain remission was observed in 67% of individuals.

- Non-invasive brain stimulation techniques include electrical methods such as transcranial direct current stimulation (tDCS) and cranial electrotherapy stimulation (CES), as well as magnetic ones like recurrent transcranial magnetic stimulation (rTMS).

- They seek to regulate pain through a direct influence on cerebral activity.

- Robust experimental findings indicate that these approaches can effectuate an instantaneous modification in neurotransmitter levels, notably the principal inhibitory neurotransmitter GABA, and precipitate enduring synaptic alterations.

- In chronic pain, analgesia is believed to arise from diminished activity in brain networks that process pain and facilitate descending pain inhibitory processes.

- Regarding nerve blocks as a therapy strategy for CPP, only two small case series have examined the efficacy of hypogastric blocks, revealing minimal effect.

- The disruption of the Lee–Frankenhauser sensory nerve plexuses through laparoscopic uterosacral nerve ablation (LUNA) was commonly employed to relieve pelvic discomfort until the release of the largest LUNA study and a meta-analysis of all LUNA studies in 2009 and 2010, respectively.

- The meta-analysis corroborated the findings of the trial, indicating that the LUNA treatment is ineffective in relieving pain.

- There is evidence indicating that women who undergo the LUNA procedure may experience greater short-term pain compared to those who do not.

- Presacral neurectomy (PSN) entails the complete transection of the presacral nerves located inside the confines of the interiliac triangle, a surgery that may be executed laparoscopically.

- The data regarding the procedure's effectiveness in alleviating pelvic pain are scarce and contradictory.

- The most extensive and recent randomized controlled research indicates that PSN may be beneficial in treating severe dysmenorrhea resulting from endometriosis.

- Laparoscopic presacral neurolysis is an alternate procedure that entails the injection of a neurolytic agent, such as phenol, to chemically obliterate the microscopic neuronal structure of the presacral nerves.

- One study provides evidence indicating that this approach may be utilized in the management of pelvic discomfort, either as a standalone treatment or as an adjuvant operation.

- Nonetheless, in the absence of additional evidence demonstrating a favorable equilibrium of both efficacy and safety, neither PSN nor neurolysis can be endorsed.

- The function of neuromodulation in the treatment of persistent pelvic pain disorders yet to be thoroughly elucidated.

- Its function in overactive bladder and fecal incontinence is, however, significantly more established.

- Available techniques encompass peripheral nerve stimulation (such as posterior tibial nerve stimulation, sacral nerve/root stimulation, and pudendal nerve stimulation) as well as spinal cord stimulation (SCS).

- Intermittent percutaneous tibial nerve stimulation (PTNS) is a minimally invasive therapeutic approach that has demonstrated a significant reduction in pain symptoms among individuals with lower urinary tract dysfunction, including urge incontinence, urgency, and/or frequency.

- PTNS may be applicable in the management of individuals with CPP who have exhausted multiple therapeutic alternatives and have no remaining options. Nonetheless, longitudinal follow-up investigations are necessary.

- Sacral neuromodulation (SNM) or sacral neurostimulation (SNS) was initially proposed as a potential treatment for CPPS in 1999 by Feler and colleagues; nevertheless, the literature remains sparse.

- The distinction between the two terms is that SNS emphasizes the activation of the nerve as the primary catalyst for the positive response, while neurostimulation may initiate the response, with the sustained long-term effect resulting from its modulatory influence on the neural system.

- Permanent sacral nerve modulation implantation was conducted in patients exhibiting a minimum of 50% symptom reduction during a temporary peripheral nerve evaluation test.

- The rate of reoperation was 25%.

- Consequently, SNM plays a function, but with a considerable complication rate.

- Pudendal neurostimulation (PNS) for refractory CPPS is believed to yield superior results in patients who have not responded to alternative treatments.

- SCS is regarded as a significant therapeutic alternative for specific types of persistent neuropathic pain that are refractory to conventional treatments.

- Its function in CPPS remains ambiguous. SCS may be efficacious for thoracolumbar afferents.

- Acquiring adequate stimulation from SCS for the sacral nerves, particularly the pudendal nerve, is challenging, hence constraining the application of this therapy in the management of CPP.

- Neuromodulatory medications are inherently complicated, making patient selection crucial for their efficacy.

- Neuromodulation should only be conducted in specialized centers equipped to offer interdisciplinary treatment.

- For persistent pain unresponsive to all other therapy modalities, deep brain stimulation (DBS) may be performed by a neurosurgeon.

- The objective is to augment activity in pain inhibitory systems, typically targeting one or more of the thalamus, periventricular gray, and periaqueductal gray.

- The motor cortex can also be activated superficially (MCS).

- Meta-analyses, primarily of case series, indicate that DBS has a long-term success rate of 46%, whereas the success rates for motor cortex stimulation (MCS) fluctuate between 40% and 75%, depending on the indication.

- Both procedures exhibit a comparatively low complication rate, with infection representing the primary danger.

- DBS is linked to a risk of cerebral hemorrhage (up to 4%), a problem not seen with motor cortex stimulation (MCS).

- No research has explicitly evaluated the effectiveness of MCS or DBS in CPP in women.

- Antidepressant and anticonvulsant medications are generally well tolerated and may be initiated by a gynecologist or primary care physician.

- Other more innovative or intrusive treatments may likely necessitate a referral to a pain management specialist.

- It is essential for gynecologists to recognize the existence of such choices to facilitate referrals for individuals resistant to normal therapies before undertaking drastic or fertility-altering surgery.

QUESTIONS

1. Antidepressant medications help in pain inhibition by altering all of the following neurotransmitters, except?

    A. Serotonin

    B. Noradrenaline

    C. Dopamine

    D. Adrenaline

2. All of the following are proposed mechanisms of action of anticonvulsant medications, except?

    A. Inhibition of voltage-gated sodium and calcium channels

    B. Interactions with the GABA system

    C. Inhibiting NMDA receptors

    D. Inhibiting monoamine oxidase enzyme

3. Which of the following side effects are most commonly seen in patients taking antidepressants and anticonvulsants?

    A. Nausea

    B. Blurred vision

    C. Insomnia

    D. Constipation

4. According to research, which of the following medications has some evidence of benefit in patients with chronic urological pelvic pain?

    A. Citalopram

    B. Amitriptyline

    C. Duloxetine

    D. Nortriptyline

5. According to research, botulinum toxin injection has evidence of benefit in which of the conditions?

    A. CPP

    B. Overactive bladder

    C. Vulvodynia

    D. Stress urinary incontinence

6. LUNA involves interrupting which of the following for pain management?

   A. Auerbach's plexus

   B. Lee–Frankenhauser nerve plexus

   C. Meissner's plexus

   D. Inferior ganglion of Andersch

7. Using DBS for management of chronic refractory pain, involves stimulation of all of the following pain-inhibiting systems, except?

   A. Thalamus

   B. Periventricular gray

   C. Periaqueductal gray

   D. Hippocampus

8. Which complication is considered to be the biggest risk of using DBS for management of chronic refractory pain?

   A. Infection

   B. Stroke

   C. Confusion and delirium

   D. Seizures

9. Regarding mechanisms by which magnetism reduces chronic refractory pain, which of the following is incorrect?

   A. Selective attenuation of neuronal depolarization through modulation of membrane resting potential

   B. Augmentation of blood circulation (possibly accelerating tissue regeneration and removing deleterious mediators)

   C. Modification of ion-binding kinetics, thereby influencing the release of cytokines and other inflammatory mediators

   D. Targeted activation of large-diameter Aβ fibers to suppress the function of small nociceptive fibers

10. According to research, what percentage of patients with CPPS reported pain remission with the use of repetitive magnetic stimulation?

    A. 20%

    B. 35%

    C. 67%

    D. 90%

11. According to existing research, which of the following techniques has shown efficacy in alleviating pain in patients with CPPS/prostatitis, not responding to routine medical therapy?

    A. LUNA

    B. PSN

    C. Laparoscopic presacral neurolysis

    D. TENS

ANSWERS

1. D
2. D
3. A
4. B

5. B
6. B
7. D
8. A

9. D
10. C
11. D

41 SIP – Umbilical Cord Blood Banking

Source: Umbilical Cord Blood Banking Scientific Impact Paper No. 2 June 2006. https://www.rcog.org
.uk/guidance/browse-all-guidance/scientific-impact-papers/umbilical-cord-blood-banking-scientific
-impact-paper-no-2/

IMPORTANT POINTS FROM THE GUIDELINE (SIP)

- Since 1996, the banking of hemopoietic stem cells (HSC) from umbilical cord blood in the UK has primarily been conducted by NHS institutions within the National Blood Service (NBS), initially financed through research and development funds and presently supported by the Department of Health.

- Women in designated maternity units in the UK are solicited during the antenatal phase and presented with the opportunity to donate cord blood to the NHS Cord Blood Bank (NCBB).

- Informed permission is secured by trained NBS personnel, and the blood is taken by qualified NBS operatives.

- These donations are forwarded to the NCBB for processing and storage for prospective use in unrelated transplantation, akin to bone marrow donations.

- The donations are evaluated for many factors, including infection markers and tissue types (human leukocyte antigen [HLA]).

- The tissue types of both unrelated cord blood and bone marrow donors are accessible for matching with any patient globally in need of hematopoietic stem cell transplantation.

- This established non-directed or altruistic cord blood banking service is distinct from the directed family or autologous cord blood storage now provided by various private companies operating in the UK.

- Commercial services provide women the option to preserve their child's cord blood hematopoietic stem cells long-term, in the event that the kid or their siblings develop a metabolic, immunological, or hematological disorder that may be treated exclusively through autologous or related cord blood stem cell transplantation.

- Furthermore, with the potential of stem cell therapy to cure or alleviate degenerative disorders, commercial cord blood banks have incorporated this prospective advantage into the justification for personal cord blood storage.

- Cord blood contains hematopoietic stem cells.

- These proliferative cells are approximately one logarithmic order lower in quantity than those derived from bone marrow or peripheral blood hematopoietic stem cell donation.

- Nonetheless, they exhibit superior proliferative and colony-forming capabilities and demonstrate heightened responsiveness to certain growth stimuli.

- Furthermore, due to their greater 'naïveté' compared to proliferative cells derived from bone marrow, they appear to generate less difficulties related to some facets of hematopoietic stem cell transplantation.

- The utilization of hematopoietic stem cells derived from umbilical cord blood has emerged as a recognized option to bone marrow transplantation, particularly for hematological, immunological, and metabolic storage diseases in pediatric and young adult populations.

- The storage of cord blood for therapeutic purposes necessitates a license from the Human Tissue Authority (HTA) in accordance with the Human Tissue Act.

- Both non-directed and directed donations for at-risk families are permissible practices.

- Insufficient data persists to endorse targeted commercial cord blood collection and stem cell storage in low-risk families.

- The prospective application of non-hematopoietic stem cells remains conjectural; yet, it is reasonable that some individuals with the financial means may desire to utilize available commercial services.

DOI: 10.1201/9781003650355-41

- Nonetheless, if this is executed, it must be conducted securely and will rely on the resources of the hospital where the delivery occurs.

- Every NHS trust or institution delivering intrapartum care must formulate a strategy addressing prenatal requests for cord blood storage via commercial sources, ensuring complete economic cost recovery.

- To prevent patients from incurring financial responsibilities by registering with commercial providers prior to informing their physicians, we recommend that this policy be disclosed to prospective patients at an early stage.

- Documented guidance outlining the hospital's policy should be provided to all patients upon booking maternity services.

- The Royal College of Obstetricians and Gynaecologists (RCOG) provides specific suggestions for NHS Trusts that choose to endorse cord blood collection.

  - There should be no modification in the standard management of the third stage.

  - To optimize safety for both the mother and newborn, collection should occur from the ex utero-detached placenta.

  - Collection must be conducted by a qualified third party, rather than the attending obstetrician or midwife, utilizing methods and facilities compliant with the European Tissues and Cells Directive.

  - The service should not be offered when the attending clinician considers it contraindicated, which likely encompasses all premature births and instances where specific contraindications, such as nuchal cord or maternal hemorrhage, are evident to the attendants.

  - The hospital's policy specifics should be accessible to all patients.

  - The NHS should evaluate an enhanced funding framework for both unrelated non-directed cord blood banking in the UK and directed donations for families with genetic disorders or those with a member suffering from an acquired disease amenable to hematopoietic stem cell transplantation, to ensure comprehensive coverage and equitable access for individuals requiring the advantages of stem cell transplantation, both presently and in the future.

- The RCOG advocates for research to enhance understanding of the short- and long-term neonatal impacts of third-stage practices.

QUESTIONS

1. Which of the following are the public cord blood banks in the United Kingdom?

    A. The Anthony Nolan Cord Blood Bank

    B. The NCBB

    C. Biovault

    D. All of the above

    E. A and B

2. Regarding public cord blood banking, which of the following statements is incorrect?

    A. Public cord blood banks adhere to the quality and safety criteria established by the HTA.

    B. They catalog their cord blood units on both national and international platforms to guarantee availability for patients globally.

    C. Women giving birth in specific hospitals where public banks operate are permitted to publicly donate cord blood.

    D. Donations to public banks necessitate an annual subscription fee, and donors receive annual compensation in return.

3. Regarding private cord blood banking, all of the following statements are true, except?

   A. They catalog their cord blood units in both national and international registries.

   B. Private cord blood banking collection takes place in the majority of UK hospitals.

   C. Private cord blood units are only utilized by the individual donor and her family members.

   D. The expectant mother choosing private banking incurs the subscription price.

4. Which of the following is the preferred site for collection of umbilical cord blood?

   A. Umbilical artery (placental side)

   B. Umbilical artery (fetal side)

   C. Umbilical vein

   D. Placental sinuses

5. What is the minimum amount of cord blood that can be collected to ensure availability of adequate cells for stem cell transplantation?

   A. 20 mL   C. 60 mL

   B. 40 mL   D. 100 mL

6. In terms of proper technique for umbilical cord blood collection, which of the following statements is correct?

   A. A minimum volume of 100 mL of cord blood is necessary to guarantee its future use for stem cell transplantation.

   B. Delayed cord clamping must be implemented.

   C. The cord blood must be harvested from the umbilical vein of a doubly clamped cord segment measuring 8–10 inches in length, adhering to appropriate sterile procedures.

   D. Blood collection must occur exclusively before separation of the placenta.

7. Which of the following is considered the major clinical indication for use of umbilical cord blood in children?

   A. Lysosomal storage disorders

   B. Severe combined immunodeficiency syndrome

   C. Acute lymphoblastic leukemia

   D. Cerebral palsy

8. What is the median total nucleated cell count of one umbilical cord blood unit?

   A. 2×10^9 C. 4×10^9

   B. 1×10^9 D. 7×10^9

9. Which of the following statements regarding umbilical cord blood is not true?

   A. It comprises hematopoietic stem cells (HSC).

   B. It has a greater quantity of proliferative cells in comparison to hematopoietic stem cell donations from bone marrow or peripheral blood.

   C. They possess significant growth potential and have a high responsiveness to colony-stimulating and growth stimuli.

   D. They result in fewer complications associated with HSC transplantation compared to cells derived from bone marrow.

10. Comparing cord blood stem cells with bone marrow stem cells, which of the following statements regarding cord blood collected stem cells is correct?

    A. Cord blood stem cells have a more limited transplantation capacity compared to bone marrow stem cells.

    B. Cord blood stem cells exhibit a reduced propensity for transplant rejection.

    C. Bone marrow stem cells can enhance immune system functionality during cancer therapy.

    D. Bone marrow stem cells can be readily harvested, cryopreserved, and stored for subsequent utilization.

11. Which of the following factors can adversely affect the amount of stem cells collected during the cord blood collection?

    A. Preterm birth

    B. When cord blood collection is done following delayed cord clamping

    C. Any maternal/fetal emergency to expedite delivery

    D. All of the above

    E. A and C

ANSWERS

1. E	5. B	9. B
2. D	6. C	10. B
3. A	7. C	11. D
4. C	8. B	

42 SIP – Use of USG and MRI to Diagnose Fetal Congenital Heart Defects (CHD)

Source: The Combined Use of Ultrasound and Fetal Magnetic Resonance Imaging for a Comprehensive Fetal Neurological Assessment in Fetal Congenital Cardiac Defects Scientific Impact Paper No. 60 May 2019. https://www.rcog.org.uk/guidance/browse-all-guidance/scientific-impact-papers/the-combined -use-of-ultrasound-and-fetal-magnetic-resonance-imaging-for-a-comprehensive-fetal-neurological -assessment-in-fetal-congenital-cardiac-defects-scientific-impact-paper-no-60/

IMPORTANT POINTS FROM THE GUIDELINE (SIP)

- Congenital heart defects (CHDs) represent the most prevalent congenital anomaly, occurring in around 5–10 per 1000 live births, and are a recognized cause of infant mortality.

- About 25% of newborns with congenital heart disease will have surgical intervention for significant abnormalities within their first year of life.

- The majority of cardiac lesions are solitary, with no accompanying congenital defects detected.

- Currently, around 50–60% of cases are identified antenatally by local and national screening programs.

- The definition of CHD varies considerably.

- CHD is characterized as a significant anatomical anomaly of the heart or intrathoracic major arteries that possesses actual or potential functional implications.

- In merely 15–30% of all instances of CHD, a cause is discovered; in the remaining cases, the etiology remains unclear.

- Chromosomal aneuploidy is a recognized etiology responsible for roughly 10% of all instances of CHD.

- The incidence of CHD in individuals with Down syndrome is roughly 45%.

- Recent decades have witnessed substantial progress in cardiothoracic surgery and cardiac care.

- The 30-day survival rates for surgical procedures exceeded 97.5%, contingent upon the intricacy of the heart disease.

- The 1-year survival rate is roughly 85%.

- In certain cardiac abnormalities, a 50–70% reduction in mortality has been shown over the past two decades.

- The enhancement in survival rates has coincided with a rise in the incidence of neurological deficits among this cohort, primarily comprising patients with transposition of the great arteries (TGA) and hypoplastic left heart (HLH).

- Robust data currently indicate that the prevalence of these abnormalities may reach 50%, underscoring the necessity to prioritize neurodevelopmental deficits as main outcomes in patients with CHD.

- The incidence and severity of neurodevelopmental delay correlate with the intricacy of congenital heart disease and specific genetic disorders.

- Neurodevelopmental delay encompasses deficits in intellect and academic performance, language (both expressive and receptive), visual construction and perception, attention, executive functioning, fine and gross motor skills, and psychosocial maladjustment.

- Numerous newborns with congenital heart disease have corrective or palliative surgery during the neonatal phase, and the utilization of cardiopulmonary bypass, deep hypothermic circulatory arrest, along with various surgical and postoperative variables, has been associated with negative neurodevelopmental outcomes.

- Chromosomal and other syndromic disorders linked to CHDs are independently correlated with compromised neurodevelopmental status.

DOI: 10.1201/9781003650355-42

- Additional genetic factors, such as the expression of neuroprotective apolipoprotein E, may influence brain damage modulation post-surgery in some patients.

- Socioeconomic and parenting factors will additionally affect subsequent intellectual development.

- However, there is a growing recognition of preoperative and prenatal brain dysgenesis, immaturity, and white matter injury in newborns with CHDs.

- Significant clinical evidence indicates neurological developmental abnormalities in these infants prior to surgery, with a stronger correlation shown in some cardiac anomalies, such as HLH.

- Infants with HLH exhibit a greater prevalence of microcephaly.

- Alongside overall delay, localized brain impairments have been noted across all areas.

- Neuroimaging studies indicate that over fifty percent of neonates with congenital heart disease, particularly those in high-risk categories such as HLH syndrome and TGA, exhibit signs of white matter brain injury, commonly referred to as ischemic lesions, white matter injury, localized stroke, and periventricular leukomalacia.

- Research utilizing magnetic resonance imaging (MRI), magnetic resonance spectroscopy, and diffusion tensor imaging (DTI) has identified brain microstructural and metabolic anomalies in fetuses both prenatally and quickly postnatally, prior to surgical intervention.

- The etiology of these changes is likely complex, involving congenital brain anomalies, intrauterine hemodynamic modifications, and acquired brain injury.

- Transabdominal scanning (TAS) and transvaginal scanning (TVS) are the primary modalities for fetal ultrasound screening and evaluation, facilitating standard visualization of fetal intracranial anatomy in both the transthalamic and transcerebellar planes, thereby allowing for the identification of anomalies such as ventriculomegaly, severe cerebellar hypoplasia, holoprosencephaly, and Arnold–Chiari malformation.

- From around 18 weeks of gestation, fetal cortical development evaluated using ultrasound roughly aligns with that determined by MRI.

- Moreover, advancements in ultrasound technologies have enhanced the visualization of fetal cerebral architecture, shown by color Doppler flow imaging and higher frequency probes.

- MRI is becoming a prominent aspect of clinical practice and has been utilized antenatally for around 20 years without any documented risks to the fetus when conducted in accordance with radiological protocols.

- Fetal MRI is a recognized, safe, and complementary method for evaluating the fetus, especially the brain, in fetal medicine.

- It provides an expanded field of vision, advantageous as pregnancy advances, and facilitates effective picture capture irrespective of fetal position or maternal size.

- MRI may be utilized to validate ultrasound findings, offer additional data regarding a suspected aberration, or identify novel abnormalities not seen by previous ultrasound, including foci of infarction and cerebellar and cortical irregularities.

- Moreover, advanced MRI technologies, such as DTI tractography for imaging and mapping white matter tracts, and connectomics for integrating structural connectivity data with functional activity, may facilitate the identification of atypical brain development and ultimately yield insights into neurodevelopmental prognosis.

- Nonetheless, it is crucial to acknowledge that MRI, despite its benefits, is not the definitive standard, and each modality possesses distinct advantages.

- Ventriculomegaly exemplifies an ultrasonography diagnosis with a multifaceted cause, including acquired damage, resulting in an associated malformation rate of 10–76%.

- The ultrasound diagnosis of ventriculomegaly is uncomplicated, although the precise identification of accompanying intracranial anomalies is more difficult.

- The primary additional anomaly overlooked by ultrasonography is agenesis of the corpus callosum.

- Additional diagnoses, such as intraventricular hemorrhage and subependymal heterotopia, frequently resulting from in utero ischemic injury, are optimally identified using MRI.

- The elimination of further irregularities using MRI might also offer reassurance to the woman.

- Proliferation problems may result from environmental damage.

- The primary worry is frequently reassessed later in gestation due to the occurrence of microcephaly (head circumference exceeding three standard deviations below the mean).

- The optimal evaluation for gyral abnormalities is conducted via MRI.

- In 2013, the inaugural in utero application of the combined techniques of ultrasound scanning and MRI, referred to as MRI ultrasound fusion, was documented.

- This proof of concept illustrated the capability of the technology to overlay real-time ultrasound scanning views over MRI pictures.

- Neuroimaging plays a crucial role in identifying injuries or developmental anomalies, necessitating subsequent examinations of these patients to ascertain the therapeutic relevance of the results.

- MRI possesses enhanced proficiency compared to ultrasonography in identifying previously undiagnosed agenesis of the corpus callosum, cerebellar anomalies, cortical irregularities such as polymicrogyria, and migration disorders including subependymal heterotopia.

- Ultrasound guidelines recommend limiting MRI examinations to fetuses with suspected abnormalities identified via ultrasound.

- The predominant fetal MRI is conducted at 1.5 T, while some facilities utilize 3 T for research and therapeutic applications.

- Image acquisition employs single-shot techniques, thereby reducing the impact of fetal and, to a lesser degree, maternal mobility on image quality.

- Image acquisition may require 20 to 60 minutes.

- T2-weighted images are the primary sequence offering superior contrast of cerebral regions.

- T1-weighted approaches are effective for verifying the presence of hemorrhage, however, they are more difficult to acquire at adequate quality.

- In a clinical context, diffusion-weighted imaging can be utilized to detect regions of acute ischemia.

- Additional sophisticated methodologies encompass DTI for evaluating tissue microstructure and cerebral connectivity, MRI spectroscopy for analyzing cerebral metabolites, and phase contrast and T2 mapping techniques for assessing fetal cerebral blood flow and oxygen extraction; however, these techniques predominantly remain within the research domain.

- Currently, prenatal and perinatal counseling emphasizes the mortality risk and cardiovascular morbidity linked to particular heart abnormalities.

- Antenatal diagnosis by ultrasound and fetal MRI, coupled with advancements in technology and image acquisition, enhances the detection of prenatal neurological disorders and their correlation with long-term neurodevelopmental outcomes.

- The antenatal diagnosis of neurological disorders may guide future investigations and inform antenatal counseling.

- Consideration should be made to multidisciplinary care involving a clinical geneticist and a neurologist, due to the range of potential neurological disorders and their effect on prognosis.

- Long-term neurodevelopment will be further impacted by other brain damage that may arise during birth or during first interventions such as septostomy and subsequent surgical procedures.

- There is a case for performing supplementary imaging examinations at successive intervals to identify both developmental changes and the emergence of lesions in this susceptible population.

- Currently, prenatal ultrasonography is the principal screening modality for infants with CHD, whereas MRI is utilized in certain cases for suspected cerebral anomalies subsequent to the initial screening.

- The efficacy of MRI in identifying anomalies undetectable by ultrasound in patients with congenital heart disease remains uncertain.

- Subsequent research in this domain may prove beneficial and has the capacity to enlighten practitioners regarding the risk of neurological morbidity associated with antenatal brain development and postnatal surgical interventions, ultimately enhancing parental counseling during the antenatal phase.

QUESTIONS

1. What is the birth prevalence of CHDs in newborns?
   A. 1/1000 live births
   B. 5–10/1000 live births
   C. 1% live births
   D. 5–10% live births

2. What percentage of CHDs are detected antenatally by national screening programs?
   A. 25%
   B. 40%
   C. 50–60%
   D. 80–90%

3. What percentage of infants born with congenital heart disease have serious defects requiring surgery during the first year of life?
   A. 25%
   B. 40%
   C. 50–60%
   D. 80–90%

4. In what percentage of all cases of CHDs is the cause identified?
   A. <10%
   B. 15–30%
   C. 45%
   D. 70%

5. Chromosomal aneuploidies are a cause of what percentage of CHDs in newborns?
   A. 10%
   B. 25%
   C. 45%
   D. 75%

6. What is the prevalence of CHDs in Down syndrome?

    A. 10%

    B. 25%

    C. 45%

    D. 75%

7. All of the following single-gene defects are associated with CHDs, except?

    A. Alagille syndrome

    B. Holt–Oram syndrome

    C. Noonan syndrome

    D. Prader–Willi syndrome

8. Which of the following regarding inheritance of non-syndromic congenital heart disease is incorrect?

    A. If one affected sibling – recurrence risk is 1–6%

    B. If two affected siblings – recurrence risk is 3–10%

    C. If one of the parents is affected – risk of inheritance is higher (about 4%)

    D. The risk is 2–3-fold higher in cases of paternal CHD than maternal CHD

9. According to a meta-analysis, to what extent does prenatal vitamin supplementation reduce the risk of congenital heart disease in the fetus?

    A. By 20%   C. By 60%

    B. By 40%   D. By 80%

10. Which of the following congenital heart diseases/syndromes are known to be linked to neurological deficits?

    A. HLH syndrome

    B. Transposition of great arteries

    C. DiGeorge syndrome

    D. All of the above

    E. A and B

11. Which of the following congenital heart diseases/syndromes has a higher prevalence of microcephaly?

    A. HLH syndrome

    B. Transposition of great arteries

    C. DiGeorge syndrome

    D. Bicuspid aortic valve

12. CHARGE syndrome includes all of the following birth defects, except?

    A. Coloboma of the eye

    B. Heart defects

    C. Atresia choanae

    D. Gastroschisis

    E. Ear abnormalities and hearing impairment (absence of semicircular canals)

13. Regarding the role of MRIs in the detection of fetal defects, which of the following statements is incorrect?

    A. It is indicated for a fetus with a suspected or proven congenital cardiac abnormality.

    B. It is indicated if there is any suspicion of fetal abnormality on ultrasonography.

    C. It aids in the identification of agenesis of the corpus callosum, cerebellar anomalies, cortical irregularities (such as polymicrogyria), and migratory disorders (such as subependymal heterotopia).

    D. The majority of fetal MRIs are conducted on three Tesla machines.

14. In terms of the different approaches in MRI, which of the following is not correctly matched with their individual assessment abilities?

    A. T2-weighted images provide excellent contrast of brain structures

    B. T1-weighted images confirm the presence of hemorrhage

    C. Diffusion-weighted imaging helps to identify areas of acute ischemia

    D. DTI assesses fetal cerebral blood flow and oxygen extraction

    E. MRI spectroscopy assesses cerebral metabolites

15. After what gestation does the fetal cortical development evaluated by ultrasound closely align with that determined by MRI?

    A. 12 weeks

    B. 18 weeks

    C. 24 weeks

    D. 28 weeks

16. All of the following white matter injuries are noted in more than 50% of fetuses born with high-risk CHDs such as HLH syndrome and TGA, except?

    A. Ischemic lesions

    B. Localized stroke

    C. Periventricular leukomalacia

    D. Cerebral atrophy

17. Which of the following is not a defect that explains 'tetralogy of Fallot'?

    A. Pulmonary stenosis

    B. Overriding pulmonary artery

    C. Ventricular septal defect

    D. Right ventricular hypertrophy

18. Ebstein's anomaly typically affects which of the following parts of the fetal heart?

    A. Pulmonary artery

    B. Tricuspid valve

    C. Mitral valve

    D. Aortic valve

19. A 34-year-old patient presents to your antenatal outpatient department (OPD) with her mid-trimester anomaly scan report. She is quite concerned and has been referred to you by her GP. Her report is suggestive of HLH syndrome. You refer her to the specialized fetal medicine department for further management. All of the following are recommended surgical options for HLHS, except?

    A. Norwood procedure

    B. Heart transplant

    C. Fontan procedure

    D. Arterial switch operation

20. Which of the following heart defects is not commonly associated with Down syndrome?

    A. Atrioventricular septal defect

    B. Ventricular septal defect

    C. Patent ductus arteriosus

    D. Truncus arteriosus

ANSWERS

1. B	8. D	15. B
2. C	9. B	16. D
3. A	10. D	17. B
4. B	11. A	18. B
5. A	12. D	19. D
6. C	13. D	20. D
7. D	14. D	

43 SIP – Uterine Natural Killer (uNK) Cells

Source: The Role of Natural Killer Cells in Human Fertility Scientific Impact Paper No. 53 December 2016. https://www.rcog.org.uk/guidance/browse-all-guidance/scientific-impact-papers/the-role-of-natural-killer-cells-in-human-fertility-scientific-impact-paper-no-53/

IMPORTANT POINTS FROM THE GUIDELINE (SIP)

- Uterine natural killer (uNK) cells constitute the predominant leukocyte population in the endometrium during implantation and have garnered significant interest regarding their function in proper implantation and early placental development.

- While numerous clinical studies indicate an elevation of peripheral blood natural killer (PBNK) cells and/or uNK cells in women experiencing recurrent miscarriage (RM) and recurrent implantation failure (RIF), a meta-analysis and systematic review did not yield definitive conclusions due to substantial heterogeneity among the studies resulting from varying methodologies employed to quantify NK cells.

- Natural killer (NK) cells were initially characterized as large granular lymphocytes capable of lysing cells without prior sensitization and not constrained by the expression of major histocompatibility complex class I molecules on target cells.

- Natural killer (NK) cells are increasingly recognized to possess functions beyond lysis, including cytokine production.

- Human NK cells are characterized by the presence of distinct cell surface markers, notably CD16 and CD56; they lack the expression of CD3, immunoglobulin, and T lymphocyte receptors.

- Natural killer (NK) cells are present in PB and several lymphoid and non-lymphoid organs.

- Two primary subsets of peripheral blood natural killer (PB NK) cells have been identified: The predominant subset, comprising over 90%, expresses CD56 at low density and CD16, designated as $CD56^{dim} CD16^+$ cells, capable of lysing target cells; conversely, approximately 10% of PB NK cells exhibit high surface expression of CD56 without CD16 expression, classified as $CD56^{bright} CD16^-$ cells.

- PB NK cells exhibit minimal or negligible cytotoxic action while secreting a substantial quantity of cytokines.

- The human endometrium harbors a significant population of natural killer (NK) cells, known as uNK cells, whose quantity and percentage relative to the total number of endometrial stromal cells fluctuate over the menstrual cycle.

- While uNK cells are seen in proliferative endometrium, their numbers significantly increase during the mid-secretory phase, making them the predominant endometrial lymphocyte population in the late secretory phase and the first trimester of pregnancy.

- uNK cells are characterized as $CD56^{bright} CD16^+$ and furthermore express CD9, a marker absent in PBNK cells.

- Unlike PB $CD56^{bright} CD16^-$ NK cells, uNK cells possess many cytoplasmic granules filled with perforin and granzyme.

- There is no firm agreement regarding the origin of uNK cells.

- Mature PB NK cells or immature precursors may infiltrate the endometrium from the bloodstream, may be in response to chemokines secreted by endometrial cells during particular phases of the menstrual cycle and pregnancy, and may be influenced by additional variables within the endometrium.

- For instance, the secretion of CXCL-12 by extravillous trophoblast (EVT) cells may draw NK cells into the decidua during pregnancy; interleukin (IL)-15, produced by the secretory endometrium and decidua, exerts a selective chemoattractant influence on PB CD16⁻ NK cells; and transforming growth factor beta 1 (TGF-β1) has been proposed to convert PB NK cells into uNK cells.

 DOI: 10.1201/9781003650355-43

- An additional proposition is that uNK cells originate from hematopoietic progenitor cells located in the endometrium.

- The elevated quantity of uNK cells in the late-secretory phase endometrium and early decidua indicates the role of progesterone.

- Despite the absence of progesterone receptor (PR) expression in uNK cells, a progesterone-mediated response may be enabled by cytokines and growth factors secreted by other endometrial cells that do express PR.

- Progesterone stimulates IL-15 production by stromal cells in the secretory phase endometrium and early pregnancy decidua.

- Macrophage inflammatory protein 1 beta, a chemoattractant for PB NK cells, is likewise increased by progesterone in human endometrial tissue.

- Various chemokines and cytokines in the endometrium may facilitate the recruitment of PBNK cells and their subsequent transformation into uNK cells.

- There is unequivocal evidence that uNK cells can multiply within the endometrium and decidua.

- Research has shown that uNK cells display the proliferation marker Ki-67, especially during the secretory phase, characterized by a rapid increase in uNK cell populations.

- Regardless of their origin, a study of PBNK cells and uNK cells within the same individual has demonstrated that uNK cells are unique from both $CD56^{dim}$ $CD16^+$ and $CD56^{bright}$ $CD16^-$ PB NK cells, warranting their classification as a separate population.

- Embryo implantation necessitates the attachment of the embryo to the luminal epithelium of the endometrium, followed by penetration of the epithelial layer and embedding within the underlying endometrial stroma.

- The invasion of trophoblast cells into the decidualized stromal cells and their subsequent differentiation into diverse cell types is crucial to the process.

- Trophoblast cells initially multiply to create cytotrophoblast columns, which expand outward to establish a cytotrophoblast shell.

- EVT cells develop within the cytotrophoblast columns into highly invasive cells that penetrate the maternal decidua, extending into the inner third of the myometrium by two separate pathways.

- Interstitial EVT invasion occurs via the decidual tissue and correlates with the degradation of the extracellular matrix (ECM).

- Conversely, the endovascular trophoblast migrates into the lumen of the spiral arteries, temporarily substituting the endothelium and ultimately remodeling the uterine spiral arteries from robust musculoelastic vessels into dilated conduits.

- The proximity of uNK cells to the invading EVT cells indicates their potential involvement in this process.

- The cytotoxic efficacy of uNK cells is diminished in comparison to PB NK cells.

- uNK cells extracted from early pregnancy decidua exhibit little cytolytic activity against fetal EVT cells, potentially attributable to the expression of human leukocyte antigen G by EVT cells.

- There is significant interest in the function of cytokines during pregnancy, with the implication that a predominance of type 2 cytokines promotes successful pregnancy, whereas type 1 cytokines are deemed harmful.

- uNK cells secrete a variety of cytokines and growth factors, including IL-1, IL-2, IL-4, IL-6, IL-8, IL-10, tumor necrosis factor alpha, granulocyte-macrophage colony-stimulating factor, TGF-1, leukemia inhibitory factor, and interferon gamma.

- uNK cells serve as a significant source of angiogenic growth factors.

- uNK cells from the secretory phase endometrium and early pregnancy decidua have been reported to produce angiogenin, angiopoietin (Ang)-1, Ang-2, vascular endothelial growth factor (VEGF)-A, VEGF-C, placental growth factor, keratinocyte growth factor, fibroblast growth factor, and platelet-derived growth factor-BB.

- There are variations in the secretory activity of uNK cells based on gestational age: cells from 12–14 weeks of gestation secrete more cytokines and fewer angiogenic factors compared to those from 8–10 weeks of gestation.

- Both interstitial trophoblast invasion and spiral artery remodeling necessitate the degradation of the extracellular matrix by proteolytic enzymes.

- uNK cells release matrix metalloproteinases (MMP)-1, MMP-2, MMP-7, MMP-9, MMP-10, tissue inhibitors of metalloproteinases (TIMP)-1, TIMP-2, TIMP-3, urokinase plasminogen activator (uPA), and the uPA receptor.

- The immunoreactivity of MMP-7 and MMP-9 by leukocytes adjacent to spiral arteries during early pregnancy has been documented.

- Spiral arteries are essential blood vessels in the non-pregnant endometrium and the pregnant decidua.

- Following menstruation, these arteries regenerate from vessel stumps in the residual endometrial stratum basalis, and research indicates that uNK cells may play a role in this process.

- uNK cells are often clustered around the spiral arteries and arterioles during early pregnancy, suggesting their involvement in facilitating vascular modifications in this period.

- The presence of elevated uNK cells in the endometrium of women experiencing reproductive failure, including infertility, RM, and pre-eclampsia, indicates their potential involvement in this pathophysiology.

- Nevertheless, the findings from multiple studies are inconsistent, and despite the use of cell count measurements in clinical practice, there is still no compelling evidence to suggest they are the cause of reproductive failure.

- The conflicting results from various studies indicate that while aberrant PB NK or uNK cell numbers may have a role in RIF, there is inadequate data to reach definitive conclusions.

- RM is characterized by the loss of three or more consecutive pregnancies, confirmed by a positive pregnancy test, prior to 24 weeks of gestation, or the loss of two or more consecutive pregnancies, defined as a nonviable intrauterine pregnancy exhibiting either an empty gestational sac or an embryo or fetus lacking fetal heart activity within the initial 12 weeks of gestation.

- In 50% of women, the etiology of recurrent loss remains unidentified, and in these individuals, a potential involvement of uNK cells has been hypothesized.

- The divergent findings from various studies indicate that PB NK or uNK cells may be implicated in RM; however, additional research is necessary for validation.

- Pre-eclampsia is characterized by insufficient remodeling of the spiral arteries, especially inside the myometrial layer.

- The findings indicating that uNK cells are crucial to spiral artery remodeling implies their potential involvement in pre-eclampsia.

- Various studies present contradictory information concerning the involvement of uNK cells in the etiology of pre-eclampsia.

- The documented rise in uNK cell quantities in RIF or RM has led to heightened demand from women with these illnesses for assessments of PB NK and uNK cell counts.

- The significance of the outcomes of these tests is constrained.

- The quantity of NK cells in PB is typically assessed by evaluating the expression of $CD56^+$ using flow cytometry.

- There is minimal agreement over the definition of a high PBNK cell count; various studies have employed thresholds ranging from 12% to 18%.

- The quantity of PBNK cells may be influenced by phases of the menstrual cycle.

- NK cell counts and activity are elevated during the periovulatory phase and diminished by the use of contraceptive pills.

- Consequently, blood samples for NK cell assessment must be collected at a certain phase of the cycle and from women not on steroid hormone therapy.

- The quantity of NK cells in the endometrium can be ascertained using either immunostaining of tissue sections or by mincing and digesting the tissue, thereafter, analyzed via flow cytometry.

- The benefit of the latter strategy is that NK cell subsets can be easily acquired.

- Endometrial tissue sample is typically performed during the mid-secretory phase, also known as the peri-implantation stage.

- The biopsy must be scheduled accurately in accordance with the luteinizing hormone spike, ideally performed 7 days after the surge.

- Intravenous immunoglobulin (IVIg) given during gestation has been utilized for the management of both RM and RIF.

- Multiple theories have been suggested about its mechanism, including the attenuation of NK cell activity and alteration of cytokine output.

- Nevertheless, the data indicates that treatment with IVIg lacks support and, due to potential major adverse effects, should be avoided.

- Glucocorticoids have been utilized in a study to address reproductive failure in women with elevated levels of uNK cells, predicated on the finding that uNK cells express the glucocorticoid receptor.

- The literature analysis concerning therapies to enhance reproductive outcomes in women with elevated NK cell counts undergoing assisted conception has underscored the lack of high-quality randomized controlled trials in this specific domain.

- Despite extensive research, the function of uNK cells in pregnancy remains ambiguous, and it is unclear if the elevated uNK cell counts observed in conjunction with aberrant pregnancy pathologies (RM, RIF, or pre-eclampsia) are actually causative or indicative of more basic endometrial issues.

- Clinicians should recognize that uNK cells differ from PBNK cells, and that assessing the latter provides limited insight into the function of uNK cells in reproductive failure, when addressing patients interested in NK cell testing.

- Routine uNK cell testing in women experiencing infertility or pursuing IVF treatment is not currently recommended.

- The use of uNK cell testing in cases of RM and RIF remains contentious and should be considered experimental until further evidence is available.

- The quantification of uNK cells must be standardized, and the definitions of 'normal' and 'high' levels should be based on established reference ranges determined from standardized methodologies.

- Women participating in uNK cell testing should be aware that there is currently no established therapeutic treatment for individuals with potentially aberrant results, but preliminary studies indicate a possible beneficial benefit of prednisolone.

QUESTIONS

1. Which of the following receptors is not expressed by human NK cells?

A. CD56

B. CD16

C. CD9

D. CD3

2. Regarding human NK cells, which of the following statements is incorrect?

   A. Human NK cells express CD56 and CD16 receptors.

   B. Over 90% of uNK cells have low-density expression of CD56 and CD16, classified as CD56^{dim} CD16$^+$ cells.

   C. Approximately 10% of PB NK cells exhibit elevated surface expression of CD56 but lacking CD16, categorizing them as CD56^{bright} CD16$^-$ cells.

   D. Uterine NK cells are characterized as CD56^{bright} CD16$^+$ and furthermore express CD9.

3. PB NK cells do NOT express which of the following receptors?

   A. CD56^{bright}

   B. CD56^{dim}

   C. CD16

   D. CD9

4. uNK cells do NOT express which of the following receptors?

   A. CD56^{bright}

   B. CD56^{dim}

   C. CD16

   D. CD9

5. uNK cells increase in number in all the following phases in the endometrium, except?

   A. Proliferative phase

   B. Mid-secretory phase

   C. Late-secretory phase

   D. First trimester of pregnancy

6. Which of the following is the proliferative marker expressed by uNK cells during the secretory phase of the menstrual cycle?

   A. P21

   B. Mini-chromosome maintenance (MCM) proteins

   C. Ki-67

   D. Proliferating cell nuclear antigen (PCNA)

7. Which of the following chemokines is not considered as a chemoattractant for uNK cells?

   A. CXCL-12 produced by EVT

   B. IL-15, produced by secretory endometrium and decidua

   C. TGF-β1

   D. Tumor necrosis factor-beta (TNF-β)

8. All of the following factors increase the number of PB NK cells, except?

   A. Peri-ovulatory period

   B. Luteal phase of menstrual cycle

   C. Use of oral contraceptive pills

   D. Any event causing acute stress

9. According to available research, what is considered to be a significantly high number of PB NK cells?

   A. >1–5%

   B. >12–18%

   C. >25–30%

   D. >40%

10. The number of NK cells in the PB is usually measured by flow cytometry testing for expression of which of the following receptors?

    A. CD16

    B. CD56

    C. CD9

    D. CD3

11. Which of the following phases of the menstrual cycle is the best time to take endometrial tissue samples to test for natural killer cells?

    A. Proliferative phase

    B. Peri-ovulatory phase

    C. Early secretory phase

    D. Mid-secretory phase (the peri-implantation period)

12. Which of the following regarding the precise timing of endometrial tissue sampling to detect natural killer cells is correct?

    A. Sample to be taken 7 days after FSH surge

    B. Sample to be taken 7 days after LH surge

    C. Sample to be taken 3 days after FSH surge

    D. Sample to be taken 3 days after LH surge

13. Which of the following conditions during pregnancy are considered to be linked with functioning of NK cells?

    A. Pre-eclampsia

    B. Fetal growth restriction

    C. Recurrent implantation failure in patients undergoing in vitro fertilization

    D. All of the above

14. NK cells belong to which of the following categories of the human immune system?

    A. Innate immunity

    B. Cell-mediated immunity

    C. Humoral immunity

    D. All of the above

    E. B and C

ANSWERS

1. D	6. C	11. D
2. B	7. D	12. B
3. D	8. C	13. D
4. B	9. B	14. A
5. A	10. B	

44 SIP – Uterine Transplantation

Source: Uterine Transplantation Scientific Impact Paper No. 65 April 2021. https://www.rcog.org.uk/guidance/browse-all-guidance/scientific-impact-papers/uterine-transplantation-scientific-impact-paper-no-65/

IMPORTANT POINTS FROM THE GUIDELINE (SIP)

- Uterine transplantation (UTx) is a prospective therapeutic option for women experiencing absolute uterine factor infertility (AUFI).
- AUFI is generally regarded as impacting 1 in 500 women of reproductive age.
- AUFI pertains to women experiencing infertility due to the absence of a uterus or the existence of a uterus that is anatomically or physiologically impaired.
- The recognized pathways to motherhood for women with AUFI encompass adoption or surrogacy, which are deemed acceptable alternatives by many.
- These options are not only linked to intricate legal, financial, cultural, ethical, and religious considerations, but they also preclude the experience of pregnancy.
- UTx offers a solution to certain challenges while enabling women with AUFI to conceive through assisted reproductive technologies and experience motherhood firsthand.
- Adoption and surrogacy do not provide the experience of pregnancy, which has been shown to be the principal incentive for 63% of women with AUFI seeking UTx.
- Although UTx entails significant physical risks, such as multiple major surgeries and the requirement for immunosuppression during the donor transplant's duration, it enables recipients to achieve pregnancy and mitigates certain legal and religious complications related to surrogacy.
- While there is no direct substitute for UTx, it is imperative to consider adoption and surrogacy during the counseling process for UTx.
- This guarantees that the consent procedure is thoroughly informed, allowing for the appropriate consideration of the increased risks associated with UTx in relation to the perceived individualized advantages.
- Potential candidates for UTx are women of reproductive age with AUFI, which may be attributed to congenital or acquired reasons.
- Typically, women with (Mayer–Rokitansky–Küster–Hauser) MRKH syndrome possess properly functioning ovaries, rendering them appropriate candidates for UTx.
- A research study evaluating attitudes of UTx among women with MRKH revealed that nearly two-thirds of participants were amenable to the treatment, fully comprehending the associated risks.
- Women eligible for UTx must meet specified preoperative criteria.
- A physiologically functional vagina of typical length (7 cm or more) is seen a requirement by several teams, hence excluding women with a neovagina.
- Women with atypical MRKH, particularly those with renal anomalies, may be eligible for UTx.
- Precautions are necessary for individuals with unilateral renal agenesis, which occurs in around 25% of instances, due to the more than 2-fold elevated risk of hypertensive problems during pregnancy, including pre-eclampsia.
- Individuals with pelvic kidneys necessitate further evaluation by magnetic resonance imaging (MRI) or computed tomography (CT) scanning to accurately locate the pelvic kidney and ascertain whether it may interfere with the eventual uterine transplantation procedure.
- Indications for hysterectomy in women of reproductive age encompass benign gynecological disorders, gynecological malignancies (such as cervical cancer), or significant postpartum hemorrhage.

DOI: 10.1201/9781003650355-44

- Caution is necessary for women undergoing UTx after prior cancer diagnoses due to the potential risk of recurrence associated with the obligatory postoperative immunosuppression.

- Consequently, further counseling is necessary for these women, and it is advisable to permit a minimum of 5 years in remission before considering them for UTx.

- Asherman syndrome, characterized by the presence of a defective endometrium in the uterus, affects up to 1.5% of women of reproductive age.

- This disorder, marked by the development of adhesions within the uterus and/or cervix, can lead to amenorrhea, recurrent miscarriage, and infertility.

- Hysteroscopic adhesiolysis can facilitate fertility restoration; nonetheless, elevated rates of infertility, miscarriage, suboptimal implantation, and aberrant placentation persist.

- UTx for Asherman syndrome should be contemplated solely in severe instances, after all alternative therapeutic modalities have been tried.

- Living donors have constituted 80% of the UTx instances conducted to date.

- From a logistical perspective, coordinating elective surgery with living donors is more straightforward than the on-call arrangement necessary for deceased donation, due to the varied variety of interdisciplinary competence required.

- The standard evaluations conducted for other solid organ transplants are also applicable to UTx donors, encompassing microbiological screening to avert the transmission of infections such as HIV, hepatitis B and C, cytomegalovirus, Epstein–Barr virus, syphilis, toxoplasma, and human T-cell lymphotropic virus.

- The utilization of living donors permits additional time for specific investigations related to UTx, which should minimally encompass a cervical smear and human papillomavirus testing, assessments to rule out sexually transmitted infections (chlamydia, gonorrhea, and trichomoniasis), and a vaginal culture to exclude *Candida* species and bacterial vaginosis.

- A transvaginal ultrasound should be performed to rule out structural problems.

- Magnetic resonance angiography or computed tomography angiography help to furnish details regarding vascular anatomy, caliber, and patency.

- The utilization of first-degree relatives may confer immunological advantages, while employing older donors is linked to additional risks.

- The likelihood of atherosclerotic changes in the pelvic arteries significantly increases with age, potentially leading to an organ of inadequate quality for implantation.

- Furthermore, before the manifestation of macroscopic or histological indicators of atherosclerosis, advancing age has been demonstrated to induce arterial inflammation, thereby heightening the risk of post-transplant graft vasculopathy.

- The primary drawback of living donors is the considerable risk posed to the donor.

- The live donor faces the risk of surgical morbidity.

- The utilization of deceased donors effectively eliminates donor risk and permits a more extensive dissection, facilitating the procurement of bigger caliber arteries, which presumably diminishes the danger of graft thrombosis.

- A possible disadvantage of utilizing deceased donors is the widespread brain-death inflammation that may affect organ quality.

- UTx involves the transplantation of the uterus, encompassing the cervix, a segment of the vagina, adjacent ligamentous, and connective tissues, along with the principal blood arteries that nourish and drain the uterus.

- Donor procedures have primarily utilized a midline laparotomy approach; however, minimally invasive surgical techniques have been suggested (both laparoscopic and robotic).

- All successful UTx surgeries have led to menstruation without the necessity for additional hormone therapy, serving as a dependable measure of uterine functionality and overall health.

- Rejection is characterized as the destruction of the donor graft by the host's immune response, which is triggered against the graft's alloantigens due to genetic disparities between the donor and recipient.

- In the UTx instances conducted to date, tacrolimus has primarily been the drug of choice, originally administered in conjunction with mycophenolate mofetil (MMF), with or without the inclusion of prednisolone.

- MMF is then discontinued prior to embryo transfer due to its teratogenic properties, typically being substituted with azathioprine.

- A recent alternate regimen employing maintenance tacrolimus and azathioprine has been implemented, showing no difference in rejection events.

- Symptoms of rejection, such as abdominal pain, fever, or vaginal discharge/bleeding, manifest only after rejection has been definitively confirmed.

- The majority of rejection episodes were well controlled with a 3-day regimen of intravenous methylprednisolone; however, severe episodes necessitated the inclusion of anti-thymocyte globulin.

- A distinctive benefit of UTx compared to other solid organ transplants is that it is temporary; once the woman's family is complete, the graft can be excised, enabling the discontinuation of immunosuppression.

- Embryo transfer was initially postponed for a minimum of 12 months postoperatively, in accordance with conventional solid organ transplant protocols.

- Recently, a duration of 6 months has been established, providing adequate time for surgical recovery and stabilization of the immunosuppressive regimen.

- Tacrolimus and azathioprine have repeatedly demonstrated safety for administration during pregnancy, with no elevated risk of congenital anomalies.

- Nevertheless, possibly teratogenic immunosuppression, such as MMF, must be discontinued at least 6 weeks before embryo transfer and substituted with an alternative drug, such as azathioprine.

- In instances when MMF is not utilized, the interval between implantation and embryo transfer may be minimized to 3 months, hence potentially decreasing cumulative exposure to immunosuppression.

- All offspring have thus far been delivered via lower segment cesarean section.

- Concerning the possible effects of tacrolimus on the fetus, there exists a minimal theoretical risk of reversible neonatal hyperkalemia and renal dysfunction, necessitating postnatal evaluation.

- Although tacrolimus is present in breast milk, the amount ingested by infants is less than 1% of the maternal dosage, and breastfeeding has not been demonstrated to elevate infant tacrolimus levels postnatally, so it is regarded as safe.

- AUFI not only leads to infertility but may also cause considerable psychological consequences.

- Over one-third of infertile women experience severe depressive symptoms and exhibit a 2-fold elevated risk of suicide.

- UTx encompasses intricate bioethical dilemmas that regulate both assisted reproductive technology and organ transplantation.

- Only women who have received comprehensive counseling and are fully informed can determine if the possible advantages of UTx surpass the considerable dangers involved with the procedure.

- Although each case should be individualized, the dangers of UTx in women with substantial medical comorbidities may surpass the possible advantages.

- Subsequent to the enactment of the Organ Donation (Deemed Consent) Act 2019, the legal framework in England regarding dead organ donation transitioned to a 'opt-out' system.

- This assumes default adult consent for organ donation unless an opt-out decision has been previously documented.

- Nonetheless, similar to other innovative transplants, uterine donation is excluded from the opt-out strategy, necessitating explicit approval from the donor's family.

- UTx is linked to considerable morbidity, encompassing three to four major surgical procedures (UTx, cesarean sections, and hysterectomy for transplant removal) and the hazards associated with transitory immunosuppression.

- Furthermore, in the cases conducted to far, nearly 30% of grafts have been excised due to problems.

- Therefore, recipients must possess strong motivation, robust support networks, access to suitable psychological therapies, and comprehensive awareness of the potential hazards involved.

- Due to the procedure's novelty, it is essential to acknowledge that long-term outcomes following UTx are currently unavailable.

- Consequently, all cases must be documented in the international registry, encompassing the monitoring of donors, recipients, and their progeny.

- As UTx transitions into clinical practice, it is imperative to establish solid governance to facilitate performance and safety monitoring, as is necessary for all innovative medicines and interventions.

QUESTIONS

1. What is the prevalence of AUFI in women of childbearing age?
    A. 1 in 200 women
    B. 1 in 500 women
    C. 1 in 1000 women
    D. 1 in 1500 women

2. To date, what percentage of uterine transplant procedures have been unsuccessful?
    A. 10%
    B. 30%
    C. 50%
    D. 70%

3. Which of the following is the primary motivating factor for women with AUFI to choose UTx over adoption/surrogacy?
    A. To experience menstruation
    B. To experience sexual satisfaction
    C. To experience pregnancy
    D. To experience parturition

4. What is the incidence of MRKH syndrome?
    A. 1 in 500
    B. 1 in 1000
    C. 1 in 2000
    D. 1 in 5000

5. In terms of specific preoperative requirements for UTx, which of the following factors is an important anatomical prerequisite?

    A. Presence of cervix

    B. Presence of a physiologically functioning and normal length vagina (measuring 7 cm or more)

    C. Presence of at least one fallopian tube

    D. Presence of at least one-half of the Müllerian duct remnant

6. What is the prevalence of unilateral renal agenesis in women with atypical MRKH syndrome?

    A. 10%

    B. 25%

    C. 30%

    D. 50%

7. What is the risk of considering UTx in women with atypical MRKH syndrome with unilateral renal agenesis?

    A. Risk of renal/ureteric injury during surgery

    B. Risk of highly complicated surgery

    C. Risk of 2-fold increase in hypertensive disorders such as pre-eclampsia

    D. Risk of transplant failure is high

8. In patients who have undergone hysterectomy due to gynecological cancers in the past, how much time should be allowed for remission before they are considered candidates for UTx?

    A. 1 year

    B. 2 years

    C. 5 years

    D. 10 years

9. What is the prevalence of Asherman's syndrome in women of reproductive age?

    A. 1 in 10,000

    B. 1 in 1000

    C. 1.5%

    D. 5%

10. Which of the following are most commonly used as potential donors for UTx?

    A. Living donors

    B. Deceased donors

    C. Tissue donors

    D. Pediatric donors

11. All of the following statements regarding living donors are true, except?

    A. First-degree relatives confer immunological advantages.

    B. The quality of the organ accessible for transplantation improves with the donor's age.

    C. A primary disadvantage of selecting living donors is the considerable danger and surgical morbidity associated with the donor.

    D. Comprehensive preoperative interdisciplinary counseling is needed.

12. Which of the following risks increase with increased age of the living donor?

    A. Atherosclerotic changes in the pelvic vessels

    B. Increased risk of post-transplant graft vasculopathy

    C. Increased risk of acute allograft rejection

    D. All of the above

13. All of the following statements regarding the use of deceased donors for UTx are true, except?

    A. It entirely eliminates risk to the donor.

    B. Facilitates more extensive dissection.

    C. It allows larger vessels to be taken with the graft.

    D. Heightens risk of graft thrombosis.

14. Which of the following is a potential disadvantage of using a deceased donor for UTx?

    A. It elevates the risk of graft thrombosis

    B. It permits more extensive dissection

    C. It is linked to systemic brain death inflammation that may affect organ quality

    D. It exhibits an increased cold ischemia time

15. What percentage of recipients subsequently need emergency hysterectomy after a UTx procedure?

    A. 5%   C. 25%

    B. 10%   D. 50%

16. What is the most common indication for emergency hysterectomy subsequent to the UTx procedure?

    A. Pelvic abscess

    B. Graft thrombosis

    C. Postoperative hemorrhage

    D. Candida-associated vasculitis of arterial anastomosis

17. What is the timeframe during which most of the emergency hysterectomies occurred after UTx?

    A. 6 months   C. 1 month

    B. 3 months   D. 15 days

18. What is the overall graft survival in cases of UTx done using living donors?

    A. 25%   C. 56%

    B. 45%   D. 75%

19. What is the overall graft survival in cases of UTx done using deceased donors?

    A. 25%   C. 56%

    B. 45%   D. 75%

20. Which of the following is a reliable indicator of uterine functionality and ongoing well-being of the graft indicating a successful UTx?

    A. Adequate uterine blood flow observed on transvaginal Doppler ultrasound postoperatively

    B. Achieving regular menstruation without the necessity for supplemental hormone therapy

    C. MRI of the pelvis confirming the correct positioning of the uterus postoperatively

    D. 3D ultrasonography with Doppler demonstrating low-resistance flow in pelvic vessels postoperatively

21. Which of the following is the preferred agent for immunosuppression after a UTx procedure?

    A. Tacrolimus

    B. Prednisolone

    C. Sirolimus

    D. Cyclosporine

22. How many months after the UTx is it acceptable to do the embryo transfer?

    A. 3 months

    B. 6 months

    C. 9 months

    D. 12 months

23. What is the minimum time before embryo transfer should the teratogenic immunosuppressive agents such as MMF be stopped or replaced by safer agents?

    A. 4 weeks

    B. 6 weeks

    C. 3 months

    D. 6 months

24. What is the potential effect of tacrolimus on the fetus?

    A. Neonatal jaundice

    B. Congenital hypothyroidism

    C. Reversible neonatal hyperkalemia

    D. Neonatal hypoglycemia

25. What is the prevalence of severe symptoms of depression in women with AUFI?

    A. >10%

    B. >30%

    C. >50%

    D. >70%

26. What is the increase in risk of suicide in women with AUFI?

    A. 2-fold

    B. 3-fold

    C. 4-fold

    D. 6-fold

ANSWERS

1. B	10. A	19. C
2. B	11. B	20. B
3. C	12. D	21. A
4. D	13. D	22. B
5. B	14. C	23. B
6. B	15. C	24. C
7. C	16. B	25. B
8. C	17. D	26. A
9. C	18. D	

45 SIP – Vitamin D in Pregnancy

Source: Vitamin D in Pregnancy Scientific Impact Paper No. 43 June 2014. https://www.rcog.org.uk/guidance/browse-all-guidance/scientific-impact-papers/vitamin-d-in-pregnancy-scientific-impact-paper-43/

IMPORTANT POINTS FROM THE GUIDELINE (SIP)

- Vitamin D and its active metabolite 1,25-dihydroxyvitamin D (1,25(OH)2 D) have traditional effects on calcium homeostasis and osseous metabolism.

- Insufficient levels of 1,25(OH)2 D hinder the intestine's ability to absorb calcium and phosphate effectively, resulting in secondary hyperparathyroidism and impaired bone mineralization, manifesting as rickets in children and osteomalacia in adults.

- Rickets is a pediatric condition resulting from vitamin D deficiency, typically manifesting several months post-delivery.

- The neonate is susceptible to hypocalcemic tetany due to maternal hypovitaminosis D.

- Calcium levels remain adequate in pregnancy despite maternal vitamin D deficiency.

- Nonetheless, when maternal calcium supply is disrupted at birth, the neonate may experience hypocalcaemia.

- The developing fetus necessitates roughly 30 g of calcium.

- The maternal gastrointestinal system adjusts and can mitigate certain vitamin D deficiencies by enhanced calcium absorption.

- Vitamin D exists in two forms. Vitamin D3 (cholecalciferol) is synthesized from the conversion of 7-dehydrocholesterol in the skin, while vitamin D2 (ergocalciferol) is generated in mushrooms and yeast.

- The active biological form of vitamin D is 1,25(OH)2 D.

- This necessitates the hydroxylation of vitamin D in the liver to produce 25(OH)D (25-hydroxyvitamin D), which subsequently undergoes renal hydroxylation to provide 1,25(OH)2 D.

- Despite its poor biological activity, 25(OH)D is the predominant form of circulating vitamin D.

- Serum 25(OH)D levels are typically considered indicative of nutritional status.

- The synthesis of 1,25(OH)2 D in the kidney is meticulously controlled by plasma parathyroid hormone (PTH) and serum calcium and phosphate concentrations.

- The engagement of 1,25(OH)2 D with nuclear vitamin D receptors affects gene transcription.

- Nuclear receptors for 1,25(OH)2 D are found in various tissues, including bone, gut, kidney, lung, muscle, and skin.

- Similar to steroid hormones, 1,25(OH)2 D functions through signal transduction pathways associated with vitamin D receptors on cellular membranes.

- Primary areas of action encompass the gut, bone, parathyroid glands, liver, and pancreatic beta cells.

- Its biological effects encompass enhanced intestinal calcium absorption, transcellular calcium transport, and the activation of gated calcium channels facilitating calcium entry into cells, including osteoblasts and skeletal muscle.

- It suppresses PTH secretion and adaptive immunity, while enhancing insulin secretion and innate immunity.

- It also suppresses cell proliferation and promotes their differentiation.

- The primary source of vitamin D in humans is the synthesis from solar radiation; thirty minutes of exposure provides 50,000 IU of vitamin D for individuals with fair skin.

DOI: 10.1201/9781003650355-45

- The dietary consumption of vitamin D contributes minimally to overall vitamin D status due to the limited natural occurrence of vitamin D in the food supply.

- Melanin absorbs ultraviolet B (UVB) radiation from sunlight and reduces cholecalciferol synthesis by a minimum of 90%.

- Pre-eclampsia and neonatal hypocalcaemia are the most common consequences of maternal hypocalcaemia, significantly linked to considerable morbidity.

- A statistical correlation between glucose intolerance and vitamin D deficiency has been shown.

- Maternal vitamin D is crucial for prenatal bone growth.

- Fetal lung development and neonatal immunological disorders, such as asthma, may be somewhat associated with maternal vitamin D levels.

- While the efficacy of maternal vitamin D supplementation in preventing these disorders remains uncertain, a strategy for addressing maternal vitamin D deficiency by supplementation and treatment is suggested.

- Maternal vitamin D levels have demonstrated a positive correlation with birthweight centile.

- In a research, mothers with vitamin D insufficiency had a 2.4-fold elevated chance of delivering a small for gestational age (SGA) infant.

- Hypovitaminosis D is linked to diminished glucose tolerance and diabetes in the general populace.

- A meta-analysis of 31 research articles indicated that vitamin D insufficiency correlates with an increased risk of gestational diabetes mellitus (GDM).

- Vitamin D insufficiency is correlated with bacterial vaginosis in pregnant women.

- Hypovitaminosis D may correlate with hypertension, pre-eclampsia, and elevated rates of cesarean sections. No randomized trials demonstrate that vitamin D treatment modifies these potential dangers.

- Vitamin D insufficiency is a significant contributor to hypocalcemic seizures in neonates and infants.

- Hypocalcemia is rather prevalent in neonates and poses a potentially serious issue.

- Mothers of infants experiencing hypocalcemic seizures exhibit a higher prevalence of vitamin D deficiency (85%) compared to mothers of infants who do not experience such seizures (50%).

- Maternal vitamin D insufficiency is a prevalent and potentially preventable cause of newborn hypocalcemia.

- Currently, there is no evidence to endorse a strategy of routine measurement followed by treatment in the general female population.

- The assessment of vitamin D in a hypocalcemic or symptomatic woman remains relevant to their care. This encompasses women with diminished calcium levels, bone pain, gastrointestinal disorders, alcohol dependency, a history of offspring with rickets, and individuals on pharmacotherapy that diminishes vitamin D levels.

- Vitamin D toxicity presents as hypercalcemia and hypercalciuria.

- The National Institute for Health and Care Excellence (NICE) guidance indicates that all pregnant and nursing women should be educated on the significance of vitamin D and should consume 10 µg of vitamin D supplements daily.

- Three classifications of vitamin D supplementation are advised.
  - Generally:
    - A daily intake of 10 µg (400 units) of vitamin D is advised for all pregnant women in accordance with national guidelines.

- High-risk women:

  - Women at high risk are recommended to consume a minimum of 1000 units daily, particularly those with heightened skin pigmentation, less sunshine exposure, or those who are socially marginalized or obese.

  - Women with elevated risk of pre-eclampsia are recommended to consume a minimum of 800 units daily in conjunction with calcium.

  - Vitamin D may be contraindicated in sarcoidosis due to potential vitamin D sensitivity, or ineffective in renal illness.

  - Insufficient renal 1-α hydroxylation requires the administration of active vitamin D metabolites, including 1α-hydroxycholecalciferol or 1,25-dihydroxycholecalciferol. In such instances, it is imperative to seek specialist medical counseling.

- Therapeutic intervention:

  - Most women with vitamin D deficiency should undergo treatment for 4–6 weeks, utilizing either cholecalciferol 20,000 IU weekly or ergocalciferol 10,000 IU biweekly, followed by normal supplementation.

  - A daily dosage of 1000 IU is likely suitable for sustaining future repletion.

  - In adults, excessive dosages of vitamin D (300,000–500,000 IU intramuscular bolus) may correlate with an elevated fracture risk, and such large doses are contraindicated during pregnancy.

QUESTIONS

1. How much calcium is required by the developing fetus during pregnancy?

   A. 10 g

   B. 20 g

   C. 30 g

   D. 50 g

2. What percentage of obese women are deficient in vitamin D?

   A. 30%

   B. 45%

   C. 60%

   D. 75%

3. Which of the following is the biologically active metabolite of vitamin D?

   A. 7-dehydrocholesterol

   B. 25(OH)D

   C. 1,25(OH)2 D

   D. 24,25-dihydroxyvitamin D (24,25(OH)2 D)

4. Which of the following molecules in the skin is converted to cholecalciferol (vitamin D3)?

   A. 7-dehydrocholesterol

   B. 25(OH)D

   C. 1,25(OH)2 D

   D. 24,25(OH)2 D

5. Serum concentration of which of the following molecules is considered to reflect the nutritional status of the body?

   A. 7-dehydrocholesterol

   B. 25(OH)D

   C. 1,25(OH)2 D

   D. 24,25(OH)2 D

6. What is considered to be the minimum required level of 25(OH)D in the body in the general population to maintain overall health?

   A. ≥10 ng/mL

   B. ≥20 ng/mL

   C. ≥30 ng/mL

   D. ≥50 ng/mL

7. According to the available research regarding the classification of vitamin D deficiency, which of the following is correctly explained?

   A. <20 ng/mL is considered as deficient

   B. 20–30 ng/mL is considered as insufficient

   C. >30 ng/mL is considered as sufficient

   D. All of the above

8. Regarding the physiology of vitamin D, which of the following statements is NOT true?

   A. Vitamin D3 (cholecalciferol) is synthesized from the conversion of 7-dehydrocholesterol in the skin.

   B. Vitamin D2 (ergocalciferol) is synthesized in mushrooms and yeast.

   C. The initial stage involves the hydroxylation of vitamin D in the kidney to produce 25(OH)D.

   D. Serum concentrations of 25(OH)D are regarded as indicative of nutritional status.

9. Which of the following is NOT a biological action of 1,25(OH)2 D?

   A. It enhances the absorption of calcium in the intestine.

   B. It enhances transcellular calcium flux and activates gated calcium channels for calcium absorption in osteoblasts and skeletal muscle.

   C. It stimulates the release of PTH.

   D. It stimulates insulin secretion.

10. Which of the following is the largest source of vitamin D in adults?

    A. Mushrooms

    B. Almonds

    C. Yeast

    D. Synthesis from solar radiation

11. How much vitamin D3 is produced by half an hour of sunlight exposure in adults with white-complexioned skin?

    A. 10,000 IU

    B. 25,000 IU

    C. 50,000 IU

    D. 60,000 IU

12. Which of the following are the most prevalent complications of maternal hypocalcemia?

    A. Pre-eclampsia

    B. Neonatal hypocalcemia

    C. Neonatal immune conditions like asthma

    D. All of the above

    E. A and B

13. To what extent does melanin pigment in dark-skinned individuals reduce the production of cholecalciferol?

    A. 30%

    B. 50%

    C. 70%

    D. 90%

14. Deficiency of maternal vitamin D increases the risk of all the following maternal complications, except?

    A. Pre-eclampsia

    B. Impaired glucose tolerance

    C. Spontaneous miscarriage

    D. Cesarean section rates

    E. Bacterial vaginosis in pregnant women

15. Deficiency of maternal vitamin D increases the risk of which of the following neonatal complications?

    A. Neonatal hypocalcemic seizures

    B. Rickets and osteoporotic fractures later in life

    C. Poor fetal lung development

    D. Childhood asthma

    E. All of the above

16. In which of the following conditions is vitamin D supplementation inappropriate/ineffective?

    A. Sarcoidosis

    B. Chronic renal disease

    C. Extreme obesity

    D. All of the above

    E. A and B

17. According to the NICE guidelines, what is the recommended daily routine supplementation dose of vitamin D required for pregnant women?

    A. 400 IU (10 µg)

    B. 800 IU (20 µg)

    C. 1000 IU (25 µg)

    D. 1200 IU (30 µg)

18. What is the recommended daily supplementation dose of vitamin D required for pregnant women at high risk of pre-eclampsia?

    A. 400 IU (10 µg) combined with calcium

    B. 800 IU (20 µg) combined with calcium

    C. 1000 IU (25 µg) combined with calcium

    D. 1200 IU (30 µg) combined with calcium

19. All of the following high-risk women are recommended to take 1000 IU of vitamin D daily, except?

    A. Women with increased skin pigmentation

    B. Women with reduced exposure to sunlight

    C. Women who are socially excluded or obese

    D. Women at high risk of pre-eclampsia

20. Which of the following food sources are considered sources of vitamin D3 in our diet?

    A. Oily fish like salmon and mackerel

    B. Fruits and green leafy vegetables

    C. Fortified food products like milk and cereals

    D. All of the above

    E. A and C

21. Based on recent research concerning the role of vitamin D in pregnancy and breastfeeding, which of the following assertions is accurate?

    A. Although research on the safety of high doses is inadequate, most experts agree that supplemental vitamin D is safe at levels up to 4000 international units per day during pregnancy or lactation.

    B. There is inadequate evidence to support widespread screening for vitamin D deficiency in pregnant women.

    C. Currently, little data exists to support vitamin D supplementation for the prevention of premature birth or pre-eclampsia.

    D. All of the above.

ANSWERS

1. C	8. C	15. E
2. C	9. C	16. E
3. C	10. D	17. A
4. A	11. C	18. B
5. B	12. E	19. D
6. B	13. D	20. E
7. D	14. C	21. D

For Product Safety Concerns and Information please contact our EU
representative GPSR@taylorandfrancis.com
Taylor & Francis Verlag GmbH, Kaufingerstraße 24, 80331 München, Germany

www.ingramcontent.com/pod-product-compliance
Lightning Source LLC
Chambersburg PA
CBHW061355210326
41598CB00035B/5994